Dental Care: Oral and Systemic Disease Prevention

Dental Care: Oral and Systemic Disease Prevention

Guest Editors

Kacper Nijakowski
Anna Surdacka

MDPI

Basel • Beijing • Wuhan • Barcelona • Belgrade • Novi Sad • Cluj • Manchester

Guest Editors

Kacper Nijakowski
Department of Conservative Dentistry
Poznan University of Medical Sciences
Poznan
Poland

Anna Surdacka
Department of Conservative Dentistry
Poznan University of Medical Sciences
Poznan
Poland

Editorial Office
MDPI AG
Grosspeteranlage 5
4052 Basel, Switzerland

This is a reprint of the Special Issue, published open access by the journal *Journal of Clinical Medicine* (ISSN 2077-0383), freely accessible at: https://www.mdpi.com/journal/jcm/special_issues/M7U5558SSN.

For citation purposes, cite each article independently as indicated on the article page online and as indicated below:

Lastname, A.A.; Lastname, B.B. Article Title. *Journal Name* **Year**, *Volume Number*, Page Range.

ISBN 978-3-7258-6582-6 (Hbk)
ISBN 978-3-7258-6583-3 (PDF)
https://doi.org/10.3390/books978-3-7258-6583-3

Contents

Preface

Oral health is strongly interconnected with general health in a bidirectional manner. Insufficient oral hygiene and dental care can exacerbate systemic diseases, while systemic conditions and their therapies often present with oral manifestations. This underscores the importance of emphasizing dental prevention and care across all age groups, from childhood to old age.

Dentists are frequently the first to recognize early signs of systemic disease. Many patients take medications that may lead to xerostomia, a common side effect with a significant impact on oral health. For this reason, regular dental examinations combined with oral hygiene guidance are indispensable as preventive measures. Moreover, the COVID-19 pandemic had a profound effect on dental practice, as the first wave necessitated radical surgical interventions for patients with toothache. This experience has reinforced the principle that prevention including prevention of oral diseases must remain a top priority.

Accordingly, this Special Issue will highlight an interdisciplinary approach to oral health and disease prevention.

Kacper Nijakowski and Anna Surdacka
Guest Editors

Journal of
Clinical Medicine

MDPI

ematic Review

ating Disorders and Dental Erosion: A Systematic Review

per Nijakowski [1,*], Jakub Jankowski [2,†], Dawid Gruszczyński [2,†] and Anna Surdacka [1]

[1] Department of Conservative Dentistry and Endodontics, Poznan University of Medical Sciences, 60-812 Poznan, Poland; annasurd@ump.edu.pl
[2] Student's Scientific Group in Department of Conservative Dentistry and Endodontics, Poznan University of Medical Sciences, 60-812 Poznan, Poland; jjankowski41@wp.pl (J.J.); dawid.j.gruszczynski@gmail.com (D.G.)
* Correspondence: kacpernijakowski@ump.edu.pl
† These authors contributed equally to this work.

Abstract: Both eating disorders and dental erosion are increasingly affecting adolescents and young adults. Thus, our systematic review was designed to answer the question: "Is there a relationship between dental erosion and eating disorders?" Following the inclusion and exclusion criteria, 31 studies were included in this systematic review (according to the PRISMA statement guidelines). Based on the meta-analysis, 54.4% of patients with bulimia nervosa and 26.7% with anorexia nervosa experienced tooth erosion. For the whole group of 1699 patients with eating disorders, erosive lesions were observed in 42.1% of patients. Bulimics were more than 10 times more likely to experience dental erosion compared to healthy individuals (OR = 10.383 [95%CI: 4.882–22.086]). Similarly, more than 16 times increased odds of tooth erosion were found in patients with self-induced vomiting (OR = 16.176 [95%CI: 1.438–181.918]). In conclusion, eating disorders are associated with an increased risk of developing erosive lesions, especially in patients with bulimia nervosa.

Keywords: eating disorders; anorexia nervosa; bulimia nervosa; dental erosion; tooth erosion

1. Introduction

Eating disorders (EDs) are serious mental and behavioural disorders that may occur alone or in combination with other mood disorders [1]. Due to the global trend towards beauty and fitness, the incidence of these disorders among adolescents and young adults is rapidly increasing [2]. Although EDs are most commonly reported in young women, they can affect people of both genders at any life stage [3,4]. The etiology of these disorders is not fully understood, but it is assumed that it is multifactorial, depending on individual (biological or psychological, including low self-esteem) and environmental (developmental or sociocultural, especially pressures in home, school, etc.) issues [2,5].

The two most common ED forms include anorexia nervosa (AN) and bulimia nervosa (BN) [1,6]. AN is mainly associated with food restriction, leading to significant underweight. Patients with AN are characterised by an impaired vision of their own body shape and extreme fear of gaining weight [7,8]. In turn, BN is more common and is usually associated with normal body weight. Patients with BN demonstrate recurrent uncontrolled binge-eating episodes which are inappropriately compensated by such behaviours as self-induced vomiting, purging or overexercising [9,10].

Due to their pathophysiology, both types affect the person's general health, as well as the oral health [11]. The first symptoms can sometimes be observed in the oral cavity [12]. In patients with EDs, the most common oral symptoms include gingivitis or periodontitis, mucosal ulcers or erythema, angular cheilitis, xerostomia, as well as dental caries or erosion [13–15].

Tooth erosion is caused by the supply of acids of non-bacterial origin [16]. Food products with a low pH (e.g., fruits, fresh juices) are most often considered as etiological factors [17]. However, internal factors such as eating disorders (especially those with recurrent vomiting) are also known to cause erosion [18]. In addition, regular physical activity with supplementation of sports drinks strongly increases the risk of dental erosion [19–21].

It is now assumed that tooth erosion has become a new dental plague in a group of adolescents and young adults [22,23]. Under the influence of acids delivered to the oral cavity, the enamel dissolves, and thus erosive lesions develop [24]. It is particularly important to prevent dental erosion and eating disorders through appropriate education and prophylaxis from an early age [25,26]. The preventive actions include the right home oral hygiene manoeuvres; e.g., the use of toothpastes with fluoride [27]. Fluoridated toothpastes provide a higher degree of remineralisation at a first acid attack [28].

Therefore, our systematic review was designed to answer the question: "Is there a relationship between dental erosion and eating disorders?".

2. Materials and Methods

2.1. Search Strategy and Data Extraction

The present systematic review was conducted up to 27 August 2023, according to the Preferred Reporting Items for Systematic Reviews and Meta-Analyses (PRISMA) statement guidelines [29], using the PubMed, Scopus and Web of Science databases. The search queries included:

- for PubMed: (eating disorders OR anorexia OR bulimia) AND ((tooth OR dental) AND erosion)
- for Scopus: TITLE-ABS-KEY(("eating disorders" OR anorexia OR bulimia) AND ((tooth OR dental) AND erosion))
- for Web of Science: TS = ((eating disorders OR anorexia OR bulimia) AND ((tooth OR dental) AND erosion)).

Records were screened according to the title, abstract and full text by two independent investigators. The studies included in this review matched all the predefined criteria according to PI(E)COS ("Population", "Intervention"/"Exposure", "Comparison", "Outcomes" and "Study design"), as reported in Table 1. A detailed search flowchart is presented in the Results section. The study protocol was registered in the international prospective register of systematic reviews, PROSPERO (CRD42023458225).

Table 1. Inclusion and exclusion criteria according to the PI(E)COS.

Parameter	Inclusion Criteria	Exclusion Criteria
Population	Patients aged from 0 to 99 years, both genders	
Intervention/Exposure	eating disorders (e.g., bulimia nervosa, anorexia nervosa)	other diseases (e.g., gastrointestinal reflux)
Comparison	not applicable	
Outcomes	prevalence of dental erosion	only severity of dental erosion or only other dental indices
Study design	case-control, cohort and cross-sectional studies	literature reviews, case reports, expert opinion, letters to the editor, conference reports
	published until 27 August 2023	not published in English

The results of the meta-analysis were presented in forest plots using the MedCalc Statistical Software, version 19.5.3 (MedCalc Software Ltd., Ostend, Belgium). The meta-analysis was performed using the subgroups of anorexia nervosa and bulimia nervosa, as well as mixed eating disorders (additionally with and without self-induced vomiting). The pooled proportions and odds ratios for the prevalence of dental erosion were calculated.

2.2. *Quality Assessment and Critical Appraisal for the Systematic Review of Included Studies*

The risk of bias in each individual study was assessed according to the "Study Quality Assessment Tool" issued by the National Heart, Lung and Blood Institute within the National Institute of Health [30]. These questionnaires were answered simultaneously by two independent investigators, and any disagreements were resolved through discussion between them. The summarised quality assessment is reported in the Results section.

The level of evidence was assessed using the classification of the Oxford Centre for Evidence-Based Medicine levels for diagnosis [31].

3. Results

3.1. *Search Strategy*

Following the search criteria, our systematic review included 31 studies, demonstrating data collected in 17 different countries from a total of 1699 participants with EDs (mainly BN and AN). Figure 1 reports the detailed selection strategy of the records. The inclusion and exclusion criteria are presented in the Materials and Methods section.

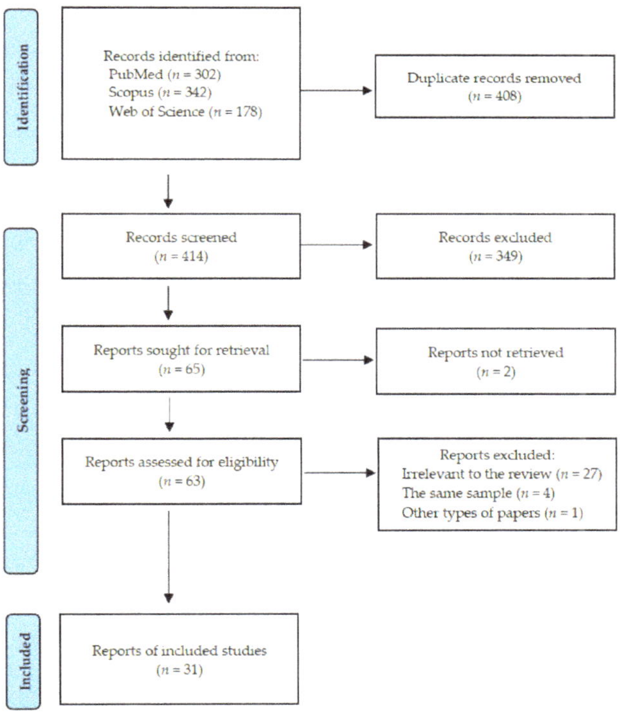

Figure 1. PRISMA flow diagram presenting search strategy.

3.2. *Characteristics of Included Studies*

As shown in Table 2, we collected data about the characteristics of each eligible study, such as the year of publication and study setting, age and gender distribution of study and control groups, diagnoses of EDs and clinical criteria for dental erosion. The vast majority of the participants were young women. Most studies had a case-control design. In terms of the types of EDs, a significant proportion were bulimics, followed by anorectics; however, some studies did not separate these subgroups to assess the oral health. Due to the very broad timeframe, the diagnostic criteria for dental erosion were very diverse, although in the latest studies, the standard was already BEWE (Basic Erosive Wear Examination).

Table 2. The characteristics of included studies.

Author	Setting	Study Group (F/M; Age)	Control Group (F/M; Age)	ED Diagnoses	Clinical Criteria for Dental Erosion
Altshuler et al., 1990 [32]	USA	40 (40/0), 23.8 ± 5.5	40 (40/0), 24.9 ± 6.1	BN	loss of enamel with exposure c dentine and/or alteration of morphology
Cavalcanti et al., 2020 [33]	Brazil	100 (100/0), mean 16.1	100 (100/0), mean 16.1	BN	based on the O'Sullivan inde
Emodi-Perlman et al., 2008 [34]	Israel	79 (79/0), 23.5 ± 3.5	48 (48/0), 24.6 ± 3.0	chronic EDs: BN (n = 29), AN (n = 24), EDNOS (n = 16), mixed-diagnosis (n = 10)	4-graded scoring system (0-nc 1-enamel, 2-dentine, 3-pulp)
Garrido-Martínez et al., 2019 [35]	Spain	59 (59/0), range 19–44	120 (120/0), range 19–44	EDs: ARFID (n = 22), AN (n = 16), BN (n = 6), EDNOS (n = 15)	the degree measured according Johansson et al. (1996)
Giraudeau et al., 2021 [36]	France	50 (48/2), mean 26.8	n/a	EDs: BN (n = 26), AN (n = 24)	BEWE scoring system using asynchronous telemedicine
Hellström, 1977 [37]	Sweden	39 (38/1), range 14–42	n/a	AN	diagnostic criteria given by Pindborg (1970) and Eccles an Jenkins (1974)
Hermont et al., 2013 [38]	Brazil	20 (20/0), range 15–18	80 (80/0), range 15–18	BN	based on the O'Sullivan inde
Hurst et al., 1977 [39]	UK	17 (14/3), range 13–33	n/a	AN	different patterns: palatal, labi or generalised
Johansson et al., 2012 [40]	Sweden	54 (50/4), mean 21.5	54 (50/4), mean 21.5	EDs: AN (n = 14), BN (n = 8), EDNOS (n = 32)	the degree measured according Johansson et al. (1996)
Jones and Cleaton-Jones, 1989 [41]	RSA	11 (11/0), 29.8 ± 8.4	22 (22/0), 28.9 ± 9.0	BN	4-graded scoring system (0-nc 1-enamel, 2-dentine, 3-pulp)
Jugale et al., 2014 [42]	India	50 (50/0), range 20–25	67 (67/0), range 20–25	EDs	perimolysis
Lifante-Oliva et al., 2008 [43]	Spain	17 (17/0), 20.1 ± 5.6	n/a	BN (n = 10), AN (n = 7)	4-graded scoring system (0-nc 1-enamel, 2-dentine, 3-pulp)
Manevski et al., 2020 [44]	Serbia	30 (28/2), 24.6 ± 4.4	30 (28/2), 24.7 ± 5.8	BN	BEWE scoring system
Milosevic et al., 1997 [45]	UK	33 (NR), mean 27.1	n/a	EDs: BN (n = 28), AN (n = 5)	TWI
Montecchi et al., 2003 [46]	Italy	80 (76/4), mean 15	n/a	AN	NR
Ohrn et al., 1999 [47]	Sweden	81 (79/2), median 25	52 (48/4), median 24	EDs: BN (n = 46), AN (n = 3), EDNOS (n = 25), mixed-diagnosis (n = 7)	classified according to a modification by Lussi et al. (19 of the system proposed by Eccles (1979)
Otsu et al., 2014 [48]	Japan	71 (71/0), mean 31.1	n/a	EDs: AN (n = 35), BN (n = 27), EDNOS (n = 3), unclear diagnosis (n = 6)	diagnostic criteria given by Japanese Society for Oral Health (1985)

Table 2. *Cont.*

Author	Setting	Study Group (F/M; Age)	Control Group (F/M; Age)	ED Diagnoses	Clinical Criteria for Dental Erosion
allier et al., 2019 [49]	France	70 (70/0), 32.1 ± 9.1	70 (70/0), 30.2 ± 4.7	AN (*n* = 36), BN (*n* = 34)	EEWE scoring system
anico et al., 2018 [50]	Argentina	65 (65/0), mean 21.6	65 (65/0), mean 23.2	EDs: BN (*n* = 46), AN (*n* = 6), EDNOS (*n* = 13)	NR
Paszynska al., 2022 [51]	Poland	117 (117/0), 14.9 ± 1.8	103 (103/0), 15.0 ± 1.8	AN	EEWE scoring system
Paszynska al., 2015 [52]	Poland	25 (25/0), 21.2 ± 3.2	44 (44/0), 25.5 ± 4.6	BN	TWI
berts and Li, 1987 [53]	USA	47 (47/0), mean 25	n/a	AN (*n* = 17), BN (*n* = 30)	erosion of maxillary palatal surfaces
Rungta and Kudpi, 2019 [54]	India	21 (21/0), range 15–17	179 (179/0), range 15–17	EDs	NR
tömaa et al., 1998 [55]	Finland	35 (35/0), 25.3 ± 6.8	105 (105/0), 25.7 ± 7.0	BN	diagnostic criteria given by Eccles and Jenkins (1974)
haughnessy al., 2008 [56]	USA	23 (23/0), 18.5 ± 2.9	n/a	AN	clinically detectable change in enamel smooth surface without evidence of dental caries
nmons et al., 1986 [57]	USA	66 (66/0), median 26	n/a	BN	clinically observable features
użycka et al., 2017 [58]	Poland	29 (NR), 18	n/a	EDs	BEWE scoring system
Szupiany-neczek et al., 2023 [59]	Poland	59 (45/14), mean 30.6	60 (45/15), mean 30.7	EDs	NR
Touyz et al., 1993 [60]	Australia	30 (30/0), mean 19.6	15 (15/0), mean 22.1	AN (*n* = 15), BN (*n* = 15)	NR
Uhlen et al., 2014 [61]	Norway	66 (63/3), mean 27.7	n/a	EDs	VEDE system
menes et al., 2010 [62]	Brazil	215 (NR) according to EAT-26, 248 (NR) according to BITE; range 12–16	n/a	EDs	NR

Legend: F, female; M, male; EDs, eating disorders; USA, the United States of America; UK, the United Kingdom; RSA, Republic of South Africa; n/a, not applicable; NR, not reported; BITE, Bulimic Investigatory Test of Edinburgh; BN, bulimia nervosa; AN, anorexia nervosa; EDNOS, eating disorders not otherwise specified; ARFID, avoidant/restrictive food intake disorder; BEWE, Basic Erosive Wear Examination; TWI, tooth wear index; VEDE, Visual Erosion Dental Examination.

3.3. *Quality Assessment of Included Studies*

Figure 2 reports the summarised quality assessment, according to the "Study Quality Assessment Tool" issued by the National Heart, Lung and Blood Institute within the National Institute of Health [30]. The most frequently encountered risks of bias were the absence of data regarding blinding (twenty-eight studies), randomisation (twenty-seven studies), sample size justification (twenty-five studies), as well as valid inclusion and exclusion criteria (twenty-one studies). The critical appraisal was summarised by adding up the points for each criterion of potential risk (points: 1—low, 0.5—unspecified, 0—high).

Ten studies (32.3%) were classified as being of "good" quality (≥80% total score) and twenty-one (67.7%) were classified as "intermediate" (≥60% total score).

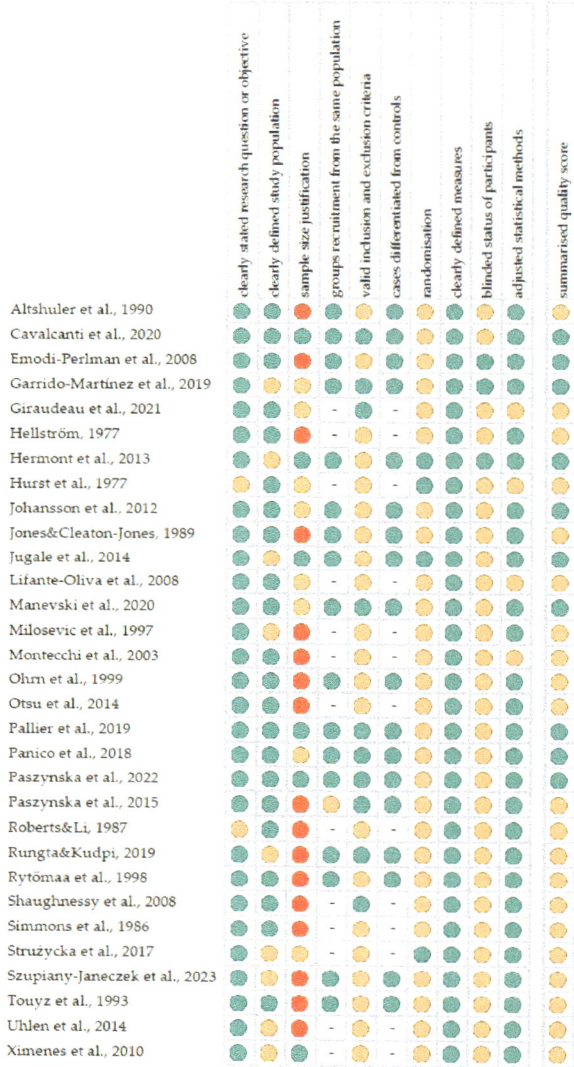

Figure 2. Quality assessment, including the main potential risk of bias (risk level: green—low, yellow—unspecified, red—high; quality score: green—good, yellow—intermediate, red—poor) [32–62].

All of the included studies had the third or fourth level of evidence (case-control or cross-sectional studies), according to the five-graded scale in the classification of the Oxford Centre for Evidence-Based Medicine levels for diagnosis [31].

3.4. Results of Meta-Analysis

As previously mentioned, most of the studies concerned bulimics. Based on the meta-analysis, it was found that more than half of the patients with BN demonstrated tooth erosion—54.4% [95%CI: 42.3–66.3]. Compared to healthy subjects, bulimics were more than 10 times more likely to experience dental erosion—OR = 10.383 [95%CI: 4.882–22.086] (Figure 3).

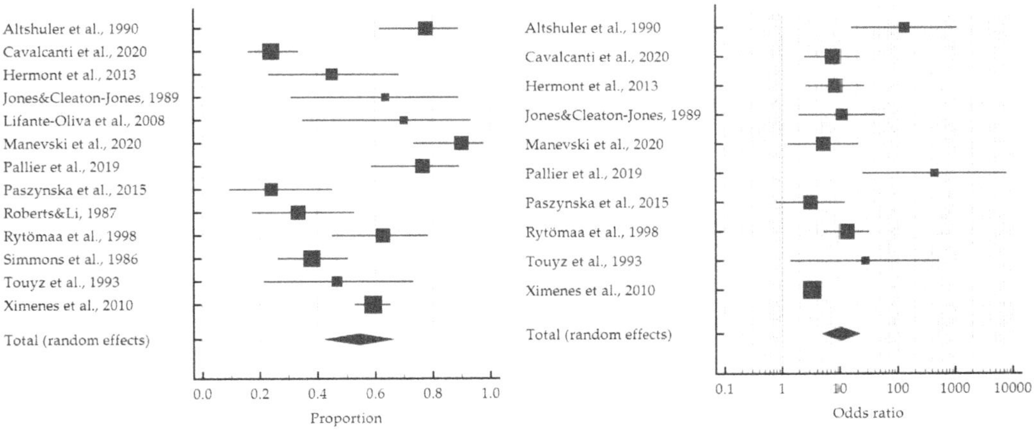

Figure 3. Forest plots presenting the summarised prevalence and odds ratio of dental erosion among patients with bulimia nervosa [32,33,38,41,43,44,49,52,53,55,57,60,62].

Analogously, more than 1/4 of the anorectic patients had erosive lesions—26.7% [95%CI: 14.5–41.1]. Only three studies compared the frequencies in anorexic and healthy individuals, similarly giving a ten times higher odds of tooth erosion—OR = 12.202 [95%CI: 2.179–68.334] (Figure 4).

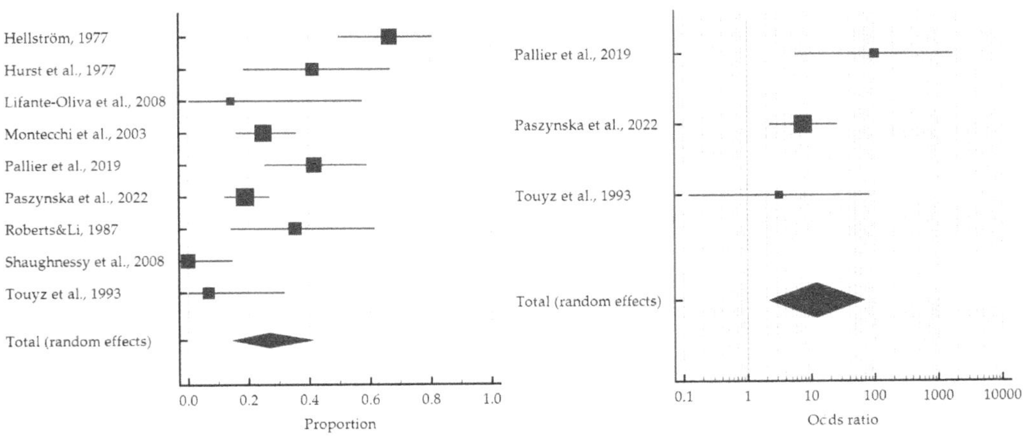

Figure 4. Forest plots presenting the summarised prevalence and odds ratio of dental erosion among patients with anorexia nervosa [37,39,43,46,49,51,53,56,60].

However, when comparing bulimics with anorectics, the former had an almost four times higher chance of erosive lesions—OR = 3.926 [95%CI: 1.153–13.365] (Figure 5).

Some of the studies did not separate subgroups of EDs for oral health outcomes. For these studies, the pooled proportion was 41.7% [95%CI: 29.1–54.9] and OR = 5.132 [95%CI: 2.571–10.246] relative to the healthy subjects (Figure 6).

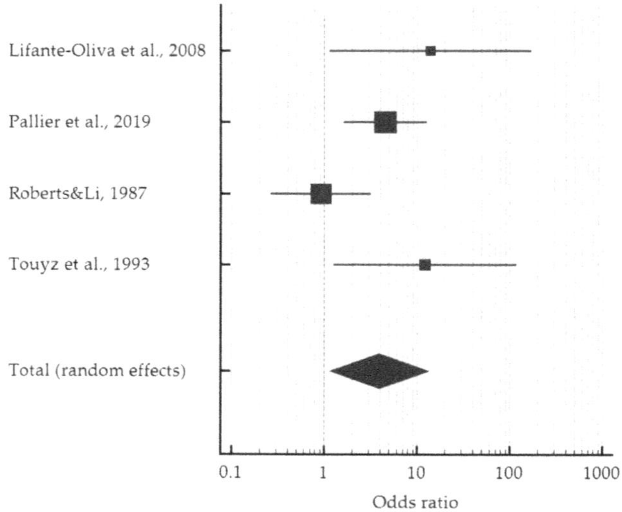

Figure 5. Forest plot presenting the odds ratio of dental erosion among patients with bulimia nervosa vs. anorexia nervosa [43,49,53,60].

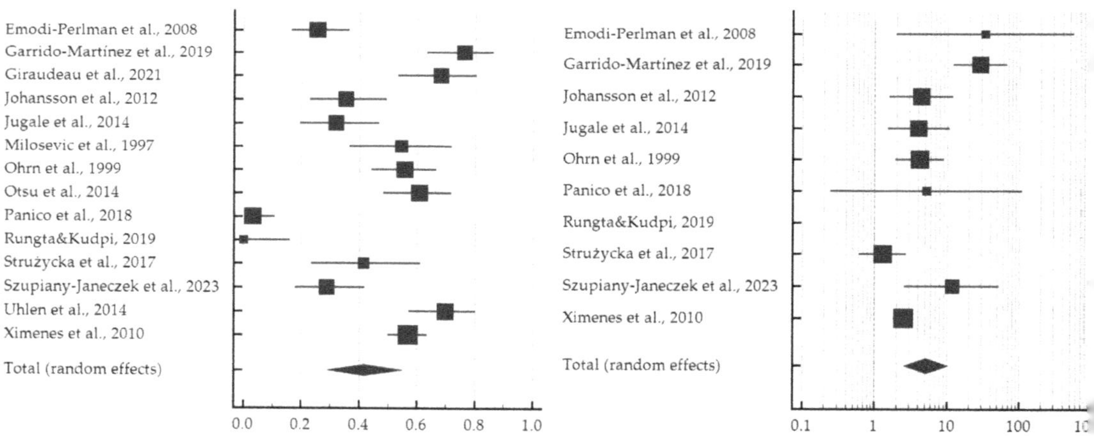

Figure 6. Forest plots presenting the summarised prevalence and odds ratio of dental erosion among other patients with eating disorders (without divided diagnoses) [34–36,40,42,45,47,48,50,54,58,59,61,62].

Interestingly, only three studies singled out self-induced vomiting. Patients with vomiting had more than 16 times higher odds to manifest erosive lesions—OR = 16.176 [95%CI: 1.438–181.918] (Figure 7).

Considering all of the included studies, the incidence of tooth erosion in patients with EDs was 42.1% [95%CI: 33.6–50.8]. In turn, the odds ratio of dental erosion for the whole group relative to the control subjects was 7.480 [95%CI: 4.456–12.556] (Figure 8).

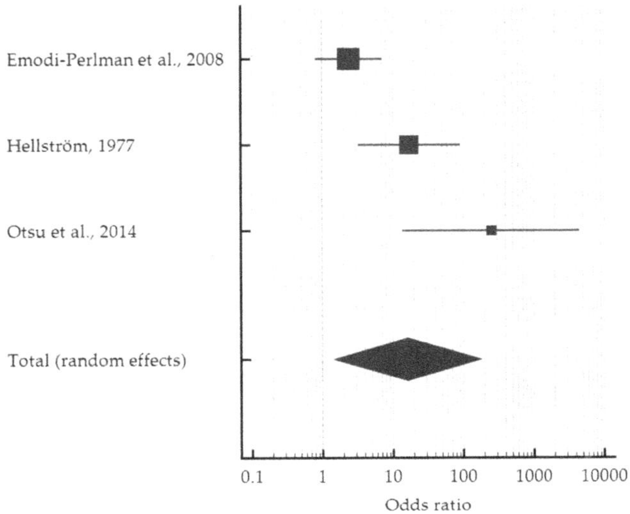

Figure 7. Forest plot presenting the odds ratio of dental erosion among patients with self-induced vomiting [34,37,48].

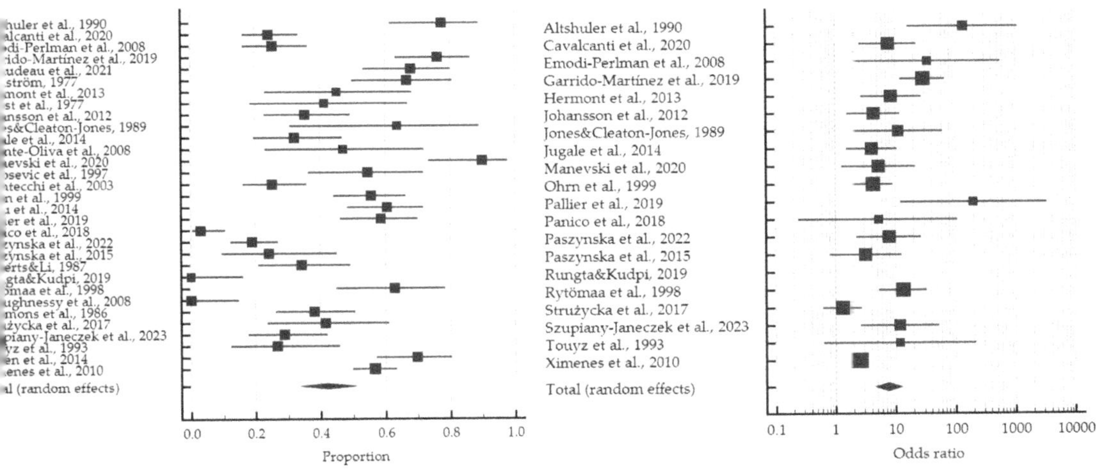

Figure 8. Forest plots presenting the summarised prevalence and odds ratio of dental erosion among all patients with eating disorders [32–62].

4. Discussion

4.1. Dental Erosion in Anorexia Nervosa

Many of the included studies considering the impact of AN on the presence of erosive lesions described patients in addiction and psychiatry hospital units, especially young women as AN is a psychosomatic disease mainly affecting this group.

In the last century, many researchers have tried to expand the knowledge regarding oral complications in AN. One of them was Hellström [37], who described 39 patients (38 females and 1 male) aged 14 to 42 years, with AN for periods ranging between 1 and 20 years. These patients were divided into two main groups: the first with vomiting patients and the second with non-vomiting patients. In the group with vomiting patients, severe lingual-occlusal erosion (perimolysis) was nearly always present, but the lingual type did not occur in the non-vomiting cases. Also, the buccal type of erosion was rare in the non-vomiting patients, but it was common in a moderate form in those with vomiting. It was pointed out that this may also be due to the longer history of vomiting with a high consumption of acid beverages. As most of the patients, especially those vomiting, showed different grades of dehydration, to relieve this, they consumed acid drops, juices and lemonade, most often at night.

Other researchers, namely Roberts and Li [53], observed that 35% of the patients with AN in their study showed palatal erosion of the maxillary anterior teeth, which was the result of frequent vomiting. These observations coincide with the study by Lifante-Oliva et al. [43], where, among young female patients with AN, erosive lesions were most often found on the palatal surfaces of the maxillary anterior teeth because these teeth were most often exposed to acidic fluids like vomit. In addition, the authors note that the development of dental erosion may be part of a cumulative process influenced by the frequency and duration of acid exposure, oral hygiene and individual vulnerability. Other factors influencing the presence, extent and advancement of erosion are the patient's age and AN duration. Therefore, prolonged exposure to the destructive effects of harmful conditions related to AN (vomiting, xerostomia) may significantly deepen or create completely new erosive lesions.

The study by Shaughnessy et al. [56] found no evidence of dental erosion, which was defined as a detectable change in the smooth enamel surface without any indication of dental caries, in any of the young women with a mean AN duration of 2.5 months. However, 26% of the participants reported a history of binge-eating or purging activity. Undoubtedly, the patients' age and the duration of their AN and vomiting—which is often related to their age—impact the extent and advancement of dental erosion in patients with EDs.

In the same year as Hellström [37], Hurst et al. [39] conducted a study on dental issues, such as erosion, in patients with AN. The study identified three factors that may cause dental problems in these patients: frequent and prolonged vomiting, an unnatural diet and the effects of wasting and dehydration during starvation. The patients were categorised into three groups—vomiters, regurgitators and non-vomiters—based on their vomiting and regurgitation history over the past three years. Like Hellström [37], the researchers noted that dental erosion was significantly more common in the vomiting and regurgitating population than in the non-vomiters. The maxillary incisors, canines and premolars showed dental erosion of the palatal surfaces, resulting in the tooth crown "shelling out". Despite the majority of the subjects consuming large amounts of fruit regularly, with a preference for citrus fruits, only two subjects displayed significant labial enamel loss due to tooth erosion. However, the researchers point out the low pH of such fruits (3–5) and the possible enamel decalcification after long-term consumption of these foods. The third factor investigated was the intraoral effects of wasting and dehydration of patients during starvation. These authors found that saliva secretion in people with AN is reduced due to starvation and the associated weight-reducing manoeuvres, which lead to the wasting and dehydration of the body. Reducing salivary flow, followed by the acid-buffering capacity of saliva, increases the risk of tooth decay in such patients, and also makes the teeth more susceptible to acid attack and erosion.

Touyz et al. [60] concluded that patients with EDs did not have lower decay incidence or salivary flow compared to the healthy subjects, but did have significantly more acidic saliva. The difference between the study groups was also visible in the frequency of dental erosion. Out of all the surfaces examined, bulimics had 6.1% of surfaces affected and anorexics had 1.0%. In this study, it was found that both anorexics and bulimics had a significantly higher number of surfaces with erosion compared to the control subjects who had no eroded surfaces.

A significant impact of vomiting on dental erosion was illustrated by Montecchi et al. [46]. They found erosive lesions in 20 of the 80 non-adult patients with AN, especially those who demonstrated vomiting several times daily. Those patients who declared daily vomiting, in addition to tooth erosion, also had carious lesions and xerostomia. Xerostomia in such cases may result from many causes, such as taking drugs that reduce salivation, which can be used in the treatment of AN, or dehydration, which is undoubtedly present after vomiting several times a day.

At present, one of the most frequently used scales by researchers to assess the erosive wear of teeth is the BEWE scoring system [16], which records the most severely affected surface in a sextant. The criteria for the grading are as follows: (0) no defect; (1) initial loss of surface texture; (2) hard tissue loss <50% of the surface area; (3) hard tissue loss ≥50% of the surface area. In a BEWE score of 2 or 3, dentine is often involved.

Paszynska et al. [51] used this scale to assess dental erosion in 220 female children (117 with AN and 113 controls). They observed a significant difference in the prevalence and severity of dental erosion between these groups. The patients had a BEWE score ≤ 2, which was discovered in 18.9% of cases, while only 2.9% of control subjects had the same score. However, no higher score ≥ 3 was identified in the control group. Erosive lesions were found more often in the patients with AN than in the controls (18.8% vs. 2.9%). In all of the healthy children, the BEWE index was ≤2, while the largest number of AN patients had BEWE 3–8, and the highest result in the AN patients was BEWE 9–13. Also, the researchers divided the AN group into subgroups: those with and without purging episodes. The anorectics without purging had significantly lower BEWE scores. Other researchers [37,46] made the same observations that patients who vomited had a greater severity of dental erosion than those who did not vomit.

Similarly, Pallier et al. [49] observed more AN patients with BEWE ≤ 2 (58.3%) compared to the controls. Overall, 16.7% of the patients with AN had BEWE ≥ 14. However, the authors noticed that the control group included females responding online for a free dental examination. They may be more dentally aware than females in the general population, which is why the BEWE score may be so low. In addition to AN patients, these researchers also examined BN patients, where a BEWE ≤ 2 was assessed in 23.5% and BEWE ≥ 14 in 20.6%. The patients with BN had significantly higher BEWE scores (>2) compared to the patients with AN (76.5% vs. 41.7%).

4.2. Dental Erosion in Bulimia Nervosa

The primary cause of dental erosion in bulimic patients is often self-induced vomiting. This results in erosive lesions on the palatal surfaces of the anterior teeth that come into contact with vomit and gastric acid. As a result, many bulimics have severe damage on these surfaces.

Simmons et al. [57] described the occurrence of dental erosion in patients with BN who self-induced vomiting at least three times a week. Their mean age was 26, and the mean disease duration was 7 years. Overall, 37.9% had significant enamel erosion, and the duration of vomiting was significantly associated with erosion. The erosion prevalence was significantly lower in those who reported vomiting for 4 years or less (24.3%) compared to those who reported vomiting for more than 4 years (55.2%).

The topic of teeth brushing immediately after every vomiting episode was also taken up in this study due to its possible impact on the progression of tooth erosion. Studies have shown that brushing one's teeth right after vomiting may not prevent erosion but could worsen it. It was found that 50% of patients who brushed their teeth immediately after vomiting had signs of erosion, indicating that brushing may promote enamel loss soon after the acid has already affected the teeth. According to the study by Otsu et al. [48], teeth brushing immediately after vomiting is not recommended. This aligns with prior research indicating that brushing after consuming acidic foods or vomiting can result in acid erosion of tooth surfaces. Additionally, brushing too soon after vomiting may strip away the tooth's outer layer, revealing the decalcified layer that requires remineralisation over time. Moreover, researchers note that to prevent dental erosion from worsening after vomiting, it is important to thoroughly rinse the mouth with water or other liquids to neutralise any acid present in the oral cavity.

Previously, such a solution was proposed by Rytömaa et al. [55]. They concluded that such action may have a positive effect in reducing tooth erosion in patients who vomit (including bulimics). Thus, bulimics can prevent tooth damage by quickly neutralizing their stomach contents with water and antacids after vomiting. This is easily achievable because they typically plan their binge eating and vomiting ahead of time.

Erosive lesions resulting from BN often have their characteristic location (as in the case of AN); this was described in the study by Altshuler et al. [32]. The presence of erosive lesions indicates a condition that has persisted for at least six months. They noted an erosion diagnosis when a tooth surface loses enamel, which exposes dentine and/or causes changes to the tooth's shape. In individuals with BN, 78% showed an average of 7.6 tooth surfaces that were eroded. There was a significant difference compared to the healthy subjects, where the mean was only 0.2 tooth surfaces. The most commonly affected area was the palatal surfaces of the anterior teeth in the maxilla. The other affected areas included the palatal and occlusal surfaces of the posterior teeth in the maxilla, as well as the lingual surfaces of the anterior teeth in the mandible. Only one individual in the control group showed signs of erosion.

Moreover, Jones and Cleaton-Jones [41] conducted a case-control study on female patients who visited a private dental office. They observed a high prevalence of erosive lesions on the buccal surfaces of the maxillary canines and first premolars, as well as on the palatal surfaces of the same teeth, but a low prevalence on the buccal surfaces of the maxillary incisors. These findings strongly suggest the presence of BN. The study also found that over 50% of the bulimic subjects had erosive defects on these teeth, with over 70% showing lesions on the labial surfaces of the central incisor and canine. Additionally, more than 40% of these patients displayed some degree of dental erosion on the lingual surfaces of the mandibular incisors. It is important to mention that, in this study, erosions were defined as "dished out" areas of enamel or enamel and dentin on the buccal or lingual surface. In addition to the location, the researchers noted the erosion depth and showed that 69% of the bulimics had tooth erosion of any stage, while only 7% of the control group had it. The control group had only enamel erosions, while the bulimic group had erosive lesions at all depths.

A more recent study by Manevski et al. [44] confirmed and summarised the speculations about the location of erosion on tooth surfaces in patients with BN. In total, 83.4% of the patients were students, which corresponds to the fact that BN is most commonly present in the university population [63]. The analysis of the tooth surfaces, based on BEWE, revealed a significant difference between the groups. The majority of the lesions in the bulimic group (43.9%) were located on the palatal/lingual surfaces, while in the control group, the lesions were predominantly found on the labial/buccal surfaces (44%). Erosive lesions on oral surfaces are linked to longer bulimia duration and more frequent vomiting, indicating repeated purging as a crucial etiological factor for dental erosion occurrence in bulimics.

A more frequent occurrence of dental erosion in bulimics was also presented in the study by Paszynska et al. [52]. The results revealed significant differences in tooth wear (TWI) between the bulimic group (24%) and the control group (9%). Only patients with BN showed a total loss of enamel and dentin (over 50% of its thickness) with a TWI score of 3. Also, in the patients with BN, the unstimulated saliva pH was significantly lower than in the healthy controls. Moreover, according to these authors, medications from the selective serotonin reuptake inhibitors, such as fluoxetine, have been proven to be effective in treating bulimic patients without causing salivary alterations.

Comparisons of AN and BN can be seen in other studies by various researchers included in our meta-analysis. As mentioned earlier, in the study by Roberts and Li [53], the AN patients showed palatal erosion of the maxillary anterior teeth. The patients with BN showed erosive lesions in the same place. However, Lifante-Oliva et al. [43] found more patients with BN who had dental erosion than patients with AN. The change in saliva secretion in these patients was also noted, which may be the reason for the increase in erosive lesions. Half of the bulimics presented decreased unstimulated saliva secretion, and 30% of them also showed a reduction in stimulated saliva secretion. In contrast, the anorectics did not demonstrate similar changes. Acidic salivary pH occurred in 20% of the BN patients and 14% of the AN patients. Roberts and Li [53] also revealed that all of the patients diagnosed with BN had a habit of frequent vomiting to control their weight. In contrast, only nearly 2/3 of the patients with AN reported the same habit. The authors pointed out that a higher incidence of erosion was not observed in the patients with BN, which could be attributed to their oral hygiene practices and rinsing habits after vomiting. They explained that patients with bulimia are more likely to adopt good oral hygiene practices and seek regular dental care, which could be the reason behind the lower incidence of erosion.

4.3. Dental Erosion in Non-Distinguished Eating Disorders

Often, the authors of the studies cited in our review did not directly distinguish individual diagnoses of Eds, but recognised them together as EDs. Undoubtedly, AN and BN have many common features, which in the context of dental erosion seem to be quite consistent because in both diseases, patients may habitually vomit. Thus, the main factor of tooth erosion in these groups is vomiting, which acidifies the oral environment.

In the study by Garrido-Martínez et al. [35], the degree of dental erosion was significantly greater in EDs. Overall, 76.3% of the ED patients had dental erosion, while in the control group, it was only 9.2%. Additionally, the groups showed a significant difference in non-stimulated salivary flow. Among the ED participants, only 28.8% had a normal salivary flow, while the others experienced reduced flow or hyposialia. However, all of the control participants, except for one, had a normal salivary flow. The ED patients had a mean non-stimulated saliva flow of 0.23 mL/min, which was significantly lower than the normal flow rate. Approximately 20.3% of the ED patients had a non-stimulated flow of less than 0.1 mL/min, indicating hyposialia.

Women with EDs showed significantly higher dental erosions than the healthy controls. This conclusion was shared by Emodi-Perlman et al. [34], who examined women hospitalised because of chronic EDs. The ED group was divided according to their habit of daily vomiting. Dental erosion occurred in 17.6% of the non-vomiting patients and 33.3% of the vomiting patients. On the other hand, in the control group, no patients had dental erosion. Similarly, Szupiany-Janeczek et al. [59] found that individuals displaying symptoms of EDs had a higher chance of experiencing dental erosions (28.81% of cases) compared to those without symptoms (3.33% of cases). Interestingly, in this study, nearly 1/4 of the study group were males.

In contrast, Rungta and Kudpi [54] did not find a statistically significant association between dental erosion and EDs. It can be assumed that the lack of a statistically significant association between dental erosion and EDs is the result of the fact that the study involved an adolescent female cohort. As mentioned earlier, the age of the patients and the ED duration in the case of dental erosion is not insignificant.

Most papers on EDs focus on dental erosions as a prominent oral symptom. However, Panico et al. [50] took a different approach. Surprisingly, only two patients with EDs had dental erosions, whereas the control group had none. The patients with EDs in this study may have maintained stricter oral hygiene, leading the authors to speculate that dental decalcification is not necessarily an early symptom of EDs.

In a study conducted by Hermont et al. [38], the occurrence of dental erosion was compared in cohorts of female adolescents with and without risk behaviour for EDs. The severe risk behaviour for EDs was significantly associated with tooth erosion (OR = 10.0, 95%CI: 2.5–39.4). The study also highlighted the role of socioeconomic factors in the concomitance of EDs and tooth erosion, showing that students from private schools proportionally presented more cases of risk behaviour for EDs. The link between symptoms of EDs and higher socioeconomic status is not just a referral artifact, but is evident in a representative community sample. Additionally, the authors concluded that adolescents with severe risk behaviour for EDs had a higher chance of tooth erosion when consuming citric fruit and ketchup and brushing their teeth shortly after eating.

4.4. Study Limitations

Undoubtedly, our systematic review with meta-analysis highlighted and summarised a significant relationship between dental erosion and EDs, considering the analyses for the specific subgroups. Among the limitations, it is certainly worth mentioning the broad timeframe of the included studies. As is well-known, the methodology and results of studies were reported differently in the past than they are now. In some previous studies, the sample size might seem relatively small. At present, EDs and dental erosion are more common among young people. The included studies also differed in the diagnostic criteria for erosive defects that have evolved over the years; however, this did not significantly affect the relationship we studied.

Among the main sources of bias, the absence of data regarding blinding, randomisation and sample size justification should be mentioned. Moreover, it should be emphasised that, in most of the studies, the participants were women, which can be explained by the fact that EDs statistically affect women more often, and among men, they are a bit of a taboo subject. Some authors also did not separate subgroups of diagnoses of patients with EDs, which concealed the factual relationships, as it can be observed that bulimics have a greater predisposition to erosion than anorectics. Similarly, only a few studies included self-induced vomiting as a confounder, allowing a comparison of the erosion risk for vomiting and non-vomiting patients. For further studies, it would be useful to look at this relationship in a multi-factor manner, considering confounding variables, which could allow for meta-regression in the future.

5. Conclusions

Eating disorders are associated with an increased risk of tooth erosion. In particular, patients with bulimia nervosa and patients with self-induced vomiting had significantly higher odds of erosive lesions. Also, more than half of bulimics experienced dental erosion.

Author Contributions: Conceptualisation, K.N.; methodology, K.N.; formal analysis, K.N., J.J. and D.G.; investigation and data curation, K.N., J.J. and D.G.; writing—original draft preparation, K.N. and J.J.; writing—review and editing, K.N. and D.G.; visualisation, K.N.; supervision, A.S. All authors have read and agreed to the published version of the manuscript.

Funding: This research received no external funding.

Institutional Review Board Statement: Not applicable.

Informed Consent Statement: Not applicable.

Data Availability Statement: Data are available on request from the corresponding author.

Conflicts of Interest: The authors declare no conflict of interest.

References

1. American Psychiatric Association. *Diagnostic and Statistical Manual of Mental Disorders DSM-5*, 5th ed.; American Psychia Association: Washington, DC, USA, 2013.
2. Treasure, J.; Duarte, T.A.; Schmidt, U. Eating Disorders. *Lancet Lond. Engl.* **2020**, *395*, 899–911. [CrossRef]
3. Stice, E.; Marti, C.N.; Rohde, P. Prevalence, Incidence, Impairment, and Course of the Proposed DSM-5 Eating Disorder Diagno in an 8-Year Prospective Community Study of Young Women. *J. Abnorm. Psychol.* **2013**, *122*, 445–457. [CrossRef]
4. Striegel-Moore, R.H.; Rosselli, F.; Perrin, N.; DeBar, L.; Wilson, G.T.; May, A.; Kraemer, H.C. Gender Difference in the Prevale of Eating Disorder Symptoms. *Int. J. Eat. Disord.* **2009**, *42*, 471–474. [CrossRef]
5. Rikani, A.A.; Choudhry, Z.; Choudhry, A.M.; Ikram, H.; Asghar, M.W.; Kajal, D.; Waheed, A.; Mobassarah, N.J. A Critique of Literature on Etiology of Eating Disorders. *Ann. Neurosci.* **2013**, *20*, 157–161. [CrossRef]
6. Sharan, P.; Sundar, A.S. Eating Disorders in Women. *Indian J. Psychiatry* **2015**, *57*, S286–S295. [CrossRef]

Porras-Garcia, B.; Ferrer-Garcia, M.; Serrano-Troncoso, E.; Carulla-Roig, M.; Soto-Usera, P.; Miquel-Nabau, H.; Fernández-Del castillo Olivares, L.; Marnet-Fiol, R.; de la Montaña Santos-Carrasco, I.; Borszewski, B.; et al. AN-VR-BE. A Randomized Controlled Trial for Reducing Fear of Gaining Weight and Other Eating Disorder Symptoms in Anorexia Nervosa through Virtual Reality-Based Body Exposure. *J. Clin. Med.* **2021**, *10*, 682. [CrossRef]
Gaudio, S.; Brooks, S.J.; Riva, G. Nonvisual Multisensory Impairment of Body Perception in Anorexia Nervosa: A Systematic Review of Neuropsychological Studies. *PLoS ONE* **2014**, *9*, e110087. [CrossRef]
Nitsch, A.; Dlugosz, H.; Gibson, D.; Mehler, P.S. Medical Complications of Bulimia Nervosa. *Cleve. Clin. J. Med.* **2021**, *88*, 333–343. [CrossRef] [PubMed]
Kim, Y.-R.; An, Z.; Kim, K.-H.; Kim, D.-M.; Hwang, B.-I.; Kim, M. Factors Associated with Underweight, Overweight, and Eating Disorders in Young Korean Women: A Population-Based Study. *Nutrients* **2022**, *14*, 1315. [CrossRef] [PubMed]
Lo Muzio, L.; Lo Russo, L.; Massaccesi, C.; Rappelli, G.; Panzarella, V.; Di Fede, O.; Kerr, A.R.; Campisi, G. Eating Disorders: A Threat for Women's Health. Oral Manifestations in a Comprehensive Overview. *Minerva Stomatol.* **2007**, *56*, 281–292. [PubMed]
Monda, M.; Costacurta, M.; Maffei, L.; Docimo, R. Oral Manifestations of Eating Disorders in Adolescent Patients. A Review. *Eur. J. Paediatr. Dent.* **2021**, *22*, 155–158. [CrossRef]
Garbin, C.A.S.; Martins, R.J.; de Melo Belila, N.; Garbin, A.J.Í. Oral Manifestations in Patients with Anorexia and Bulimia Nervosa: A Systematic Review. *J. Public Health* **2020**, *28*, 765–771. [CrossRef]
Lo Russo, L.; Campisi, G.; Di Fede, O.; Di Liberto, C.; Panzarella, V.; Lo Muzio, L. Oral Manifestations of Eating Disorders: A Critical Review. *Oral Dis.* **2008**, *14*, 479–484. [CrossRef]
Presskreischer, R.; Prado, M.A.; Kuraner, S.E.; Arusilor, I.-M.; Pike, K. Eating Disorders and Oral Health: A Scoping Review. *J. Eat. Disord.* **2023**, *11*, 55. [CrossRef] [PubMed]
Bartlett, D.; Ganss, C.; Lussi, A. Basic Erosive Wear Examination (BEWE): A New Scoring System for Scientific and Clinical Needs. *Clin. Oral Investig.* **2008**, *12* (Suppl. 1), S65–S68. [CrossRef] [PubMed]
Mehta, L.K.; Hegde, A.; Thomas, A.; Virdi, M.S. Acidogenic Potential of Packaged Fruit Juices and Its Effect on Plaque and Salivary pH. *Int. J. Clin. Pediatr. Dent.* **2019**, *12*, 312–317. [CrossRef] [PubMed]
Valena, V.; Young, W.G. Dental Erosion Patterns from Intrinsic Acid Regurgitation and Vomiting. *Aust. Dent. J.* **2002**, *47*, 106–115. [CrossRef]
Butera, A.; Gallo, S.; Pascadopoli, M.; Scardina, G.A.; Pezzullo, S.; Scribante, A. Home Oral Care Domiciliary Protocol for the Management of Dental Erosion in Rugby Players: A Randomized Clinical Trial. *J. Clin. Med.* **2022**, *11*, 4893. [CrossRef]
Nijakowski, K.; Walerczyk-Sas, A.; Surdacka, A. Regular Physical Activity as a Potential Risk Factor for Erosive Lesions in Adolescents. *Int. J. Environ. Res. Public. Health* **2020**, *17*, 3002. [CrossRef]
Nijakowski, K.; Zdrojewski, J.; Nowak, M.; Podgórski, F.; Surdacka, A. Regular Physical Activity and Dental Erosion: A Systematic Review. *Appl. Sci.* **2022**, *12*, 1099. [CrossRef]
Johansson, A.-K.; Omar, R.; Carlsson, G.E.; Johansson, A. Dental Erosion and Its Growing Importance in Clinical Practice: From Past to Present. *Int. J. Dent.* **2012**, *2012*, 632907. [CrossRef] [PubMed]
Skalsky Jarkander, M.; Grindefjord, M.; Carlstedt, K. Dental Erosion, Prevalence and Risk Factors among a Group of Adolescents in Stockholm County. *Eur. Arch. Paediatr. Dent.* **2018**, *19*, 23–31. [CrossRef]
Buzalaf, M.A.R.; Hannas, A.R.; Kato, M.T. Saliva and Dental Erosion. *J. Appl. Oral Sci.* **2012**, *20*, 493–502. [CrossRef] [PubMed]
Chan, A.S.; Tran, T.T.K.; Hsu, Y.H.; Liu, S.Y.S.; Kroon, J. A Systematic Review of Dietary Acids and Habits on Dental Erosion in Adolescents. *Int. J. Paediatr. Dent.* **2020**, *30*, 713–733. [CrossRef]
Buzalaf, M.A.R.; Magalhães, A.C.; Rios, D. Prevention of Erosive Tooth Wear: Targeting Nutritional and Patient-Related Risks Factors. *Br. Dent. J.* **2018**, *224*, 371–378. [CrossRef] [PubMed]
Ludovichetti, F.S.; Signoriello, A.G.; Colussi, N.; Zuccon, A.; Stellini, E.; Mazzoleni, S. Soft Drinks and Dental Erosion during Pediatric Age: A Clinical Investigation. *Minerva Dent. Oral Sci.* **2022**, *71*, 262–269. [CrossRef]
Ludovichetti, F.S.; Zambon, G.; Cimolai, M.; Gallo, M.; Signoriello, A.G.; Pezzato, L.; Bertolini, R.; Mazzoleni, S. Efficacy of Two Toothpaste in Preventing Tooth Erosive Lesions Associated with Gastroesophageal Reflux Disease. *Appl. Sci.* **2022**, *12*, 1023. [CrossRef]
Page, M.J.; McKenzie, J.; Bossuyt, P.; Boutron, I.; Hoffmann, T.; Mulrow, C.D.; Shamseer, L.; Tetzlaff, J.; Akl, E.; Brennan, S.E.; et al. The PRISMA 2020 Statement: An Updated Guideline for Reporting Systematic Reviews. *Int. J. Surg.* **2020**, *88*, 105906. [CrossRef]
NHLBI, NIH. Study Quality Assessment Tools. Available online: https://www.nhlbi.nih.gov/health-topics/study-quality-assessment-tools (accessed on 22 August 2020).
OCEBM. Levels of Evidence. Available online: https://www.cebm.net/2016/05/ocebm-levels-of-evidence/ (accessed on 22 August 2020).
Altshuler, B.D.; Dechow, P.C.; Waller, D.A.; Hardy, B.W. An Investigation of the Oral Pathologies Occurring in Bulimia Nervosa. *Int. J. Eat. Disord.* **1990**, *9*, 191–199. [CrossRef]
Cavalcanti, A.L.; Andrade, N.M.; Brandt, L.M.T.; Fernandes, L.H.F.; Toscano, R.L.; Auad, S.M.; Buldur, B.; Cavalcanti, A.F.C. Risk Behaviors for Eating Disorders among Brazilian Female Adolescents. *Open Dent. J.* **2020**, *14*, 7–12. [CrossRef]

34. Emodi-Perlman, A.; Yoffe, T.; Rosenberg, N.; Eli, I.; Alter, Z.; Winocur, E. Prevalence of Psychologic, Dental, and Temp mandibular Signs and Symptoms among Chronic Eating Disorders Patients: A Comparative Control Study. *J. Orofac. Pain* **2** *22*, 201–208. [PubMed]
35. Garrido-Martínez, P.; Domínguez-Gordillo, A.; Cerero-Lapiedra, R.; Burgueño-García, M.; Martínez-Ramírez, M.-J.; Gór Candela, C.; Cebrián-Carretero, J.-L.; Esparza-Gómez, G. Oral and Dental Health Status in Patients with Eating Disorder Madrid, Spain. *Med. Oral Patol. Oral Cir. Bucal* **2019**, *24*, e595–e602. [CrossRef] [PubMed]
36. Giraudeau, N.; Camman, P.; Pourreyron, L.; Inquimbert, C.; Lefebvre, P. The Contribution of Teledentistry in Detecting To Erosion in Patients with Eating Disorders. *Digit. Health* **2021**, *7*, 20552076211019250. [CrossRef] [PubMed]
37. Hellström, I. Oral Complications in Anorexia Nervosa. *Scand. J. Dent. Res.* **1977**, *85*, 71–86. [CrossRef]
38. Hermont, A.P.; Pordeus, I.A.; Paiva, S.M.; Abreu, M.H.N.G.; Auad, S.M. Eating Disorder Risk Behavior and Dental Implicati among Adolescents. *Int. J. Eat. Disord.* **2013**, *46*, 677–683. [CrossRef]
39. Hurst, P.S.; Lacey, L.H.; Crisp, A.H. Teeth, Vomiting and Diet: A Study of the Dental Characteristics of Seventeen Anor Nervosa Patients. *Postgrad. Med. J.* **1977**, *53*, 298–305. [CrossRef]
40. Johansson, A.-K.; Norring, C.; Unell, L.; Johansson, A. Eating Disorders and Oral Health: A Matched Case-Control Study. *Eu Oral Sci.* **2012**, *120*, 61–68. [CrossRef]
41. Jones, R.R.; Cleaton-Jones, P. Depth and Area of Dental Erosions, and Dental Caries, in Bulimic Women. *J. Dent. Res.* **1989** 1275–1278. [CrossRef]
42. Jugale, P.V.; Pramila, M.; Murthy, A.K.; Rangath, S. Oral Manifestations of Suspected Eating Disorders among Women of 20 Years in Bangalore City, India. *J. Health Popul. Nutr.* **2014**, *32*, 46–50.
43. Lifante-Oliva, C.; López-Jornet, P.; Camacho-Alonso, F.; Esteve-Salinas, J. Study of Oral Changes in Patients with Eating Disorc *Int. J. Dent. Hyg.* **2008**, *6*, 119–122. [CrossRef]
44. Manevski, J.; Stojšin, I.; Vukoje, K.; Janković, O. Dental Aspects of Purging Bulimia. *Vojnosanit. Pregl.* **2020**, *77*, 300–307. [Cross
45. Milosevic, A.; Brodie, D.A.; Slade, P.D. Dental Erosion, Oral Hygiene, and Nutrition in Eating Disorders. *Int. J. Eat. Disord.* **1** *21*, 195–199. [CrossRef]
46. Montecchi, P.P.; Custureri, V.; Polimeni, A.; Cordaro, M.; Costa, L.; Marinucci, S.; Montecchi, F. Oral Manifestations in a Grou Young Patients with Anorexia Nervosa. *Eat. Weight Disord. EWD* **2003**, *8*, 164–167. [CrossRef] [PubMed]
47. Ohrn, R.; Enzell, K.; Angmar-Månsson, B. Oral Status of 81 Subjects with Eating Disorders. *Eur. J. Oral Sci.* **1999**, *107*, 157– [CrossRef] [PubMed]
48. Otsu, M.; Hamura, A.; Ishikawa, Y.; Karibe, H.; Ichijyo, T.; Yoshinaga, Y. Factors Affecting the Dental Erosion Severity of Patie with Eating Disorders. *Biopsychosoc. Med.* **2014**, *8*, 25. [CrossRef]
49. Pallier, A.; Karimova, A.; Boillot, A.; Colon, P.; Ringuenet, D.; Bouchard, P.; Rangé, H. Dental and Periodontal Health in Ad with Eating Disorders: A Case-Control Study. *J. Dent.* **2019**, *84*, 55–59. [CrossRef]
50. Panico, R.; Piemonte, E.; Lazos, J.; Gilligan, G.; Zampini, A.; Lanfranchi, H. Oral Mucosal Lesions in Anorexia Nervosa, Buli Nervosa and EDNOS. *J. Psychiatr. Res.* **2018**, *96*, 178–182. [CrossRef]
51. Paszynska, E.; Hernik, A.; Slopien, A.; Roszak, M.; Jowik, K.; Dmitrzak-Weglarz, M.; Tyszkiewicz-Nwafor, M. Risk of De Caries and Erosive Tooth Wear in 117 Children and Adolescents' Anorexia Nervosa Population-A Case-Control Study. *Fr Psychiatry* **2022**, *13*, 874263. [CrossRef]
52. Paszyńska, E.; Słopień, A.; Węglarz, M.; Linden, R.W.A. Parotid Salivary Parameters in Bulimic Patients—A Controlled Clin Trial. *Psychiatr. Pol.* **2015**, *49*, 709–720. [CrossRef]
53. Roberts, M.W.; Li, S.H. Oral Findings in Anorexia Nervosa and Bulimia Nervosa: A Study of 47 Cases. *J. Am. Dent. Assoc.* 1 **1987**, *115*, 407–410. [CrossRef]
54. Rungta, N.; Kudpi, R. Evaluation of Eating Disorders Using "scoff Questionnaire" among Young Female Cohorts and Its Der Implications-an Exploratory Study. *J. Orofac. Sci.* **2019**, *11*, 27–31. [CrossRef]
55. Rytömaa, I.; Järvinen, V.; Kanerva, R.; Heinonen, O.P. Bulimia and Tooth Erosion. *Acta Odontol. Scand.* **1998**, *56*, 36–40. [CrossR [PubMed]
56. Shaughnessy, B.F.; Feldman, H.A.; Cleveland, R.; Sonis, A.; Brown, J.N.; Gordon, C.M. Oral Health and Bone Density Adolescents and Young Women with Anorexia Nervosa. *J. Clin. Pediatr. Dent.* **2008**, *33*, 87–92. [CrossRef]
57. Simmons, M.S.; Grayden, S.K.; Mitchell, J.E. The Need for Psychiatric-Dental Liaison in the Treatment of Bulimia. *Am. J. Psychia* **1986**, *143*, 783–784. [CrossRef] [PubMed]
58. Strużycka, I.; Lussi, A.; Bogusławska-Kapała, A.; Rusyan, E. Prevalence of Erosive Lesions with Respect to Risk Factors i Young Adult Population in Poland-a Cross-Sectional Study. *Clin. Oral Investig.* **2017**, *21*, 2197–2203. [CrossRef] [PubMed]
59. Szupiany-Janeczek, T.; Rutkowski, K.; Pytko-Polończyk, J. Oral Cavity Clinical Evaluation in Psychiatric Patients with Eat Disorders: A Case-Control Study. *Int. J. Environ. Res. Public. Health* **2023**, *20*, 4792. [CrossRef] [PubMed]
60. Touyz, S.W.; Liew, V.P.; Tseng, P.; Frisken, K.; Williams, H.; Beumont, P.J. Oral and Dental Complications in Dieting Disorders. *J. Eat. Disord.* **1993**, *14*, 341–347. [CrossRef] [PubMed]
61. Uhlen, M.-M.; Tveit, A.B.; Stenhagen, K.R.; Mulic, A. Self-Induced Vomiting and Dental Erosion--a Clinical Study. *BMC C Health* **2014**, *14*, 92. [CrossRef] [PubMed]

Ximenes, R.; Couto, G.; Sougey, E. Eating Disorders in Adolescents and Their Repercussions in Oral Health. *Int. J. Eat. Disord.* **2010**, *43*, 59–64. [CrossRef]
Mehler, P.S.; Rylander, M. Bulimia Nervosa—Medical Complications. *J. Eat. Disord.* **2015**, *3*, 12. [CrossRef]

Journal of
Clinical Medicine

Systematic Review

Relationship between Prostate Inflammation and Periodontal Disease—A Systematic Review and Meta-Analysis

Pablo Ortíz de Urbina Comerón [1], Álvaro Zubizarreta-Macho [1,2,*], Ana Belén Lobo Galindo [2], José María Montiel-Company [3], María-Fernanda Lorenzo-Gómez [1,4] and Javier Flores Fraile [1]

1 Department of Surgery, Faculty of Medicine and Dentistry, University of Salamanca, 37008 Salamanca, Spain; pabloortizdeurbina@usal.es (P.O.d.U.C.); mflorenzogo@yahoo.es (M.-F.L.-G.); j.flores@usal.es (J.F.F.)
2 Department of Implant Surgery, Faculty of Health Sciences, Alfonso X el Sabio University, 28691 Madrid, Spain; alobogal@hotmail.com
3 Department of Stomatology, Faculty of Medicine and Dentistry, University of Valencia, 46010 Valencia, Spain; jose.maria.montiel@uv.es
4 Servicio de Urología del Hospital, Universitario de Salamanca, 37007 Salamanca, Spain
* Correspondence: alvaro.zubizarreta@usal.es

Abstract: The aim of this systematic review and meta-analysis was to analyze the association between periodontal disease and prostate inflammation with a null hypothesis stating that periodontal disease does not increase the incidence of prostate inflammation. Materials and methods: A systematic literature review and meta-analysis of longitudinal observational cohort and case-control studies that evaluated the odds ratio or hazard ratio and confidence interval was undertaken based on the Preferred Reporting Items for Systematic Reviews and Meta-Analyses (PRISMA) recommendations (2020). A total of four databases were consulted in the literature search: PubMed-Medline, Scopus, Embase, and Web of Science. After eliminating duplicated articles and applying the inclusion criteria, seven articles were selected for the qualitative and quantitative analyses. Results: Four observational cohort studies and three observational cohort case-control studies were included in the meta-analysis. The four observational cohort studies were combined using the random effects model to estimate a hazard ratio of 1.32 with a confidence interval of 95% between 0.87 and 1.77. The meta-analysis presented high heterogeneity (Q test = 56.1; p value < 0.001; I^2 = 94.9%). Moreover, the three observational case-control studies were combined using the random effects model to estimate an odds ratio of 1.62 with a confidence interval of 95% between 1.41 and 1.84. The meta-analysis presented high heterogeneity (Q test = 1.07; p value = 0.782; I^2 = 0%). Conclusions: The incidence of periodontal disease does not increase the risk of the incidence of prostate inflammation.

Keywords: periodontitis; prostatitis; prostate specific-antigen; odds ratio; hazard ratio

1. Introduction

Previous studies have suggested that inflammation of the dental supporting tissues and inflammation of the prostate gland could share a common etiology and reciprocally influence their incidence. This would indicate that dentists can influence the development and establishment of prostate diseases, since by controlling periodontal disease, they can prevent the appearance of prostate diseases.

In addition, Barone et al. (2023) reported a bacterial etiology of 5–10% of all prostatic inflammation and highlighted bacterial reduction as the most efficacious treatment approach to treating prostatitis [1]. Furthermore, De Luca et al. (2020) reported that granulomatous prostatitis, which is considered an uncommon (3.3%) chronic prostate inflammation with an autoimmune etiology, has shown an association with psoriasis (another autoimmune disease). This fact could demonstrate that certain pathologies may have a common etiology that leads to their establishment and development [2].

Prostatic inflammation or prostatitis is considered one of the most common prostate pathologies, with a prevalence of 11% in people under 50 years of age [3]. In addition, it was described as a "pathology" by the National Institutes of Health (NIH) in 1995, considering its multifactorial etiology [4].

Inflammation of the prostate gland is a condition that must be taken into consideration since it can sometimes lead to the development of prostate cancer. Additionally, benign prostatic hyperplasia is a common condition of the prostate gland, which is usually diagnosed incidentally during digital rectal examination and is confirmed by ultrasound-guided transrectal biopsy, as well as by prostate-specific antigen (PSA) levels [5].

In recent years, the molecular characterization of oral microbiota has facilitated the detection of 700 bacterial species or biotypes with the capability of colonizing the tissues in the oral cavity. However, a healthy individual harbors between approximately 150 and 200 different bacterial species, of which between 10 and 30 can cause periodontal diseases (PD) [6]. Subgingival bacterial counts show that a healthy individual harbors 103 colony-forming units (CFUs), whereas individuals with established PD can harbor up to 108 CFUs [7]. These types of infections are responsible for damaging tooth support tissues [8–10].

Periodontal diseases are characterized by their high prevalence. Epidemiological studies indicate that between 5 and 20% of the population suffers from advanced forms of periodontitis [11,12]. The etiopathogenesis of periodontal disease is strongly associated with the formation of dental plaque. Dental plaque is a complex polymicrobial biofilm model, whose process initiates with the introduction, establishment, and growth of primary colonizing bacteria on teeth, such as *Streptococcus oralis*.

Longitudinal clinical trials have shown that adequate control of bacterial plaque can prevent periodontitis and that the withdrawal of oral hygiene mechanisms is accompanied by an increase in bacterial plaque and the onset of this disease [13–15].

Previous studies have suggested a possible relationship between periodontal pathology and prostate inflammation, since multiple typical oral pathogens of periodontitis—*Porphyromona gingivalis*, *Fusobacterium nucleatum*, *Actinomyces actinomycetemcomitans*, *Treponema denticola*, and *Escherichia coli*—have also been found in cultures extracted from prostate disorders [16]. Therefore, this fact highlights the relevance of oral health as an integral part of the general health and well-being of patients. Moreover, some theories have been developed to explain the relationship between periodontal inflammation and prostate disease, such as the distant migration of oral microbial agents via the hematogenous route. This hypothesis was verified by Estemalik et al. (2017), who carried out DNA tests using dental plaque and prostatic fluids, finding the presence of at least one bacterial biotype in both tests in 64.7% of samples. This finding further highlighted the critical role of microbial flora in human health and disease [17].

Additionally, another possibility could be an association with the presence of certain proinflammatory cytokines of periodontal origin, which would cause a state of chronic inflammatory weakness that could stimulate the appearance of systemic disorders. Some of these cytokines are interleukins (ILs) (IL-1β, IL-6 and IL-8; tumor necrosis factor-α (TNF-α); interferon-γ). The possible inflammatory affectation by cytokines could explain abacterial prostatitis.

Finally, another hypothesis theorizes that the inflammatory response of the prostate gland is caused by a local increase in PSA levels, which could occur distantly, even in the periodontium. The generation of PSA in the periodontium tissues would imply the systemic alteration of pro-inflammatory mediators, establishing a dysfunction of these mediators.

Therefore, previous longitudinal clinical trials have shown that adequate control of bacterial plaque can prevent periodontitis and secondarily prostate inflammation and that the withdrawal of oral hygiene mechanisms is accompanied by an increase in bacterial plaque and the onset of this disease [11–13]. Many authors emphasize the importance of oral hygiene techniques to prevent the formation of bacterial biofilm [18].

The aim and rationale of this systematic review and meta-analysis were to analyze and compare the association between the incidence of periodontal disease and the risk of increased incidence of prostate inflammation, with a null hypothesis (H_0) stating that periodontal disease does not increase the incidence of prostate inflammation.

2. Materials and Methods

2.1. Study Design

This bibliographic search was conducted following PRISMA (Preferred Reporting Items for Systemic Reviews and Meta-Analyses; http://www.prisma-statement.org) guidelines for systematic reviews and meta-analyses (INPLASY registration number: INPLASY202350030; DOI number: 10.37766/inplasy2023.5.0030). The review also fulfilled the PRISMA 2020 Checklist [19].

2.2. Focused Question

The PECO (population, exposition, comparison, outcome) question was: 'Do men exposed to periodontal disease have a higher risk of suffering prostate inflammation?' with the following components: population: men affected by periodontal disease and prostate inflammation; exposition: periodontal disease and prostate inflammation; comparison: men not affected by periodontal disease and prostate inflammation; and outcomes: prostate inflammation.

2.3. Databases and Search Strategy

An electronic search was conducted in the following databases and gray literature: PubMed; Scopus; Embase; and Web of Sciences (A.Z.-M.; J.M.M.-C.). The search covered all the literature published internationally up to May 2023. The search included seven medical subject heading (MeSH) terms: 'periodontitis'; 'prostatitis'; 'prostate-specific antigen'; 'odds ratio'; and 'hazard ratio'. The Boolean operators applied were ('OR' and 'AND'). The search terms were structured as follows: '((periodontitis OR periodontal disease) AND (prostatitis OR prostate-specific antigen)) AND (odds ratio OR hazard ratio)'. Two researchers (A.Z.-M; J.F.F.) conducted the database searches in duplicate independently. Titles and abstracts were selected by applying inclusion and exclusion criteria.

2.4. Study Selection

Titles and abstracts were selected by two authors (A.B.L.G.; J.M.M.-C.), applying inclusion and exclusion criteria.

Inclusion criteria: longitudinal observational cohort and case-control studies. No restriction was placed on the year of publication or language.

Exclusion criteria: systematic reviews of the literature, clinical cases, case series with up to 5 patients and editorials; studies that include women or men under 18 years of age; and studies with samples of 5 or fewer patients. The following data were extracted from each article by two authors (P.O.d.U.C.; A.Z.-M.): author and year of publication; title and journal in which the article was published; sample size (n); follow-up time, odds ratio or hazard ratio; and confidence interval. Studies that analyzed the incidence risk of periodontal disease and prostate inflammation were included in the systematic review and meta-analysis.

2.5. Data Extraction and Study Outcomes

Data extraction was conducted in duplicate (P.O.d.U.C.; J.M.M.-C.) using predefined Excel spreadsheets and accounting for the following items: author and year, study type, sample size, follow-up in months, odds ratio or hazard ratio, and 95% confidence intervals.

2.6. Methodological Quality Assessment

The risk of bias in the studies selected for review was assessed by two authors (J.F.F.; P.O.d.U.C.) using the Newcastle–Ottawa scale for methodological quality assessment of longitudinal observational cohort and case-control studies. The Newcastle–Ottawa scale consists of three items that evaluate selection, comparisons, and results [20]. The level of agreement between evaluators was determined using Kappa scores.

2.7. Quantitative Synthesis—Meta-Analysis

The statistical data collection and analysis were conducted by two authors (A.Z.-M.; J.M.M.-C.). The studies included in the meta-analysis were combined using a random effects model with the maximum likelihood method used for effect size estimation as the odds ratio or hazard ratio. Heterogeneity between the combined studies was assessed using the Q test (p-value < 0.05) and was quantified using the I^2. Heterogeneity was considered to be slight if it was between 25 and 50%, moderate between 50 and 75%, and high if > 75%. The existence of statistical significance was assessed using the Z test (p-value < 0.05). Meta-analyses were represented with forest plots. Publication bias was assessed using the trim-and-fill adjustment method and represented with funnel plots.

3. Results

3.1. Flow Diagram

The initial electronic search identified 24 articles in PubMed, 37 in Web of Sciences, 16 in Embase, 12 in Scopus, and none in gray literature. Of the total 89 works, 26 were discarded as duplicates. After reading the titles and abstracts, a further 42 were eliminated leaving a total of 21. A further 14 were rejected as they failed to fulfill the following inclusion criteria: they did not include survival rate data, or they did not include a hazard ratio, odds ratio, or confidence interval. A final total of seven articles were included in the qualitative synthesis. Seven articles were included in the quantitative synthesis as these included all the data and variables required (Figure 1).

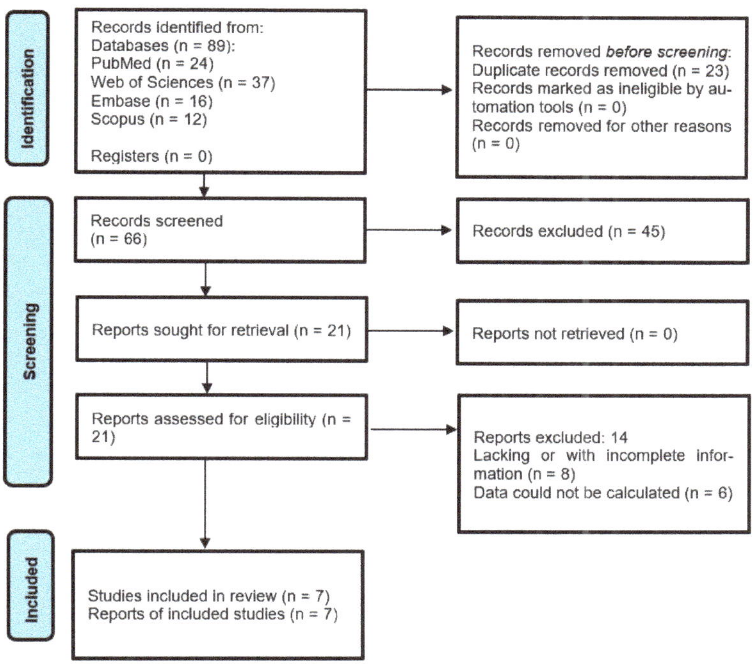

Figure 1. Preferred Reporting Items for Systematic Reviews and Meta-Analyses (PRISMA) flow diagram.

3.2. Qualitative Analysis

Of the seven articles included, four were longitudinal observational studies (cohort studies) [21–24] and three were cross-sectional observational clinical studies (case-control studies) [25–27] (Table 1).

Table 1. Qualitative analysis of articles included in the systematic review.

Author/Year	Study Design	N_Control Group	HN_Control Group	IC_Control Group
Michaud et al., 2008 [21]	Cohort	48,275	0.89	0.71–1.10
Huang et al., 2019 [23]	Cohort	38,092	2.11	1.63–2.73
Michaud et al., 2016 [22]	Cohort	19,933	1.17	0.94–1.47
Lee et al., 2017 [24]	Cohort	1235	1.5	1.05–2.10
Wu et al., 2019 [25]	Case-control	2171	1.81	0.76–4.34
Hujoel et al., 2003 [27]	Case-control	5240	0.49	0.19–1.26
Boland et al., 2013 [26]	Case-control	1240	1.5	1.05–2.10

3.3. Quality Assessment

The results of the methodological quality assessment were performed by one author (A.Z.-M.) using the Newcastle–Ottawa scale and are shown in Tables 2 and 3. The Newcastle–Ottawa scale obtained scores between 6 and 8, indicating high methodological quality and low risk of bias.

3.4. Quantitative Analysis

3.4.1. Hazard Ratio of Prostate Inflammation in Patients Affected by Periodontal Disease

Four studies, in which only two showed a significant association, were combined using the random effects model and the maximum likelihood method to estimate a hazard ratio = 1.32 and with a 95% confidence interval between 0.87 and 1.77, indicating the absence of significance. Periodontal disease increases the risk of prostatitis by 1.32 times, although it is not significant. The meta-analysis presented high heterogeneity; a Q test = 56.1 with a p value < 0.001 and I^2 = 94.9%. (Figure 2).

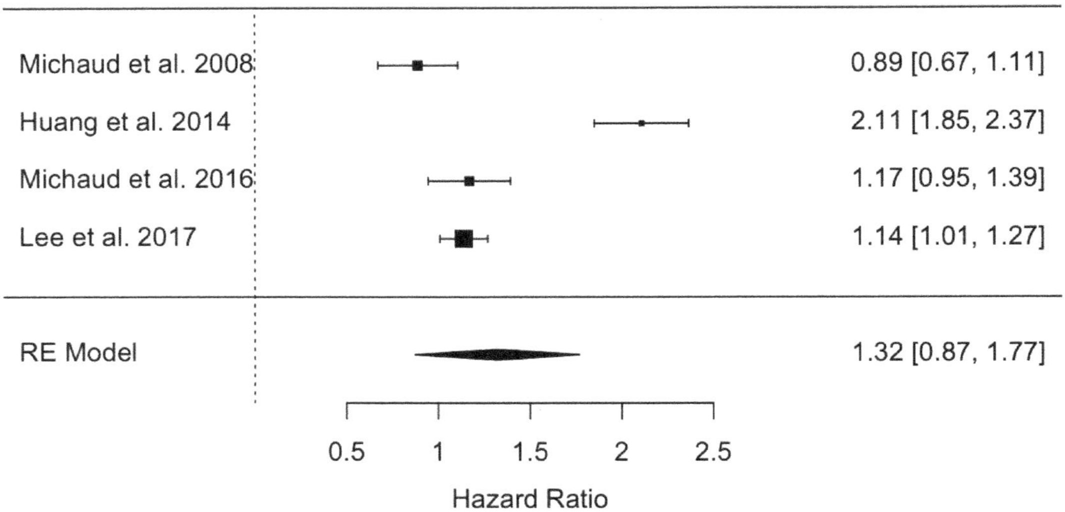

Figure 2. Forest plot of the hazard ratio meta-analysis of prostatitis in periodontal patients versus non-periodontal patients [21–24].

Table 2. Assessment of methodological quality of observational cohort studies, according to the Newcastle–Ottawa scale.

Author/Year	Selection				Comparability		Outcome			Total
	Representative of the Exposed Cohort	Selection of External Control	Ascertainment of Exposure	Outcome of Interest Not Present at the Start of the Study	Main Factor	Additional Factor	Assessment of Outcomes	Sufficient Follow-Up Time	Adequacy of Follow-Up	
Michaud et al., 2008 [21]	*		*	*			*	*	*	6/9
Huang et al., 2019 [23]	*	*	*	*	*		*	*	*	8/9
Michaud et al., 2016 [22]	*		*	*			*	*	*	6/9
Lee et al., 2017 [24]	*		*	*			*	*	*	6/9

*: Means that the response is affirmative.

Table 3. Assessment of methodological quality of observational case-control studies, according to the Newcastle–Ottawa scale.

Author/Year	Selection				Comparability		Outcome			Total
	Representative of the Exposed Cohort	Selection of External Control	Ascertainment of Exposure	Outcome of Interest Not Present at the Start of the Study	Main Factor	Additional Factor	Assessment of Outcomes	Sufficient Follow-Up Time	Adequacy of Follow-Up	
Boland et al., 2013 [26]	*		*	*			*	*	*	6/9
Wu et al., 2019 [25]	*		*	*			*	*	*	6/9
Hujoel et al., 2003 [27]	*		*	*			*	*	*	6/9

*: Means that the response is affirmative.

3.4.2. Odds Ratio of Prostate Inflammation in Patients Affected by Periodontal Disease

Three studies were combined using the random effects model and the maximum likelihood method to estimate an odds ratio = 1.62 and with a 95% confidence interval between 1.41 and 1.84, indicating the existence of a statistical significance. The ratio between periodontal disease and healthy periodontal tissue is 1.6 times higher in patients with prostatitis. The meta-analysis did not present heterogeneity (Q test = 1.07; p value = 0.782; and I^2 = 0%) (Figure 3).

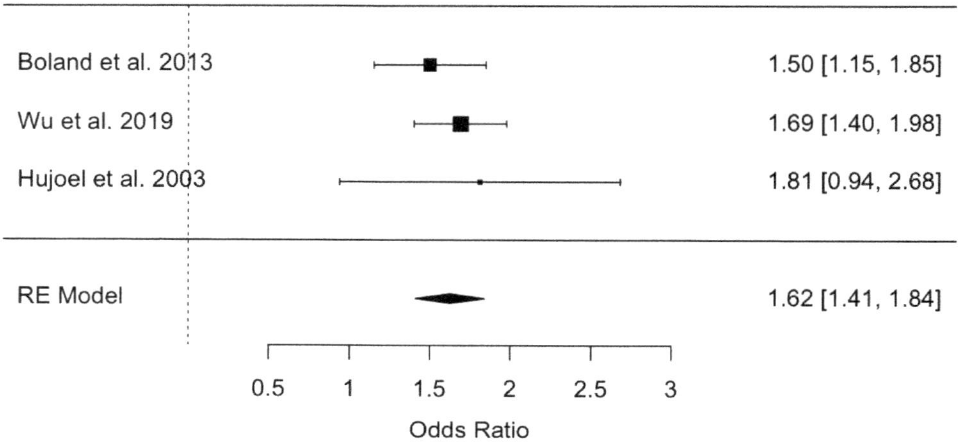

Figure 3. Forest plot of the odds ratio meta-analysis of prostatitis in periodontal patients versus non-periodontal patients [25–27].

3.5. Publication Bias

Publication bias was assessed using the Regression Test for Funnel Plot Asymmetry using a mixed-effects model, thus for the HR Test for Funnel Plot Asymmetry meta-analysis, z = 1.2326, p = 0.2177 (Figure 4), whereas for the OR meta-analysis Test for Funnel Plot Asymmetry, z = 0.2515, p = 0.8014 (Figure 5). Both results indicate the absence of publication bias.

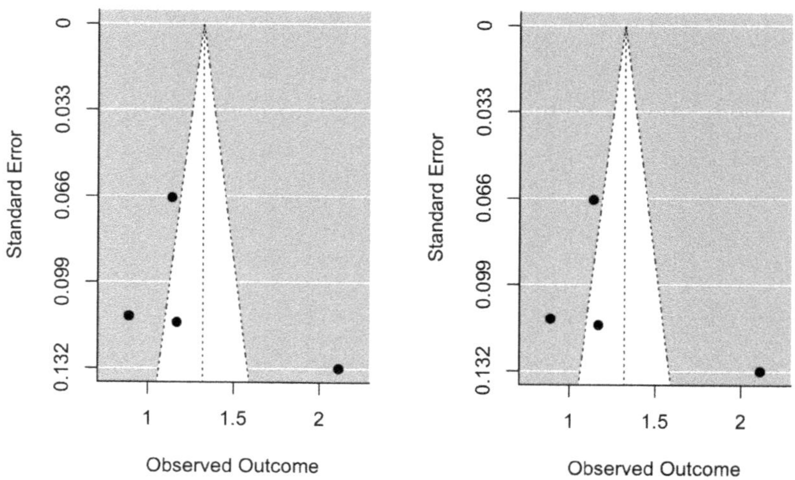

Figure 4. Initial hazard ratio funnel plot and after trim-and-fill adjustment.

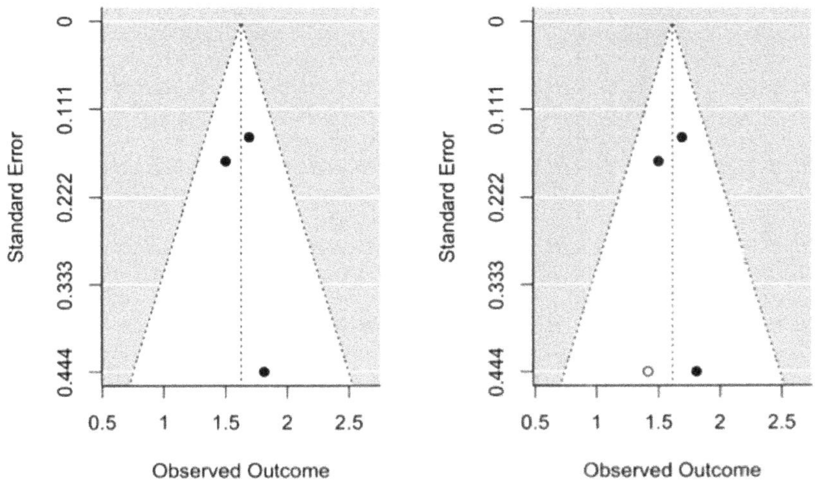

Figure 5. Initial odds ratio funnel plot and after trim-and-fill adjustment.

4. Discussion

The results obtained in the present study accept the null hypothesis (H_0) stating that periodontal disease does not increase the incidence of prostate inflammation.

Previous studies found a relationship between periodontitis and prostatitis [28,29], specifically in moderate-severe periodontitis, due to greater probing depths (LAC), worse plaque index (PI) values and worse bleeding rates, and higher prostate-specific antigen (PSA) levels ($\geq$4 ng/mL), possibly due to oral microbiome biotypes (*Treponema denticola, P. gingivalis* and *Tanarella forsythea*). In addition, most of the patients (95%) with both pathologies have previously been affected by chronic bacterial prostatitis [30]. Therefore, Joshi et al. (2010) highlighted periodontal therapy as an adjunctive treatment for the control and management of chronic prostatitis. Non-surgical periodontal treatment consists of mechanical debridement of supra- and infra-gingival bacterial biofilm and subsequent instruction in oral hygiene maintenance techniques [31]. Furthermore, the clinical diagnosis of chronic prostatitis is characterized by difficulty urinating completely or painful urination, constant urinary incontinence, pain in the penis and/or testicles, and fever; therefore, emphasis should be placed on early diagnosis and the elimination of associated factors [32].

In addition, PD has also been linked to other systemic pathologies such as atherosclerotic valve disease, premature births, diabetes mellitus, chronic renal failure, and pulmonary infections [33]. Specifically, the oral cavity acts as a reservoir for microorganisms that may reach the prostate gland through metastatic infections, dissemination of bacterial toxins, and/or immune alterations, which can cause prostate damage once they cross the intraepithelial tissue of the prostate gland [34]. This migration could lead to the establishment of a new neoplastic transformation. Indeed, it would be associated with Gram-negative bacteria, the predominant etiological agents in periodontitis and in categories I and II of prostatitis.

Moreover, Liu et al. (2015) suggested that the presence of chronic prostatitis and periodontitis could inhibit self-healing and, therefore, maintain both diseases in the chronic inflammatory phase [35]. In addition, Endo M (2017) proposed avoiding bacterial reinfection by prescribing antibiotic treatment for 15 days to eliminate the residual bacterial load from the original infection [36]. Most of the authors agreed with applying a non-surgical periodontal treatment to achieve an improvement in PSA levels, especially in patients affected with a moderate-severe prostate pathology. However, the reduction in PSA levels does not exempt us from performing prostate biopsies that could report other prostate alterations [37].

Although most studies highlighted the beneficial effect of periodontal treatment on the reduction of PSA levels, Kruck et al. (2017) showed that supra- and infra-gingival biofilm debridement alongside adequate instruction in oral hygiene techniques was not enough to significantly reduce PSA levels, probably due to the limited number of PSA measurements and the prostatitis classification of the selected patients [38]. However, Alwithanami et al. (2015) concluded that periodontal treatment for 4–8 weeks led to a significant reduction in PSA levels, compared with the control group; specifically, 21 out of 27 patients experienced a significant decrease in PSA levels [39]. Likewise, Fang et al. (2021) performed a randomized clinical trial and did not find an association between the oral microbiome and prostate changes; however, the manipulation of the microbial composition could effectively prevent the establishment of periodontal and systemic pathology [40]. Alwithanami et al. (2015) also reported that it may not only be the disease that is involved in the deterioration of the state of the prostate gland since the loss of teeth would also be a relevant factor in the development of prostatitis and the subsequent development of prostate cancer. For all these reasons, the establishment of periodontal therapy was suggested as a required treatment to improve dental health and reduce high PSA levels [37]. However, periodontal therapy with oral hygiene instructions is not considered an ideal treatment choice for all studies, since—as demonstrated in those patients with abacterial prostatitis—it may not have plausible effects at the PSA level. In addition, secondary bacterial infections could demonstrate chronic maintenance of asymptomatic prostatitis through chronic pelvic pain syndrome [41].

Additionally, Fu et al. (2021) stated that diabetes mellitus could lead to the development of gingivitis and subsequent periodontitis, which would likely become chronic. The prostate could consequently be affected, leading to prostatitis and benign prostatic hyperplasia and/or prostate cancer. Many risk and environmental factors have been associated; however, the development of prostatitis in patients with periodontitis is up to 4.6 times more likely than in patients without periodontitis [39].

Therefore, it is essential to highlight periodontal treatment, specifically in patients with unfavorable LAC, PI, and gingival index values [29]. Since the oral cavity constitutes a microbial reservoir for Gram-positive and Gram-negative bacteria, it is possible that the reduction of the bacterial load would consequently produce a distant reduction of multiple Gram-negative bacteria which could reduce the high levels of PSA and therefore the concomitant immune and inflammatory responses that could be present locally or systemically.

The relationship between periodontitis and prostatitis has been widely described in previous studies. Additionally, various studies have highlighted the incidence of periodontal disease with other systemic diseases such as cardiovascular diseases, acute myocardial infarctions, diabetes mellitus, adverse effects of pregnancy, respiratory disorders, osteoporosis, obesity, malnutrition, rheumatoid arthritis, and a wide variety of cancers.

However, the scant published scientific evidence is not enough to define in greater depth the advantages and disadvantages of periodontal therapy in patients with chronic prostatitis. Therefore, it is quite pertinent that further randomized clinical trials are carried out to confirm the association of periodontal disease with chronic prostatitis.

The authors report that the reduced number of articles included in this systematic review and meta-analysis could be considered a limitation; therefore, we encourage researchers to perform further and better-designed clinical studies with higher quality.

5. Conclusions

Meta-evidence suggests that the incidence of periodontal disease does not increase the risk of incidence of prostate inflammation; however, more clinical studies are necessary to confirm this statement.

Author Contributions: Conceptualization, P.O.d.U.C. and Á.Z.-M., design, J.F.F.; data acquisition, P.O.d.U.C. and J.F.F.; formal analysis, A.B.L.G.; statistical analysis, Á.Z.-M. and J.M.M.-C.; review and editing, P.O.d.U.C., M.-F.L.-G. and J.F.F. All authors have read and agreed to the published version of the manuscript.

Funding: This research received no external funding.

Institutional Review Board Statement: Not applicable.

Informed Consent Statement: Not applicable.

Data Availability Statement: Data available on request due to restrictions, e.g., privacy or ethical.

Conflicts of Interest: The authors declare no conflict of interest.

References

1. Barone, B.; Mirto, B.F.; Falcone, A.; Del Giudice, F.; Aveta, A.; Napolitano, L.; Del Biondo, D.; Ferro, M.; Busetto, G.M.; Manfredi, C.; et al. The Efficacy of Flogofilm® in the Treatment of Chronic Bacterial Prostatitis as an Adjuvant to Antibiotic Therapy: A Randomized Prospective Trial. *J. Clin. Med.* **2023**, *12*, 2784. [CrossRef]
2. De Luca, L.; Crocetto, F.; Barone, B.; Creta, M.; Pesce, S.; Aveta, A.; Campanino, M.R.; Imbimbo, C.; Longo, N. Granulomatous prostatitis mimicking prostate cancer in a patient with psoriatic arthritis: A case report. *Future Sci* **2020**, *6*, FSO591. [CrossRef] [PubMed]
3. Arnold, M.; Karim-Kos, H.E.; Coebergh, J.W.; Byrnes, G.; Antilla, A.; Ferlay, J.; Renehan, A.G.; Forman, D.; Soerjomataram, I. Recent trends in incidence of five common cancers in 26 European countries since 1988: Analysis of the European Cancer Observatory. *Eur J Cancer.* **2015**, *51*, 1164–1187. [CrossRef] [PubMed]
4. Flores-Fraile, M.C.; Padilla-Fernández, B.Y.; Valverde-Martínez, S.; Marquez-Sanchez, M.; García-Cenador, M.B.; Lorenzo-Gómez, M.F.; Flores-Fraile, J. The Association between Prostate-Specific Antigen Velocity (PSAV), Value and Acceleration, and of the Free PSA/Total PSA Index or Ratio, with Prostate Conditions. *J. Clin. Med.* **2020**, *9*, 3400. [CrossRef]
5. Polackwich, A.S.; Shoskes, D.A. Chronic prostatitis/chronic pelvic pain syndrome: A review of evaluation and therapy. *Prostate Cancer Prostatic Dis.* **2016**, *19*, 132–138. [CrossRef] [PubMed]
6. Kolenbrander, P.E.; Palmer, R.J., Jr.; Rickard, A.H.; Jakubovics, N.S.; Chalmers, N.I.; Díaz, P.I. Bacterial interactions and successions during plaque development. *Periodontol. 2000* **2006**, *42*, 47–79. [CrossRef] [PubMed]
7. Marsh, P.D. Controlling the oral biofilm with antimicrobials. *J. Dent.* **2010**, *38* (Suppl. 1), S11–S15. [CrossRef]
8. Socransky, S.S.; Haffajee, A.D. Evidence of bacterial etiology: A historical perspective. *Periodontol. 2000* **1994**, *5*, 7–25. [CrossRef]
9. Haffajee, A.D.; Socransky, S.S. Introduction to microbial aspects of periodontal biofilm communities. development and treatment. *Periodontol. 2000* **2006**, *42*, 7–12. [CrossRef]
10. Paster, B.J.; Olsen, I.; Aas, J.A.; Dewhirst, F.E. The breadth of bacterial diversity in the human periodontal pocket and other oral sites. *Periodontol. 2000* **2006**, *42*, 80–87. [CrossRef]
11. Albandar, J.M.; Rams, T.E. Global epidemiology of periodontal diseases: An overview. *Periodontol. 2000* **2002**, *29*, 7–10. [CrossRef] [PubMed]
12. Quirynen, M.; Teughels, W.; De Soete, M.; van Steenberghe, D. Topical antiseptics and antibiotics in the initial therapy of chronic adult periodontitis: Microbiological aspects. *Periodontol. 2000* **2002**, *28*, 72–90. [CrossRef] [PubMed]
13. Socransky, S.S.; Haffajee, A.D. The bacterial etiology of destructive periodontal disease: Current concepts. *J. Periodontol.* **1992**, *63* (Suppl. 4), 322–331. [CrossRef] [PubMed]
14. Bascones, A.; Morante, S.; Mateos, L.; Mata, M.; Poblet, J. Influence of additional active ingredients on the effectiveness of non-alcoholic chlorhexidine mouth washes: A randomized controlled trial. *J. Periodontol.* **2005**, *76*, 1469–1475. [CrossRef] [PubMed]
15. Corbet, E.F.; Davies, W.I. The role of supragingival plaque in the control of progressive periodontal disease. A review. *J. Clin. Periodontol.* **1993**, *20*, 307–313. [CrossRef] [PubMed]
16. Matsumoto, S.; Matsuda, M.; Takekawa, M.; Okada, M.; Hashizume, K.; Wada, N.; Hori, J.; Kita, M.; Iwata, T.; Kakizaki, H. Association between Chronic Periodontal Disease and Lower Urinary Tract Symptoms in Both Sexes. *Low. Urin. Tract Symptoms* **2015**, *7*, 17–21. [CrossRef]
17. Estemalik, J.; Demko, C.; Bissada, N.F.; Joshi, N.; Bodner, D.; Shankar, E.; Gupta, S. Simultaneous Detection of Oral Pathogens in Subgingival Plaque and Prostatic Fluid of Men with Periodontal and Prostatic Diseases. *J. Periodontol.* **2017**, *88*, 823–829. [CrossRef]
18. Davies, R.M. Toothpaste in the control of plaque/gingivitis and periodontitis. *Periodontol. 2000* **2008**, *48*, 23–30. [CrossRef]
19. Liberati, A.; Banzi, R.; Moja, L. Measuring the impact of evidence: The Cochrane systematic review of organized stroke care. *Intern. Emerg. Med.* **2009**, *4*, 507–510.
20. Lo, C.K.; Mertz, D.; Loeb, M. Newcastle-Ottawa Scale: Comparing reviewers' to authors' assessments. *BMC Med. Res. Methodol.* **2014**, *14*, 45. [CrossRef]

21. Michaud, D.S.; Liu, Y.; Meyer, M.; Giovannucci, E.; Joshipura, K. Periodontal disease, tooth loss, and cancer risk in male he professionals: A prospective cohort study. *Lancet Oncol.* **2008**, *9*, 550–558. [CrossRef] [PubMed]
22. Michaud, D.S.; Kelsey, K.T.; Papathanasiou, E.; Genco, C.A.; Giovannucci, E. Periodontal disease and risk of all cancers am male never smokers: An updated analysis of the Health Professionals Follow-up Study. *Ann. Oncol.* **2016**, *27*, 941–947. [Cross [PubMed]
23. Huang, Y.; Michaud, D.S.; Lu, J.; Carter, H.B.; Platz, E.A. The association between clinically determined periodontal dis and prostate-specific antigen concentration in men without prostate cancer: The 2009–2010 National Health and Nutri Examination Survey. *Cancer Causes Control* **2019**, *30*, 1293–1300. [CrossRef] [PubMed]
24. Lee, J.H.; Kweon, H.H.; Choi, J.K.; Kim, Y.T.; Choi, S.H. Association between Periodontal disease and Prostate cancer: Results 12-year Longitudinal Cohort Study in South Korea. *J. Cancer* **2017**, *8*, 2959–2965. [CrossRef] [PubMed]
25. Wu, L.; Li, B.H.; Wang, Y.Y.; Wang, C.Y.; Zi, H.; Weng, H.; Huang, Q.; Zhu, Y.J.; Zeng, X.T. Periodontal disease and risk of ber prostate hyperplasia: A cross-sectional study. *Mil. Med. Res.* **2019**, *6*, 34. [CrossRef] [PubMed]
26. Boland, M.R.; Hripcsak, G.; Albers, D.J.; Wei, Y.; Wilcox, A.B.; Wei, J.; Li, J.; Lin, S.; Breene, M.; Myers, R.; et al. Discover medical conditions associated with periodontitis using linked electronic health records. *J. Clin. Periodontol.* **2013**, *40*, 474– [CrossRef]
27. Hujoel, P.P.; Drangsholt, M.; Spiekerman, C.; Weiss, N.S. An exploration of the periodontitis-cancer association. *Ann. Epiden* **2003**, *13*, 312–316. [CrossRef]
28. Boyapati, R.; Swarna, C.; Devulapalli, N.; Sanivarapu, S.; Katuri, K.K.; Kolaparthy, L. Unveiling the Link between Prostatitis Periodontitis. *Contemp. Clin. Dent.* **2018**, *9*, 524–529. [CrossRef]
29. Muhsin, J.M.; Al-Sayyid, M.M. The possible Connection of periodontal diseases (PD) with cardiovascular disease (CVD) prostatitis in sample of Iraqi patients. *Muthanna Med. J.* **2019**, *6*, 1–12. [CrossRef]
30. da Silva, A.P.B.; Alluri, L.S.C.; Bissada, N.F.; Gupta, S. Association between oral pathogens and prostate cancer: Building relationship. *Am. J. Clin. Exp. Urol.* **2019**, *7*, 1–10.
31. Joshi, N.; Bissada, N.F.; Bodner, D.; Maclennan, G.T.; Narendran, S.; Jurevic, R.; Skillicorn, R. Association between periodo disease and prostate-specific antigen levels in chronic prostatitis patients. *J. Periodontol.* **2010**, *81*, 864–869. [CrossRef] [PubM
32. Coker, T.J.; Dierfeldt, D.M. Acute Bacterial Prostatitis: Diagnosis and Management. *Am. Fam. Physician.* **2016**, *93*, 114– [PubMed]
33. Hajishengallis, G. Periodontitis: From microbial immune subversion to systemic inflammation. *Nat. Rev. Immunol.* **2015**, 30–44. [CrossRef]
34. Kulhánová, I.; Bray, F.; Fadhil, I.; Al-Zahrani, A.S.; El-Basmy, A.; Anwar, W.A.; Al-Omari, A.; Shamseddine, A.; Znaor, Soerjomataram, I. Profile of cancer in the Eastern Mediterranean region: The need for action. *Cancer Epidemiol.* **2017**, *47*, 125– [CrossRef] [PubMed]
35. Liu, C.; Han, G.; Chen, J.; Yi, S.; Feng, X. Effect of periodontitis on rats with chronic bacterial prostatitis. *Anticancer. Res.* **2015**, 22–30.
36. Endo, M.; Yoshida, F.; Mori, M.; Nakano, M.; Morimura, T.; Ohno, Y.; Komura, M. Role of Helicobacter pylori in causing repea Reinfection from Oral cavity in Chronic Prostatitis. *Arch. Surg. Clin. Res.* **2018**, *2*, 5–12. [CrossRef]
37. Sanz, M.; Herrera, D.; Kebschull, M.; Chapple, I.; Jepsen, S.; Beglundh, T.; Sculean, A.; Tonetti, M.S. EFP Workshop Participa and Methodological Consultants. Treatment of stage I–III periodontitis-The EFP S3 level clinical practice guideline. *J. C Periodontol.* **2020**, *47* (Suppl. 22), 4–60, Erratum in *J. Clin. Periodontol.* **2021**, *48*, 163. [CrossRef]
38. Kruck, S.; Hennenlotter, J.; Amend, B.; Geiger, M.; Filipova, E.; Neumann, T.; Stühler, V.; Schubert, T.; Todenhöfer, T.; Rausch et al. Chronic Periodontitis Does Not Impact Serum Levels of Prostate-specific Antigen. *Anticancer. Res.* **2017**, *37*, 3163–3 [CrossRef]
39. Alwithanani, N.; Bissada, N.F.; Joshi, N.; Bodner, D.; Demko, C.; MacLennan, G.T.; Skillicorn, R.; Ponsky, L.; Gupta, S. Periodo Treatment Improves Prostate Symptoms and Lowers Serum PSA in Men with High PSA and Chronic Periodontitis. *Dentis* **2015**, *5*, 284–288. [CrossRef]
40. Fang, C.; Wu, L.; Zhao, M.J.; Deng, T.; Gu, J.M.; Guo, X.P.; Li, C.; Li, W.; Zeng, X.T. Periodontitis Exacerbates Benign Prost Hyperplasia through Regulation of Oxidative Stress and Inflammation. *Oxid. Med. Cell. Longev.* **2021**, *2021*, 2094665. [Cross
41. Fu, E.; Cheng, C.M.; Chung, C.H.; Lee, W.C.; Chen, W.L.; Sun, G.H.; Chien, W.C. Association of chronic periodontitis w prostatic hyperplasia and prostatitis: A population-based cohort study in Taiwan. *J. Periodontol.* **2021**, *92*, 72–86. [CrossR [PubMed]

Journal of
Clinical Medicine

MDPI

tematic Review

ral Manifestations of Crohn's Disease: A Systematic Review

ría Pilar Pecci-Lloret, Emma Ramirez-Santisteban, Adraz Hergueta-Castillo, Julia Guerrero-Gironés *
Ricardo Elías Oñate-Sánchez

Gerodontology and Special Care Dentistry Unit, Morales Meseguer Hospital, Faculty of Medicine, IMIB-Arrixaca, University of Murcia, 30008 Murcia, Spain; mariapilar.pecci@um.es (M.P.P.-L.); emma.ramirezs@um.es (E.R.-S.); adraz.hergueta@um.es (A.H.-C.); reosan@um.es (R.E.O.-S.)
* Correspondence: julia.guerrero@um.es

Abstract: Crohn's disease (CD) is a chronic inflammatory intestinal condition that can affect the entire gastrointestinal tract. It is characterized by its clinical heterogeneity and irregularities in its course. The etiology and pathogenesis are not well established, so it is difficult to establish an early diagnosis and an effective treatment plan. The objective of this systematic review was to present a qualitative synthesis of the studies referring to the oral manifestations of CD. This systematic review was carried out following the PRISMA guide. Research was conducted in the Pubmed, Web of Science, Scopus, Scielo, and Cocrahne Library databases on 23 February 2023, and updated on 1 September 2023. Articles published between 2012 and 2023 were selected. Articles that analyzed the oral manifestation of CD patients and met the established search terms. In addition, the quality of all the selected studies was analyzed following the CARE guidelines for case reports and the STROBE scale for observational studies. A total of 19 articles were included in this review that met the inclusion criteria. Regarding the oral manifestation of CD, oral ulcers, angular cheilitis, and gingivitis stand out. Periodontitis and vegetative pyostomatitis were the least representative manifestations. The most prevalent locations were lips, mucosa, and gingivae. Ulcers, gingivitis, and angular cheilitis are the most frequent oral manifestations in patients with CD. Their early identification and possible relationship with the disease are important for an early diagnosis and an adequate treatment plan.

Keywords: Crohn's disease; oral manifestations; oral lesions; systematic review

1. Introduction

Crohn's disease (CD) is described as a chronic inflammatory bowel disease, mainly affecting the lower gastrointestinal tract, with the ileocolonic region being the most affected. It is characterized by periods of remission and exacerbation. It is incurable and has a disabling course due to the development of various complications. In addition, it involves the skin, the musculoskeletal system, and the eyes [1–4].

In terms of epidemiology, CD affects men and women equally. Its age of onset has a bimodal distribution, with a peak between 20 and 40 years of age and a second peak between 50 and 60 years of age. The disease's incidence and prevalence have increased significantly worldwide [3].

Crohn's disease is of unknown etiology, is associated with an altered immune response, and has a strong genetic association. Whole genome studies revealed that when the NOD-2 receptor (a microbial recognition protein expressed on monocytes, macrophages, dendritic cells, and paneth cells) is mutated, an alteration of the patient's immune response occurs and is directed towards the bacterial flora of the gut, being related to the development of CD [2,5–7].

In addition to the genetic susceptibility of patients, the interaction with environmental factors has to be present. CD appears to be the result of an alteration in the commensal microbiota of the gut. This may be altered by diet, drug use, smoking, or infectious processes. The most relevant would be Mycobacterium avium paratuberculosis (MAP), or measles virus. In addition, recent studies link the use of toothpaste or a history of appendectomy as environmental factors related to the disease. On the other hand, it has been shown that breastfeeding or contact with animals in childhood may be protective factors against the disease. However, there is no causal relationship between the above-mentioned factors and the development of the disease [2,3,5,6].

The presentation of the disease is very heterogeneous, with many subtypes. Initially, the most frequent presentation is purely inflammatory. In the final presentation, intestinal fibrosis is found, leading to intestinal strictures and fistulas. There is a 50% chance of developing perianal fistulas within 20 years of the initial diagnosis [8,9].

The main symptoms that raise suspicion of Crohn's disease are abdominal pain and chronic diarrhoea leading to weight loss, observed in 60–70% of patients. Depending on the type of diarrhoea emitted by the patient, the area that is most affected may be suspected. If the diarrhoea is large in volume, the involvement is more likely to be located in the ileum, whereas if the diarrhoea is smaller and mucus and blood are present, the colon is possibly the area most affected [2,6,9].

Oral manifestations are common in Crohn's disease and may present as the first symptom. Early symptoms include aphthous ulcers, redness, edema, and pain. They are predominantly located on the mucosa, lips, and tongue. The presence of lesions in the cavity was associated with an exacerbation of the disease. There are specific and non-specific manifestations. The difference lies in the non-caseating inflammation and granulomatous substrate in the case of specific manifestations. Specific manifestations include ulcers and lips with granulomatous changes or Miescher cheilitis. Sometimes indurated polypoid tumours can be observed on the buccal mucosa in their specific form. Non-specific manifestations include oral aphthous ulcers, erythema nodosum, and a variety of neutrophilic dermatoses [1,2,10].

Treatment of CD is primarily aimed at achieving sustained clinical and endoscopic remission. It is important to interrupt the destructive course of the disease, which, if prolonged, can lead to intestinal failure and associated complications. It should be individualised for each patient [5].

Finally, it is important to emphasise the importance of early and accurate diagnosis and subsequent appropriate treatment. There is a high risk of malignancy for people with Crohn's disease for small bowel, colorectal, and mucinous carcinoma arising from perianal fistulas [9].

Currently, CD is a chronic intestinal disease of unknown aetiology, but with patients with high genetic susceptibility and involvement of various environmental factors, some of which have no proven scientific evidence. There is variability in its clinical presentation, ranging from intestinal and extraintestinal manifestations to associated autoimmune disorders. This makes a diagnosis and choice of treatment difficult.

There are several oral clinical manifestations that appear as early signs of the disease and that are essential to detect in order to identify the disease as early as possible. This leads to an improvement in the patient's prognosis and quality of life. Therefore, there is a need for a multidisciplinary team for its management that is aware of the most characteristic manifestations, and in this case, at the oral level. There is a lack of scientific knowledge on the subject to date. Thus, the aim of this systematic review was to present a qualitative synthesis of various studies concerning the oral manifestations of Crohn's disease.

2. Materials and Methods

2.1. Declaration and Protocol

This systematic review was conducted according to the PRISMA guide, an acronym for "Preferred Reporting Items for Systematic Reviews and Meta-Analyses". In addition to the regulations of the Final Degree Projects of the University of Murcia. It was registered in PROSPERO with registration number CRD42022377915.

2.2. Inclusion and Exclusion Criteria

The criteria for the inclusion of articles were the following: (i) articles published between the last 10 years (2012 and 2023); (ii) articles analysing and identifying oral manifestations present in CD patients; (iii) articles published in English or Spanish; (iv) any type of research article.

Exclusion criteria were as follows: (i) articles published more than 10 years ago; (ii) articles that provided information about inflammatory bowel diseases in a generalised way and did not study the oral manifestations of CD; (iii) articles in a language other than English or Spanish; (iv) systematic reviews or literature reviews.

In order to establish the inclusion criteria, the PICO model should be followed:

Population/problem (P): Patients with Crohn's disease; Intervention (I); Comparison/control (C): Healthy patients; Outcome (O): Oral manifestations present in patients with Crohn's disease.

So, the PICO question is: What are the oral manifestations of patients with Crohn's disease?

2.3. Search Strategy

2.3.1. Sources of Information

In order to search for information on the topic proposed for this systematic review, an exhaustive search was carried out in the following databases: Pubmed, Web of Science, Scopus, Scielo, and Cocrahne Library.

This search was carried out on 23 February 2023 and updated on 1 September 2023.

2.3.2. Search Terms

The terms used for the search were obtained from the Mesh (Medical Subject Heading) thesaurus. Those referring to Crohn's disease are "Crohn's disease", "Crohn's", "Crohn's", "inflammatory bowel disease", and "bowel disease." Those referring to oral manifestations are "Oral manifestation" and "oral lesion". Boolean operators ("AND" and "OR") were used to relate the mentioned terms to each other. The following table shows the results obtained from the search performed (Table 1).

Table 1. Search fields.

Database	Search Field	Results
Medline (PubMed)	1# "Crohn's disease" OR "Chron's" OR "Crohn" OR "inflammatory bowel disease" OR "bowel disease".	103,567
	2# "oral manifestation" OR "oral lesion".	9302
	1# AND 2#	220
Web of Science	1# "Crohn's disease" OR "Chron's" OR "Crohn" OR "inflammatory bowel disease" OR "bowel disease".	136,376
	2# "oral manifestation" OR "oral lesion".	6826
	1# AND 2#	196
SCOPUS	1# "Crohn's disease" OR "Chron's" OR "Crohn" OR "inflammatory bowel disease" OR "bowel disease".	153,087
	2# "oral manifestation" OR "oral lesion".	11,159
	1# AND 2#	298
Scielo	1# "Crohn's disease" OR "Chron's" OR "Crohn" OR "inflammatory bowel disease" OR "bowel disease".	617
	2# "oral manifestation" OR "oral lesion".	1065
	1# AND 2#	1
Cochrane Library	1# "Crohn's disease" OR "Chron's" OR "Crohn" OR "inflammatory bowel disease" OR "bowel disease".	8479
	2# "oral manifestation" OR "oral lesion".	278
	1# AND 2#	2

2.3.3. Selection of Studies

The studies obtained in the search process were entered into the Endnote Analytics bibliographic manager. After that, the manager discarded duplicate articles, and other duplicate articles not identified by the manager were manually discarded.

Subsequently, a first selection of articles was made on the basis of their titles. The abstract of the articles selected by title was read, and a second selection was made. Finally, the selected articles were read in full text and checked for compliance with the inclusion and exclusion criteria.

2.3.4. Data Extraction

For the bibliometric analysis, the years of publication, authors, city, and journals were taken into account. To summarise the methodology of the studies, a summary table was drawn up with the following data: type of studies; most frequent manifestations; most frequent location in the oral cavity.

2.3.5. Quality Analysis

The quality of the studies included in this systematic review was analyzed by two reviewers (ERS and MPPL). Any discrepancies were decided by involving a third reviewer (JGG). Use was made of the CARE guideline for clinical cases, which sets out a series of recommendations on the quality of clinical cases. It is composed of 30 items, 11 of which refer to the different parts that make up a clinical case (title, keywords, abstract, introduction, patient information, clinical findings, dates, diagnostic evaluation, therapeutic intervention, follow-up and results, discussion, patient perspective, and informed consent). Each of these was marked with a positive tick (✔) when the requirement was met and a cross (✗) as negative when the requirement was not met. The attached table shows the 30 items contained in the CARE guide that were followed for our analysis. In the case of control, cross-sectional, cohort, and prospective studies, the guide used was the modified STROBE scale (Strengthening the Reporting of Observational Studies in Epidemiology), which establishes the necessary recommendations for what an observational study should include. It is composed of 11 items that refer to the parts of the studies mentioned (material, methods, and results). Studies with 9 to 11 items were selected as low bias; those with 6–8 were considered moderate bias; those with less than 5 were considered high bias. The same methodology as above was applied.

3. Results

3.1. Selection of Studies and Flow Diagram

The results of the selection are shown in Figure 1. After the exhaustive database search, a total of 717 references were obtained, of which 220 were from Medline, 298 from Scopus, 196 from Web of Science, 2 from Cocrahne Library, and 1 from Scielo.

Later, 178 articles were discarded using the Endnote bibliographic manager. Subsequently, another 248 duplicate references not detected by the manager were eliminated, resulting in a total of 498 articles. Next, 452 articles that did not cover the topic of study were eliminated by title and abstract. Thus, 46 references were evaluated in full text, discarding 24 of them and finally obtaining 22 valid articles.

3.2. Bibliometric Analysis

The studies resulting from the search were distributed by year of publication, country of publication, and journal of publication. With regard to the year of publication, the continuous publication of articles on the subject is perceived, with an increase in the year 2021. The years 2019 and 2020 are the years with the lowest publication rate. Concerning the country of publication, the highest prevalence of published studies is found in the United States with seven articles, followed by Italy with four published articles. For the rest of the countries mentioned, one publication per country was found. There are a wide variety of journals that include articles related to CD and its oral manifestations, the most prominent being BMJ, which, in addition to case reports, also published a case control, and Wiley Clinical, which includes 2 case reports.

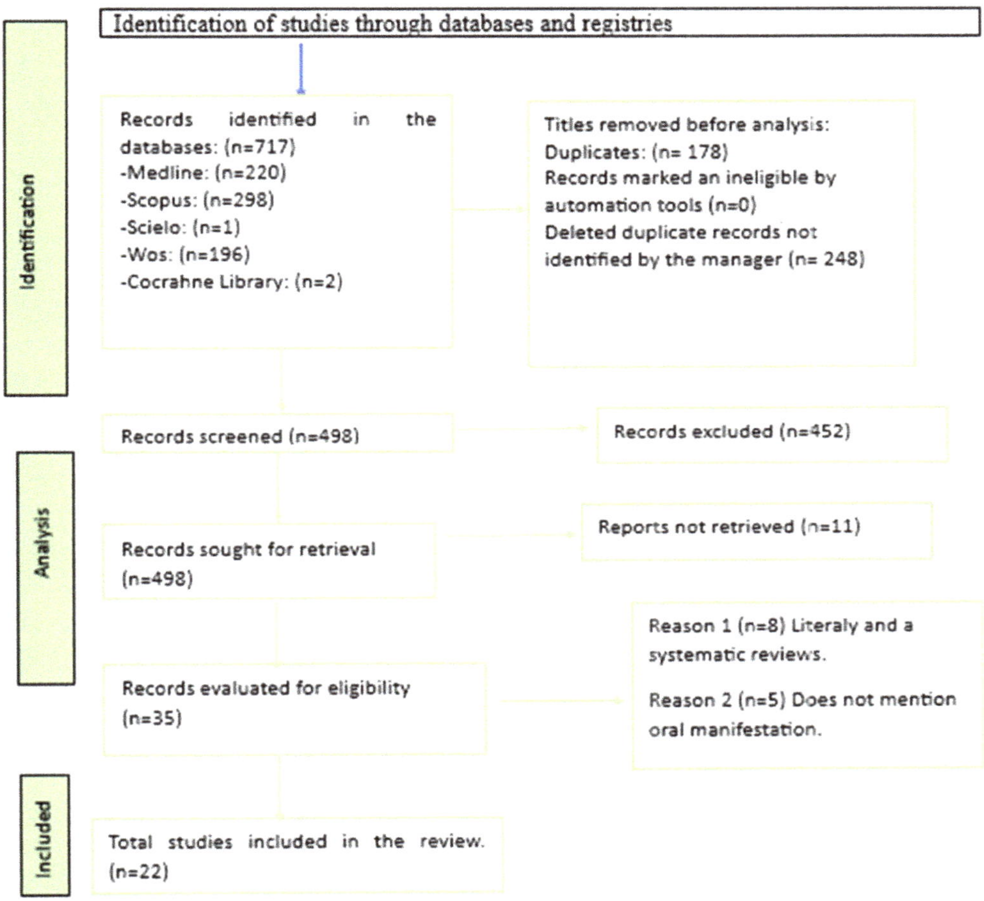

Figure 1. Flowchart diagram.

3.3. Results of Data Extraction

The results of the extraction are represented in Table 2, where the different categories mentioned above and the significance of the association of oral manifestations as a clinical part of CD can be observed.

Table 2. Description of the variables differentiated for each of the articles examined.

Author	Study Type	Participants Number	Age	Oral Manifestations	Location	Treatment	Developments	Anatomical Diagnosis	Differential Dx
Katarzyna Szczeklik et al., 2012 [11]	Prospective Study	95	-------	Glossitis, ulcers, canker sores, aphthae, gingivitis and angular cheilitis	Tongue, gingiva and mucosa	Mesalazine, azathioprine, corticosteroids, tumour necrosis factor	----------	----------	----------
Nicolas Bruscino et al., 2012 [12]	Clinical Case	1	12 y	Perioral erythema, vesicles, pustules, crusts and swelling	Lower lip	Mercaptopu-rina	4 years	Non-caseating granulomas, lymphocytes and plasma cell infiltrate	----------
Stephan R. Vavricka et al., 2013 [13]	Case Control	113	40 y	Gingivitis, periodontitis, ulcers, leukoplakia and angular cheilitis	Lips, gums, palate and tongue	Thiopurines Anti-TNF therapy	----------	----------	----------
Hamid Salek et al., 2013 [14]	Clinical Case	1	64 y	Painful cobblestone ulcers	Oral and labial mucosa	Topical corticosteroids	30 years	Granulomatous inflammation	Orofacial granulomatosis, vegetating pyostomatitis, chronic non-specific ulcers, fungal infection, tuberculosis and pemphigus.
Carolina ciacci et al., 2014 [15]	Clinical Case	1	23 y	Granulomatous cheilitis	Lowerlip	Infliximad	----------	Inflammatory tissue with non-caseating granulomatous inflammation	----------
Raimund HM Preidl et al., 2014 [16]	Clinical Case	1	36 y	Perimandibular swelling, Dysphagia, and pain	Mandibular posterior region	Prednisolone Adalimumab	----------	Granulomatous inflammatory reaction with necrosis	----------

Table 2. *Cont.*

Author	Study Type	Participants Number	Age	Oral Manifestations	Location	Treatment	Developments	Anatomical Diagnosis	Differential Dx
Bn Padmavathi et al., 2014 [17]	Clinical Case	1	34 y	Angular cheilitis, Swelling and hyperplasia	Lips and buccal mucosa	----------------	13 years	Presence of diffuse lymphocytes and clusters with scattered fibrotic aggregates of non-caseating granuloma	Sarcoidosis Orofacial granulomatosis
G gale et al., 2015 [18]	Cohort study	29	32 and 7 y	Swelling, erythema, enlargement gingival and pain	Lips, mucosa and gingiva	----------------	----------	Non-caseating granulomas with multinucleated giant cells, lymphoedema and lymphocytic infiltration	Orofacial granulomatosis
Victoria L. Woo, 2015 [10]	Clinical Case	1	6 y	Pain, bleeding, erythema and ulcers	Gum	Mesalamine Azathioprine	7 months	Fibrous connective tissue with lymphocytes and plasma cells+ non-caseating granulomas	Sarcoidosis Orofacial Granulomatosis
Henedina Antunes et al., 2015 [19]	Clinical Case	1	17 y	Painful ulcers and cheilitis	----------	Prednisolone Azathioprine	2 months	Lymphoplasmacytic infiltrate and epitheloid granulomas	Orofacial Granulomatosis
Bryce L. Desmond et al., 2016 [20]	Clinical Case	1	17 y	Granulomatous cheilitis of the inf. lip	Lip inf.	Azathioprine	--------	Granulomatous dermatitis with lymphocytes + plasma cells	Idiopathic granulomatous cheilitis
Saede atarbashi-moghadam et al., 2016 [21]	Clinical Case	1	39 y	Pain, halitosis ulcers and exophytic pustules	Gingiva and mucosa	Mezalanin and Azeram	1 month	Intraepithelial clefts and acantholysis	Pemphigus vulgaris and vegetans

Table 2. *Cont.*

Author	Study Type	Participants Number	Age	Oral Manifestations	Location	Treatment	Developments	Anatomical Diagnosis	Differential Dx
Tavares dos Santos et al., 2017 [22]	Clinical Case	1	------	Solitary lesions, blackberry lesions and erosions	Gum	Azathioprine and mesazalin	---------	Pseudoepitheliomatous hyperplasia with microabscesses + Granulomatous tissue with lymphocytic infiltrate	Fungal infection and syphilis
Ashley Eckel et al., 2017 [23]	Clinical Case	1	15 y	Pain, gingival bleeding, swelling and ulcers	Palate, cheeks and retromolar area	Corticosteroids	1 month	Discrete non-caseating granulomas, sialodenitis and plasmacytosis	Infectious diseases, drug reactions, nutritional
Anu Haarano et al., 2018 [24]	Transversal study	46	-------	Amygular cheilitis, ulcers, erythema, swelling	Mucosa, gingiva, lips, palate and floor of the mouth	Anti-TNF therapy, Azathioprine, 5-aminosalicylic acid and methotrexate.	----------	------------------------	Orofacial granulomatosis
Saverio Capodiferro et al., 2019 [25]	Clinical Case	1	12 y	Gingivitis, fissures and angular cheilitis	Gums, lips and mucosa	Anti-inflammatories and immuno-suppressants	----------	Non-caseating granulomas	---------------
Miray Karakoyun et al., 2019 [26]	Clinical Case	1	16 y	Inflammation and ulcers	Lip and mucosa.	Methylprednisolone and mesalazine Azathioprine	3 months	-------------------------	----------------
Mei Li Huang et al., 2020 [27]	Clinical case	1	11 y	Sores, swelling, cracking and tooth mobility	Oral mucosa and lips	Metronidazole, Infliximab Mercaptopurine	----------	--------------------------	----------------
Mohammad S. Alrasdan et al., 2021 [28]	Clinical Case	1	23 y	Canker sores	Buccal mucosa, uvula, pillars of the fauces and oropharynx	Adalimumab Prednisolone Azathioprine	3 months	Diffuse granulomatous inflammation	---------------

Table 2. Cont.

Author	Study Type	Participants Number	Age	Oral Manifestations	Location	Treatment	Developments	Anatomical Diagnosis	Differential Dx
Sol de Boyang et al., 2021 [29]	Cohort study	18	-------	Caries, Periodontitis and bleeding	Teeth and periodontium	------------------	-----------	----------------------	--------------
Franncesca Giaccaglia et al., 2021 [30]	Clinical Case	1	15 y	Erythema, inflammation and angular cheilitis	Gums and lips	Adalimumab Infliximad	-----------	Inflammatory infiltration of submucosal lymphocytes and monocytes+ granulomatous aggregates	Sarcoidosis Granulomatosis orofacial
Colin E. McCorkle et al., 2021 [31]	Clinical Case	1	27 y	Gingival irritation and swelling of the lip	Lips and chin	Adalimumab Prednisona	4 months	Non-caseating submucosal granulomatous inflammation + lymphoid infiltrate	Sarcoidosis, Vasculitis, Neoplasms

The results obtained are shown in Table 2. As can be seen, most of them are clinical cases, with a single patient in all of them. There are fewer observational studies, but they contain a larger volume of patients, with a maximum of 113 patients [13].

The age of the patients in the studies varied. Patients ranged in age from 6 to 64 years of age [10,14]. It should be noted that most of them were in their early twenties [15,19,20,28].

All of them had oral lesions. The evolution of these lesions is unknown in some cases, but in the cases in which it was known, the minimum duration was 1 month [21,23]. The clinical case with the longest evolution of the lesions was 30 years old [14].

The most prevalent oral manifestations were angular cheilitis, oral ulcers, and gingivitis, as well as pain, dysphagia, halitosis, bleeding, and inflammation. Periodontitis and vegetating pyostomatitis were the least representative manifestations.

Regarding their location, the lips, mucosa, and gingiva are the places where most of them were found. However, some patients are shown with lesions at the level of the floor of the mouth, posterior mandible, palate, or even the uvula. Some of the cases presented were diagnosed with CD at the time of the oral manifestations, while others were diagnosed with CD as a result of the oral manifestations. The described lesions were examined microscopically, and the findings were summarised as diffuse non-caseating granulomatous inflammation with lymphocytic infiltrate and the presence of multinucleated giant cells, monocytes, and plasma cells.

In several patients, a differential diagnosis of the oral manifestations presented was necessary. The most repeated diseases were orofacial granulomatosis, sarcoidosis, and pemphigus. Tuberculosis, syphilis, vasculitis, or infectious diseases were mentioned as possible diagnoses before determining the final diagnosis of CD.

Finally, the medication administered to patients was mainly directed at CD and not at the oral manifestations. In the same way that it improved the course of the disease, it reduced the symptoms at the oral level, and in many cases, the manifestations found disappeared. We highlight the administration of immunosuppressants (azathioprine) and monoclonal antibodies (infliximab and adalimumab) as first-line treatments.

3.4. Quality Assessment

The quality of the clinical cases was assessed using the CARE guideline [32] (Table 3). The quality of the studies was medium, as many of them did not meet items 8b, 9c, 10c, 10d, and 12 referring to therapeutic intervention, follow-up, outcomes, and patient perspective. Only items 6–8 referring to timing, clinical findings, and diagnostic assessment were fulfilled by all items [10,12,14,17,23,25,28,30,31].

The articles were evaluated, after which a percentage was established for each of them, with the highest percentage achieved being 83.33%, followed by 76.66% [16,26]. The clinical cases with a higher bias have a lower percentage, and in this case, their value is 23.33% [12]

In the case of observational studies, the modified STROBE scale was used (Table 4). The quality of the studies was moderate with a high bias [11,13,24,29]. Item 5 was not met by any of the studies, while items 1 and 7 were met by all of them (Table 4).

Table 3. Results of the analysis of observational studies.

	Vavricka et al., 2013 [13]	Haarano et al., 2018 [24]	Boyang et al., 2021 [29]	Gale et al., 2014 [18]	Szczeklik et al., 2012 [11]
1	✔	✔	✔	✔	✔
2	✗	✔	✔	✗	✗
3	✗	✗	✗	✗	✗
4	✗	✗	✗	✗	✗
5	✔	✔	✔	✔	✔
6	✔	✔	✗	✔	✗
7	✔	✔	✔	✔	✔
8	✔	✗	✗	✗	✗
9	✔	✔	✔	✔	✗
10	✔	✔	✗	✔	✗
11	✔	✗	✗	✗	✔
nal puntuation	8	7	5	6	4
Risk of bias	moderate	moderate	high	moderate	high

Table 4. Results of the quality analysis of the clinical cases.

	McCorkle et al., 2021 [31]	Desmond et al., 2016 [20]	HM Preidl et al., 2014 [16]	Ciacci et al., 2014 [15]	Eckel et al., 2017 [23]	L. Woo 2015 [10]	Bruscino et al., 2012 [12]	Antunes et al., 2015 [19]	Capodiferro et al., 2019 [25]	Dos Santos et al., 2017 [22]	Atarbashi-moghada 2016 [21]	Karakoyun et al., 2019 [26]	Salek et al., 2013 [14]	Huang et al., 2020 [27]	Padmavathi et al., 2014 [17]	Giaccaglia et al., 2021 [30]	Alrasdan et al., 2021 [28]	Dos Santos et al., 2017 [22]	Atarbashi-moghadam 2016 [21]
1	✗	✔	✔	✔	✗	✔	✗	✗	✗	✗	✗	✔	✗	✗	✗	✔	✔	✗	✗
2	✔	✗	✔	✔	✗	✗	✗	✗	✔	✔	✔	✔	✔	✔	✗	✔	✔	✔	✔
3a	✔	✔	✔	✔	✔	✔	✗	✗	✔	✔	✔	✔	✔	✔	✔	✔	✔	✔	✔
3b	✔	✔	✔	✔	✔	✔	✗	✗	✔	✔	✔	✔	✔	✔	✔	✗	✗	✔	✔
3c	✗	✗	✔	✔	✔	✗	✗	✗	✔	✔	✔	✔	✔	✔	✔	✔	✗	✔	✔
3d	✔	✔	✔	✔	✔	✔	✗	✗	✔	✔	✔	✔	✔	✔	✔	✔	✔	✔	✔
4	✔	✗	✔	✔	✔	✔	✗	✗	✗	✔	✗	✔	✔	✔	✔	✔	✔	✔	✗
5a	✔	✔	✔	✔	✔	✔	✔	✔	✔	✔	✔	✔	✔	✔	✔	✔	✔	✔	✔
5b	✔	✔	✔	✔	✔	✔	✔	✗	✔	✔	✔	✔	✔	✔	✔	✔	✔	✔	✔
5c	✔	✔	✔	✔	✔	✔	✗	✔	✗	✔	✔	✔	✔	✔	✗	✔	✔	✔	✔
5d	✔	✗	✔	✗	✗	✔	✗	✗	✗	✔	✔	✗	✔	✔	✗	✔	✔	✔	✔
6	✔	✔	✔	✔	✔	✔	✔	✔	✔	✔	✔	✔	✔	✔	✔	✔	✔	✔	✔
7	✔	✔	✔	✔	✔	✔	✔	✔	✔	✔	✔	✔	✔	✔	✔	✔	✔	✔	✔
8a	✔	✔	✔	✔	✔	✔	✔	✔	✔	✔	✔	✔	✔	✔	✔	✔	✔	✔	✔
8b	✗	✗	✗	✗	✗	✗	✗	✗	✗	✗	✗	✗	✗	✗	✗	✗	✗	✗	✗
8c	✔	✗	✗	✗	✔	✔	✗	✔	✗	✗	✔	✗	✔	✔	✔	✔	✔	✗	✔
8d	✗	✗	✗	✗	✗	✗	✗	✗	✗	✗	✗	✔	✗	✗	✗	✗	✗	✗	✗
9a	✔	✔	✔	✔	✔	✔	✔	✔	✔	✔	✔	✔	✔	✔	✗	✔	✔	✔	✔
9b	✗	✗	✔	✔	✗	✗	✗	✔	✗	✔	✗	✔	✔	✗	✗	✗	✔	✔	✗
9c	✗	✗	✗	✗	✗	✗	✗	✗	✗	✗	✗	✗	✗	✗	✗	✗	✔	✗	✗
10a	✔	✔	✔	✔	✔	✔	✔	✔	✔	✔	✔	✔	✔	✔	✔	✔	✔	✔	✔
10b	✔	✔	✔	✔	✔	✔	✗	✗	✗	✔	✔	✔	✔	✔	✗	✗	✔	✔	✔
10c	✔	✗	✔	✔	✗	✗	✗	✗	✗	✗	✗	✗	✗	✗	✗	✗	✗	✗	✗
10d	✗	✗	✔	✗	✗	✗	✗	✗	✗	✗	✗	✗	✗	✗	✗	✗	✗	✗	✗
11a	✔	✔	✔	✔	✔	✔	✗	✔	✔	✔	✔	✔	✔	✔	✔	✔	✔	✔	✔
11b	✔	✔	✔	✔	✔	✔	✗	✗	✔	✔	✔	✔	✔	✔	✔	✔	✔	✔	✔
11c	✗	✗	✗	✔	✗	✗	✗	✔	✗	✔	✔	✔	✔	✔	✔	✔	✔	✔	✔
11d	✔	✔	✔	✔	✔	✔	✗	✗	✔	✔	✔	✔	✔	✔	✔	✔	✔	✔	✔
12		✗	✔	✔	✗	✔	✗	✗	✗	✗	✗	✗	✗	✗	✗	✗	✗	✗	✗
13	✔	✗	✔	✔	✗	✗	✗	✔	✗	✗	✗	✔	✗	✔	✗	✗	✗	✗	✗
Total	22	16	25	24	17	20	7	12	15	21	20	23	22	22	16	20	22	21	20
%	73.33%	53.33%	83.33%	80%	56.66%	66.66%	23.33%	40%	50%	70%	66.66%	76.66%	73.33%	73.33%	53.33%	66.66%	73.33%	70%	66.66%

4. Discussion

The results of this systematic review indicate that all selected studies showed oral manifestations of CD.

Oral manifestations are part of the extraintestinal manifestations of CD. It is vitally important to know about them and the prevalence in which they occur. In the adult population, lesions are found in around 0–9%, while in children, they appear in around 50–80% of patients and may precede severe intestinal involvement in up to 42% of the latter [23,28,30,31]. Rarely have cases been reported where oral involvement was unique and unaccompanied by intestinal disease [14].

The oral cavity is recognised as a useful part of the gastrointestinal tract in the diagnostic procedure for CD. Thus, dentists play an important role in the early diagnosis of the disease and subsequent improvement in both quality of life and prognosis, especially in the paediatric population, with a major impact on growth, puberty, and emotional development [25,33].

Oral involvement can take two forms: specific, including diffuse lip and oral swelling, cobblestoning of the oral mucosa, linear and serpiginous ulcers, and mucogingivitis. In the paediatric population, these types of lesions are more common, with mucogingivitis and ulcers being predominant, and they are non-specific, differentiated from the previous ones by the lack of granulomas when observed microscopically. These include aphthous ulcers, angular cheilitis, and glossitis. It should be noted that these ulcers are sometimes not part of the disease process but are secondary to nutritional deficiencies caused by the course of the disease [10,11,15,17,20,24,27,28,31].

Periodontitis and vegetating pyostomatitis are non-specific manifestations that only some articles classify as such [23,27,30]. CD is one of the systemic conditions affecting the periodontium. Recent studies have speculated that CD is likely to induce periodontitis by changing its oral microbiota and subsequent inflammatory response [27,29].

A 2012 study by Szczeklik et al. [11] found a higher prevalence of periodontitis in patients with CD. One year later, a case-control study conducted by Dr. Stephan Vavircka et al. [13] affirms the previous findings and provides that, in addition to the higher prevalence, the disease behaves with greater severity and extension, both in the adult population. Recently, the first case of a girl with CD presenting with periodontal disease and advanced bone loss has been described [11,27].

In addition, it is important to recognise vegetating piostomatitis. A very specific marker of CD, it is a very rare oral disorder characterised by white or yellow pustules affecting the oral cavity on an erythematous base, which, when ruptured, take the form of a snail's footprint [14,21].

Regarding the location of the lesions mentioned, there is a predominance of lesions on the mucosa, especially on the lower lips and gums. Lesions are present in other less common locations, such as the soft palate, uvula, tongue, and pillars of the fauces [10–17,19–28,30,31].

Finally, it can be concluded that the most predominant oral manifestations of CD are mucosal cobblestoning, the presence of linear ulcers, granulomatous cheilitis of the lips, with a predominance of the lower lip, and mucogingivitis. However, some less conspicuous but indicative lesions are found, such as vegetating pyostomatitis or periodontitis in some cases.

As well described, mucosal cobblestoning is significant in CD. Macroscopically in the intestine, one can observe the onset of small focal ulcers that coalesce to form longitudinal, serpiginous ulcers, giving the cobblestone appearance mentioned at the oral level. Microscopically, we find chronic patchy and transmural inflammation, with an increase in plasma cells and lymphocytes, discontinuous irregularity of the crypts, but without rupture of the crypts, and the presence of non-caseating granulomas in the lamina propria. In oral biopsies of the reported cases, plasma cell and lymphocyte infiltrate and the presence of non-caseating granulomas of the lamina propria and submucosa were found in most of them [6,10,12,14–17,19,20,22,23,25,28,30,34].

It is important to note that the presence of non-caseating granulomas is specific and may fit various diagnoses such as orofacial granulomatosis, although according to Colin E. McCorkle et al. [31], author of one of the selected studies, orofacial granulomatosis is a sign of an underlying process and not a definitive diagnosis as described by other authors [10,14,17,19,24,30]. Therefore, it could be suggested that oral ulcers share histology and appearance with intestinal ulcers.

The presenting symptomatology is varied. In many of the articles mentioned, the patient presented with pain, mostly caused by ulcers. Others presented with lip enlargement, gingival irritation, dry lips, and cracking. The proportion of asymptomatic patients was high, which complicates the early diagnosis of the disease, as the user attended the doctor when the lesion was very evident. Sometimes, oral symptomatology was accompanied by intestinal symptoms such as diarrhoea, weight loss, abdominal pain, and general malaise [10,12,14,15,17–21,23,24,26–28,31]. There are several treatments for CD, but the most widespread is pharmacological. We highlight the use of aminosalicylates, corticosteroids, immunomodulators, and biological therapy [10–16,19–28,30,31]. Most patients with oral lesions were treated with systemic therapy; only three cases were reported where lesions were treated with topical corticosteroids. Two of them received only topical corticosteroid rinses, showing marked improvement in symptomatology and eventually remission. The author of the third case, Victoria Woo et al. [10], notes that the patient received azathioprine and aminosalicylates in addition to topical treatment, which also improved intestinal symptoms. Saede Atarbashi-Moghadam et al. [21] stress the importance of using local treatment in the absence of systemic symptomatology but note that it has limited success [14,17,21,26]. In several articles mentioned, patients were treated with immunosuppressants and corticosteroids [10–14,16,19,20,22–28,31]. The results were very good, as there was an improvement in oral and gastrointestinal lesions. Long-term use of immunosuppressants can present severe complications for the patient. Harim Tavares dos Santos et al. [22] report a rare case of paracoccidioidomycosis in a woman with CD on long-term azathioprine treatment who presented with a blackberry lesion on the palate. The use of immunosuppressants leads to a series of complications, including fungal infection, virus, leukopenia, or worsening of the periodontal status and overgrowth in the case of mercaptopurine, according to Mei Li huang et al. [12,20,25,27,30].

Finally, biologic therapy is one of the most effective and accepted therapies for CD. The most widely used are Adalimumab, infliximab, and ustekinumab [11,13,15,16,24,26–28,31]. Patients treated with Adalimumab, in the articles selected for this study, have been the group with the most complications and recurrence of symptoms [16,28,31].

Preidl et al. [16] report a case of osteonecrosis of the jaw in a patient with CD after a course of bisphosphonate therapy and current treatment with Adalimumab. In other case reports, some correlation between patients with osteonecrosis of the jaw and biologic therapy can be seen [35]. It is still unclear whether biologic therapy interferes with bone physiology, bone turnover, and long-term wound repair.

This review has limitations, as do the other published articles. Limitations in the selection of the studies included in the systematic review have to be considered. Most of the articles selected were case reports of medium quality. With respect to the observational studies chosen, they were smaller in number and highly biased. Thus, the articles are biased, which is a drawback for the presentation of good-quality articles.

The main limitation of this review is the number of patients. Most of the proposed articles are clinical case reports of a single patient. In the case of observational studies, the number of patients reaches a maximum of 113, but only 69 of them had CD. Even in one of them, the oral examination was not performed by dentists [13]. Moreover, in most of them, the follow-up of the patient after the healing of the lesions was not described.

As mentioned earlier in this review, knowledge of the oral manifestations of patients with CD and collaboration between gastroenterologists and dentists will help in the early diagnosis of the disease and subsequent improvement in both the prognosis and quality of life of patients, as has already been seen with other diseases and their oral manifestations [36].

5. Conclusions

CD is a chronic, relapsing inflammatory bowel disease with uncertain pathogenesis. The aetiology is speculated to be multifactorial and involves genetic, environmental, immune, and microbial factors. It affects the entire gastrointestinal tract, but lesions predominate in the terminal ileum and colon. It is relapsing, and there is currently no cure for it.

Based on the results obtained in this systematic review, we can conclude that:

- CD presents with oral manifestations. Some oral lesions develop silently and go unnoticed by the patient. Others become established, causing pain and incapacitating the patient in their normal life, sometimes accompanied by gastrointestinal symptoms.
- Oral involvement in CD patients has been reported in 0.5% to 37% of cases. The length of time in the mouth is not well defined, as in some patients the lesions go unnoticed and in others there are recurrences.
- The most representative oral manifestations of CD are mucogingivitis (especially in the paediatric population), angular cheilitis, serpiginous and linear ulcers, and cobblestone-like mucous membranes.
- Visualisation of oral manifestations of CD plays an important role in the early diagnosis of CD, as they are sometimes the first sign of the disease or oral and intestinal lesions are found simultaneously.

More studies with better quality are needed to corroborate the results obtained in this work.

Author Contributions: Conceptualization, E.R.-S. and A.H.-C.; methodology, E.R.-S., M.P.P.-L. and R.E.O.-S.; formal analysis, E.R.-S., M.P.P.-L. and J.G.-G.; data curation, E.R.-S. and M.P.P.-L.; writing—original draft preparation, E.R.-S., J.G.-G. and A.H.-C.; writing—review and editing, M.P.P.-L.; supervision, M.P.P.-L., J.G.-G. and R.E.O.-S. All authors have read and agreed to the published version of the manuscript.

Funding: This research received no external funding.

Conflicts of Interest: The authors declare no conflict of interest.

erences

Reszczyńska, M.; Poniewierka, E.; Waśko-Czopnik, D.; Paradowski, L. Crohn's disease in the upper gastrointestinal tract. Own experience and review of the literature. *Gastroenterol. Rev./Przegląd Gastroenterol.* **2011**, *6*, 23–29. [CrossRef]

Ruocco, E.; Cuomo, A.; Salerno, R.; Ruocco, V.; Romano, M.; Baroni, A. Crohn's disease and its mucocutaneous involvement. *Skinmed* **2007**, *6*, 179–185. [CrossRef] [PubMed]

O'Neill, I.D.; Scully, C. Biologics in oral medicine: Oral Crohn's disease and orofacial granulomatosis. *Oral Dis.* **2012**, *18*, 633–638. [CrossRef] [PubMed]

Yamamoto-Furusho, J.-K. Enfermedad de Crohn: Diagnóstico y tratamiento. *Rev. Gastroenterol. México* **2013**, *78*, 68–70. [CrossRef] [PubMed]

Baumgart, D.C.; Sandborn, W.J. Crohn's disease. *Lancet* **2012**, *380*, 1590–1605. [CrossRef] [PubMed]

Ballester Ferré, M.P.; Boscá-Watts, M.M.; Mínguez Pérez, M. Crohn's disease. *Med. Clin.* **2018**, *151*, 26–33. [CrossRef] [PubMed]

Peña, A.S. El significado de las mutaciones de CARD15 en la enfermedad de Crohn: La contribución española. *Rev. Española Enfermedades Dig.* **2007**, *99*, 563–569. [CrossRef] [PubMed]

Adler, J.; Rangwalla, S.C.; Dwamena, B.A.; Higgins, P.D. The prognostic power of the NOD2 genotype for complicated Crohn's disease: A meta-analysis. *Off. J. Am. Coll. Gastroenterol. ACG* **2011**, *106*, 699–712. [CrossRef]

Rubbino, F.; Greco, L.; di Cristofaro, A.; Gaiani, F.; Vetrano, S.; Laghi, L.; Bonovas, S.; Piovani, D. Journey through Crohn's Disease Complication: From Fistula Formation to Future Therapies. *J. Clin. Med.* **2021**, *10*, 5548. [CrossRef]

Woo, V.L. Oral Manifestations of Crohn's Disease: A Case Report and Review of the Literature. *Case Rep. Dent.* **2015**, *2015*, 830472. [CrossRef]

Szczeklik, K.; Owczarek, D.; Pytko-Polończyk, J.; Kęsek, B.; Mach, T.H. Proinflammatory cytokines in the saliva of patients with active and non-active Crohn's disease. *Pol. Arch. Med. Wewnętrznej* **2012**, *122*, 200–208. [CrossRef] [PubMed]

Bruscino, N.; Arunachalam, M.; Galeone, M.; Scarfi, F.; Maio, V.; Difonzo, E.M. Lip swelling as initial manifestation of Crohn's disease. *Arch. Dis. Child.* **2012**, *97*, 647. [CrossRef] [PubMed]

13. Vavricka, S.R.; Manser, C.N.; Hediger, S.; Vögelin, M.; Scharl, M.; Biedermann, L.; Rogler, S.; Seibold, F.; Sanderink, R.; Attin, T.; Periodontitis and gingivitis in inflammatory bowel disease: A case-control study. *Inflamm. Bowel Dis.* **2013**, *19*, 2768–2777. [Cross [PubMed]
14. Salek, H.; Balouch, A.; Sedghizadeh, P.P. Oral manifestation of Crohn's disease without concomitant gastrointestinal involven *Odontology* **2014**, *102*, 336–338. [CrossRef] [PubMed]
15. Ciacci, C.; Bucci, C.; Zingone, F.; Iovino, P.; Amato, M. Buccal localization of Crohn's disease with long-term infliximab ther A case report. *J. Med. Case Rep.* **2014**, *8*, 397. [CrossRef] [PubMed]
16. Preidl, R.H.M.; Ebker, T.; Raithel, M.; Wehrhan, F.; Neukam, F.W.; Stockmann, P. Osteonecrosis of the jaw in a Crohn's dis patient following a course of Bisphosphonate and Adalimumab therapy: A case report. *BMC Gastroenterol.* **2014**, *14*, 6. [Cross
17. Padmavathi, B.; Sharma, S.; Astekar, M.; Rajan, Y.; Sowmya, G. Oral Crohn's disease. *J. Oral Maxillofac. Pathol. JOMFP* **2014** (Suppl. S1), S139–S142.
18. Gale, G.; Ostman, S.; Rekabdar, E.; Naluai, A.T.; Hogkil, K.; Hasseus, B.; Saalman, R.; Jontell, M. Characterisation of a Swe cohort with orofacial granulomatosis with or without Crohn's disease. *Oral Dis.* **2015**, *21*, E98–E104. [CrossRef]
19. Antunes, H.; Patraquim, C.; Baptista, V.; Silva Monteiro, L. Oral manifestations of Crohn's disease. *BMJ Case Rep.* **2015**. [Cross
20. Desmond, B.L.; Thomas, R.S.; Howerter, S.S. Case Report: Crohn's Disease Presenting as Granulomatous Cheilitis. *J. D Dermatol.* **2016**, *15*, 251–252.
21. Atarbashi-Moghadam, S.; Lotfi, A.; Atarbashi-Moghadam, F. Pyostomatitis Vegetans: A Clue for Diagnosis of Silent Cro Disease. *J. Clin. Diagn. Res.* **2016**, *10*, Zd12–Zd13. [CrossRef] [PubMed]
22. Dos Santos, H.T.; de Andrade, B.A.B.; Fernandes, D.; Travassos, D.C.; Bufalino, A. Chronic paracoccidioidmycosis in a wo with Crohn Disease. *Dermatol. Online J.* **2017**, *23*, 13030/qt1gp8z9gx. [CrossRef]
23. Eckel, A.; Lee, D.; Deutsch, G.; Maxin, A.; Oda, D. Oral manifestations as the first presenting sign of Crohn's disease in a pedia patient. *J. Clin. Exp. Dent.* **2017**, *9*, e934–e938. [CrossRef] [PubMed]
24. Haaramo, A.; Alapulli, H.; Aine, L.; Tuokkola, J.; Saarnisto, U.; Roine, R.P.; Pitkäranta, A.; Kolho, K.L. Oral and Otorhinolary logical Findings in Adults Who Were Diagnosed with Pediatric Onset Crohn's Disease: A Controlled Study. *J. Clin. Gastroent* **2019**, *53*, e269–e275. [CrossRef] [PubMed]
25. Capodiferro, S.; Maiorano, E.; Limongelli, L.; Tempesta, A.; Favia, G. Cheilitis and gingivitis as first signs of Crohn's disease pediatric patient. *Clin. Case Rep.* **2019**, *7*, 387–388. [CrossRef] [PubMed]
26. Karakoyun, M.; Tasci, E.K.; Sezak, M.; Yasar, B.E.; Cetin, F. Orofacial Crohn's Disease: A Case Report. *J. Pediatr. Res.* **201** 353–355. [CrossRef]
27. Huang, M.L.; Wu, Y.Q.; Ruan, W.H. A rare case of pediatric Crohn's disease and alveolar bone loss: A report and review. *Tr Pediatr.* **2020**, *9*, 720–725. [CrossRef]
28. Alrashdan, M.S.; Safadi, R.A. Crohn's disease initially presenting with oral manifestations and managed with ustekinuma case report. *Spec. Care Dent.* **2021**, *41*, 634–638. [CrossRef]
29. Sun, B.; Liu, B.; Gao, X.; Xing, K.; Xie, L.; Guo, T. Metagenomic Analysis of Saliva Reveals Disease-Associated Microbiota Patients with Periodontitis and Crohn's Disease-Associated Periodontitis. *Front. Cell. Infect. Microbiol.* **2021**, *11*, 719411. [Cross
30. Giaccaglia, F.; Tomasin, M.; Angelini, A.; Bacci, C. Gingival manifestation of Crohn's disease in a paediatric patient: A case re *Oral Surg.* **2022**, *15*, 573–576. [CrossRef]
31. McCorkle, C.E.; Seethala, R.R.; Gillman, G.S. An uncommon case of lip swelling: Granulomatous cheilitis associated with Cro disease. *Am. J. Otolaryngol.* **2021**, *42*, 102897. [CrossRef]
32. Gagnier, J.J.; Kienle, G.; Altman, D.G.; Moher, D.; Sox, H.; Riley, D. The CARE guidelines: Consensus-based clinical case re guideline development. *J. Clin. Epidemiol.* **2014**, *67*, 46–51. [CrossRef]
33. Bertl, K.; Tsakos, G.; Pandis, N.; Bogren, A.; Burisch, J.; Stavropoulos, A. Health-related quality of life aspects of the 'Periodon prevalence in ulcerative colitis and Crohn's disease' (PPCC) cohort. *J. Clin. Periodontol.* **2023**. [CrossRef]
34. Carrasco-Avino, G. Histología en la Enfermedad Inflamatoria Intestinal. *Rev. Médica Clínica Condes* **2019**, *30*, 283–298. [Cross
35. Ebker, T.; Rech, J.; von Wilmowsky, C.; Neukam, F.W.; Stockmann, P. Fulminant course of osteonecrosis of the jaw in a rheumat arthritis patient following oral bisphosphonate intake and biologic therapy. *Rheumatology* **2013**, *52*, 218–220. [CrossRef]
36. Valentini, G.; D'Agostino, S.; Ferrara, E.; Dolci, M. Patients-Reported Oral Manifestations in Coeliac Disease and Inflammat Bowel Diseases: An Italian Survey. *Oral* **2023**, *3*, 316–324. [CrossRef]

Journal of
Clinical Medicine

MDPI

iew

ɛriodontitis and Depressive Disorders: The Effects of ntidepressant Drugs on the Periodontium in Clinical and ·eclinical Models: A Narrative Review

niano Taccardi [1], Alessandro Chiesa [1], Carolina Maiorani [1,*], Alessia Pardo [2,*], Giorgio Lombardo [2], drea Scribante [1,3], Silvia Sabatini [4] and Andrea Butera [1]

1 Unit of Dental Hygiene, Section of Dentistry, Department of Clinical, Surgical, Diagnostic and Pediatric Sciences, University of Pavia, 27100 Pavia, Italy; damiano.taccardi01@universitadipavia.it (D.T.); alessandro.chiesa@hotmail.it (A.C.); andrea.scribante@unipv.it (A.S.); andrea.butera@unipv.it (A.B.)

2 Section of Oral and Maxillofacial Surgery, Department of Surgical Sciences, Dentistry, Gynecology and Pediatrics, University of Verona, 37124 Verona, Italy; giorgio.lombardo@univr.it

3 Unit of Orthodontics and Pediatric Dentistry, Section of Dentistry, Department of Clinical, Surgical, Diagnostic and Pediatric Sciences, University of Pavia, 27100 Pavia, Italy

4 Department of Surgical, Medical, Dental and Morphological Sciences, University of Modena and Reggio Emilia, 41124 Modena, Italy; silviasabatini01@gmail.com

* Correspondence: carolinamaiorani@outlook.it (C.M.); alessia.pardo@univr.it (A.P.)

Abstract: Background/Objectives: Several psychological conditions, including stress and depression, can adversely affect oral health; in fact, antidepressants, commonly used to treat depressive disorders, may have conflicting effects on the periodontal status of individuals. The aim of this review was to determine the effects of antidepressants on the periodontium. **Methods:** A literature search was conducted using electronic databases, Pubmed/MEDLINE, Cochrane Library, focusing on the use of antidepressants and their effects on periodontal health in animals or humans. **Results**: Seventeen articles have been included with the use of amitriptyline (two studies), desipramine (one study), imipramine (two studies), desvenlafaxine (one study), fluoxetine (six studies), venlafaxine (three studies) and tianeptine (two studies). One study evaluated several categories of antidepressants, such as selective serotonin reuptake inhibitors (SSRI), serotonin-norepinephrine reuptake inhibitors (SNRI), tricyclic, atypical and monoamine oxidase inhibitors (MAO). Most trials showed improvements in periodontal health, especially with fluoxetine, but also with imipramine, desipramine, desvenlafaxine and tianeptine; on the contrary, worsening of clinical periodontal indices and increased loss of alveolar bone were reported with venlafaxine. **Conclusions**: This review suggests that in the presence of comorbidity between periodontitis and depression, pharmacological treatment with SNRIs, SSRIs and mixed antidepressants is associated with improvement in periodontal parameters, except for venlafaxine. Healthcare professionals (especially oral and mental health professionals) should investigate proper adherence to medication therapy in patients with a history of periodontitis and depression. Further clinical trials are needed to confirm these results.

Keywords: antidepressant; periodontitis; inflammation; neuroinflammation; systematic diseases

1. Introduction

Periodontal disease is a problem that affects the worldwide population: global cases of severe periodontitis were reported to be approximately 1.1 billion in 2019, an increase of 99% from 1990 to 2019, and this is attributable to population growth and increased ageing [1]. It affects almost 40% of the world's population [2].

Periodontitis is a chronic inflammatory disease of multifactorial etiology associated with dysbiotic plaque biofilms that progressively weaken and destroy the oral tissues supporting the tooth within the alveolar bone [3–5]. Periodontitis can be successfully treated with various therapies, such as mechanical or manual instrumentation, which aim to remove the bacterial biofilm, reduce bleeding on probing and promote healing of the oral tissues [6–9].

Recent evidence suggests that there may be several mechanisms linking poor oral health to mental and affective disorders; poor oral hygiene and periodontal disease may lead to low-grade chronic systemic inflammation, which is considered a risk factor for neuropsychiatric disorders [10–13]. It is well known that oral bacteria can enter the bloodstream by damaging the gums, and if the blood–brain barrier is weakened, they can also enter the brain via pro-inflammatory mediators; periodontal disease can also indirectly affect the central nervous system [14–17]. People with anxiety or depression have been found to have a higher incidence of tooth decay and loss, and people with bipolar disorder have been found to have a higher risk of periodontitis: contributing factors include poor oral hygiene and diet, tobacco use, alcohol and psychostimulants [18–21].

Affective disorders are psychopathological disorders characterized by a change in the individual's general activity, with alterations at an emotional level, mood and motivation, which manifest themselves in a reduction in functioning at a personal, work and social situations [22].

The DSM-5, a statistical and diagnostic manual of mental disorders, differentiates mood disorders into two distinct categories: depressive disorders and bipolar disorders. Major depressive disorder, also called endogenous depression, manifests itself mainly with a depressed mood, lack of motivation and vital energy, poor concentration ability, guilt, insomnia or hypersomnia, psychomotor slowing or agitation, apathy or loss of interest, and finally, suicidal ideation or attempts [22–24]. Unlike depressive disorders, which are characterised by a single polarity (i.e., the mood disorder is manifested only in the depressive variant), in bipolar disorders we observe the presence of manic or hypomanic episodes alternating with depressive episodes. In mania or hypomania, the mood is defined as "expanded", elevated, euphoric: a patient before a manic episode may show logorrhea, acceleration of thought content, reduced need for sleep, psychomotor activation, up to and including excessive expenditure, and uninhibited behaviour [24,25]. This disorder is manifested by a sense of grandeur, decreased need for sleep, logorrhea, accelerated thinking, other distractibility, a significant increase in daily activities and excess risky activities. The diagnostic criteria for major depressive disorder are met when five of the above symptoms occur simultaneously for two weeks and cause clinically significant distress to the individual; for bipolar disorder, however, at least three of the above symptoms may occur for at least four days [25,26].

Currently, depression is the most common mental illness in the world: the number of cases from 1990 to the present has increased by 49.86% (from 172 to approximately 258 million in 2017), with major depressive disorder reported as the most widespread in the population [27]. Furthermore, the World Health Organization (WHO) indicates that this specific depressive disorder will become the leading cause of disability worldwide by 2030 [28]. Worldwide, the incidence of mood disorders is second only to that of anxiety disorders, affecting a large proportion of the world's population. In Italy, according to the European Study on the Epidemiology of Mental Disorders, the lifetime prevalence of major depression and dysthymia is 11.2%. Thus, it is relatively common to develop a mood disorder over the course of a lifetime. It is also likely that some changes in Western society will favour a greater prevalence of these disorders [22–24,29].

Periodontal disease and depressive disorders have several risk factors in common, including smoking and lifestyle. Both are highly prevalent pathologies in their respective areas of concern: having a mental disorder results in reduced self-care and a potential increase in periodontal disease [30–33].

In a preclinical in vivo study, periodontitis and subsequent experimental depression were induced in a group of rats: the group in which both periodontitis and depression were induced (periodontitis was induced by inoculating P. gingivalisATCC W83 K1 and F. nucleatum DMSZ 20482 by oral gavage). The rat group with Nucleatum DMSZ 20482 by oral gavage, while depression was induced by introducing a series of different stressors that changed daily (two stressors/day)), showed significantly greater alveolar bone loss at the level of the bifurcation than the non-depressed groups with induced periodontitis. *Fusobacterium nucleatum* has been found in the frontal cortex of mice with periodontally induced depression [34].

Starting from preclinical studies on animal models, other studies have tried to investigate the associations between these pathologies in subjects with periodontitis compared to healthy individuals. A study comparing approximately 50,000 healthy subjects vs. 12,000 with periodontitis demonstrated that subjects with periodontitis were more likely to develop depression within 10 years of follow-up, indicating periodontitis as a risk factor for depression later, regardless of other associated comorbidities such as sex and age [35]; not only could periodontal disease be a risk factor for affective disorders: depression could also be a risk factor for periodontal disease, indicating a two-way link [36].

A recent meta-analysis, published in the *Journal of Clinical Periodontology* in 2021, indicated the plausibility of a bidirectional depression–periodontitis association, dividing the possible mechanisms involved into three aspects: behavioural, biological/physiological and bacteriological aspects [37].

Depressed subjects tend to engage in riskier behaviours, which can worsen oral health and predispose them to periodontitis [33–38]. Periodontitis is one of the main causes of edentulism in the population, which can compromise the contour and aesthetics of the face [39]. Periodontal disease significantly affects the patient's quality of life and masticatory function, as well as worsens self-confidence: all of these factors can predispose periodontal patients to a significant worsening of mood, with an increased risk of depression [40–45].

Individuals with depression report increased levels of certain inflammatory production factors, including interleukin-6 (IL-6), tumour necrosis factor (TNF)-alpha, interleukink-10 (IL-10), as well as several soluble receptors and interleukin antagonists and cytokines, such as the soluble IL-2 receptor, IL-13 and IL-1 receptor antagonist [46–48]. From here, the hypothesis of "inflammatory depression" was born, a real subtype of depression, which identifies mechanisms that act as catalysts/amplifiers of responses: bad eating habits, stress and sedentary lifestyle [49]. In contrast, among the possible protective factors against the development of depression, probiotics have been proposed and studied as adjuvants in the non-surgical treatment of periodontitis [49–51].

Therefore, individuals with depression and periodontitis appear to share an alteration in the production of various pro-inflammatory factors (IL-1, IL-6, TNF-α), which, on the one hand, increases the individual's systemic inflammatory load [52] and, on the other hand, increases neuroinflammation [53,54]. Cortisol-related stress is also associated with periodontitis [55]. In fact, cortisol could be differentiated into different forms of periodontitis: subjects with aggressive periodontitis had higher cortisol levels than subjects with chronic periodontitis [56]. Cortisol, resulting from the incorrect functioning of the hypothalamic–pituitary–adrenal (HPA) axis, induces endocrine and cerebral changes, increasing vulnerability to the development of depressive pathologies. Therefore, by increasing its serum production, it can cause the reduction in cellular trophism of neurons and the inhibition of neurogenesis mechanism [57], all of which seem to significantly predispose subjects to mental pathology [58]. Similarly, "inflammatory depression" induces a functional alteration of the HPA axis with increased secretion of pro-inflammatory cytokines such as IL-6 and TNF-α; the latter are in turn associated with the development of periodontitis [37,47,52,54,59]. Therefore, depression and periodontitis share a potential bidirectionality in the etiology and maintenance of pathology [60].

Virulence factors of some periodontal disease pathogens can overcome the blood–brain barrier and negatively influence the physiology of the brain via glial cells, which are mediators of various neural signals [61,62].

Antidepressants are widely used in the population, particularly in the periodontal population: subjects with periodontitis are more likely to take antidepressant drugs when compared to healthy patients [63]. Although the various anti-inflammatory functions of these drugs are well known in the literature, acting also at the level of systemic inflammation and enhancing the individual's immune response [64–66], the literature seems to be divided on their effects at the periodontal level, except for one study where it was found that the use of antidepressants could protect against periodontal disease, noting a lower loss of clinical attachment; the explanation of this effect is unclear [67]. However, other studies in the literature mention some factors at the oral level, such as bacterial infections and accumulation of bacterial biofilm, which favour the development of periodontal disease [68,69].

Therefore, the aim of this study was to determine the periodontal effects of the antidepressant drugs most commonly used to treat different forms of depression, as there are few studies focused on researching the periodontal effects of these drugs.

2. Materials and Methods

2.1. Hypothesis

Are there any periodontal effects of antidepressant drugs? What are the effects of antidepressants at the periodontal level?

2.2. Eligibility Criteria

The following inclusion criteria guided the analysis of the studies:

Study type. Clinical and preclinical studies in patients or animals, i.e., randomised, blind/double-blind clinical trials, case–control, cross-sectional, cohort and observational studies and reviews;

Type of participants. Patients or animals with experimentally induced periodontitis and/or depression;

Type of interventions. Pharmacological treatments for all clinical and subclinical forms of depression. Changes in parameters of periodontal inflammation and diagnosis of periodontitis; changes in laboratory and genetic study variables (serum biomarker titration and gene expression tests);

Type of results. Determination of positive and negative effects of antidepressants at the periodontal level.

Only studies that met all the inclusion criteria were included. However, the following exclusion criteria were considered: articles published before 2005, in vitro studies, studies evaluating inflammatory parameters in oral pathologies other than periodontal disease (because the focus of this review is periodontal disease), studies in which the comparator molecule is used to treat pathologies associated with depression, such as anxiety disorders (benzodiazepines and beta-blockers), and articles on peri-implantitis and implant loss.

2.3. Search Strategy

The population, intervention, comparison, outcome (PICO) model was used to perform this narrative review through research of studies identified in electronic databases, Pubmed/MEDLINE and the Cochrane Library. Initially, all study abstracts were taken into consideration, and all studies that met the inclusion criteria and evaluated changes in periodontal parameters in clinical or pre-clinical models using antidepressant drugs were reviewed and analysed.

We performed the search using the following keywords: "antidepressant and periodontitis"; "antidepressant and periodontal disease"; "antidepressant and periodontal health"; "antidepressant and periodontal status"; and "antidepressant and periodontal inflammation".

2.4. Screening and Selection of Articles

The electronic search yielded 130 results, which were examined to determine whether the inclusion and exclusion criteria were met; all duplicates emerging from the different searches were removed (one authors).

In the first phase, the results (abstracts) were filtered based on the use of pharmacological treatments for all clinical and subclinical forms of depression; all those that did not evaluate changes in the parameters of periodontal inflammation or met the eligibility criteria were discarded. Authors (all) continued with the reading of the articles included.

After reading the selected articles, all those that had not reported the results required by the criteria for inclusion of this review, or which evaluated other oral epidemiological factors and indices other than periodontal health were removed (three authors).

2.5. Risk of Bias and Results

One author was involved in the analysis of the articles included and evaluated the results according to the PICO model. Two other authors were commissioned to evaluate the quality of the included studies, following the full reading of the articles [69].

3. Results

The main results of these studies are shown in Table 1.

Table 1. Results of studies [66–68,70–83].

Study	Study Design and Population	Presence of Periodontitis/Depression at t0	Comparison Groups and Pharmacological Administration	Tested Parameters/Analyses Conducted	Outcome
Hakam et al., 2022 [66]	Retrospective study conducted on humans	Presence of periodontitis; no diagnosis of depression (users and non-users of antidepressants)	Group 1 (user group): subjects who use antidepressants; Group 2 (non-user group): subjects who do not use antidepressants.	Variables obtained: type of antidepressant, age, sex, smoking, mild systemic diseases, CAL, BL	Antidepressant use was associated with significantly better BL and CAL in patients with periodontitis. Analysing pharmacological classes separately, SSRI (selective serotonin reuptake inhibitor) users and users of multiple pharmacological classes had lower BL and CAL than non-users.
Bey et al., 2020 [67]	Case–control study on humans	Absence of periodontitis/presence of depression at t0	Group 1: control group diagnosed as depressed at the first visit; Group 2: depressed patients taking fluoxetine 20 mg/day; Group 3: patients taking venlafaxine 75 mg/day.	DI, CI, PPD, CAL	Fluoxetine and venlafaxine are associated with a worsening of periodontal parameters, when compared with the group not taking antidepressant drugs.
Majeed et al., 2024 [68]	Case–control study conducted on humans	Absence of periodontitis/diagnosis of depression at t0	Group 1: Subjects identified by a psychiatrist as having a mental illness (control) after presenting to the psychiatry outpatient department (OPD); Group 2: patients who are taking venlafaxine; Group 3: patients who are taking fluoxetine.	CAL, PPD, CI, DI	Antidepressants can be a risk factor for periodontal health, with an increase in periodontal parameters, as these drugs can put periodontal tissues at risk.
Hasan et al., 2019 [70]	RCT on humans	Periodontitis at t0/no depression	Group 1 (control group): standard periodontal therapy; Group 2: periodontal therapy + amitriptyline gel; Group 3: periodontal therapy + amitriptyline mouthwash.	PD, AL, tooth mobility; PI, GI, BOP; saliva sample collection and estimation of TNF-α, PGE2 and NO	Improvement in periodontal parameters in the amitriptyline + gel/mouthwash group compared to the 1 standard therapy group.
Hassan et al., 2022 [71]	Experimental study on rats	No periodontitis/no depression at t0	Control group: distilled water; Test group: 10 mg per day per kg of amitriptyline.	Radiographic analysis (CBCT), histomorphometric analysis, anti-OPN and H&E immunohistochemical staining	Amitriptyline worsened periodontal destruction and increased the expression of anti-OPN in periodontal tissues, reducing bone mineral density.

Table 1. *Cont.*

Study	Study Design and Population	Presence of Periodontitis/Depression at t0	Comparison Groups and Pharmacological Administration	Tested Parameters/Analyses Conducted	Outcome
Branco-de-Almeida et al., 2020 [72]	Experimental study on rats	Induced periodontitis/no depression at t0	Group 1 (control group): rats without ligation (saline); Group 2 (ligation group): rats with induced periodontitis treated with saline solution; Group 3 (ligation + desipramine group): rats with ligation-induced periodontitis treated with desipramine (20 mg/kg/day).	RNA isolation and gene expression of IL-1β, iNOS, COX-2, MMP-9 and TIMP-1; zymography to evaluate MMP-9 activity	Desipramine reduced alveolar bone loss by modulating gene expression of inflammatory markers.
Li et al., 2022 [73]	Experimental study on rats	Induced periodontitis/no depression at t0	Group 1: control group; Group 2: control group with aSMase (acid sphingomyelinase) inhibition; Group 3: periodontitis group; Group 4: periodontitis group with aSMase (acid sphingomyelinase) inhibition; Group 5: MetS group (metabolic syndrome); Group 6: MetS group (metabolic syndrome) with aSMase (acid sphingomyelinase) inhibition; Group 7: periodontitis and MetS (metabolic syndrome) group; Group 8: periodontitis and MetS (metabolic syndrome) group with aSMase (acid sphingomyelinase) inhibition.	Metabolic measurements, micro-computed tomography and bone volume fraction analysis, acid phosphatase staining, histological tissue processing and pathological evaluation, cell cultures to evaluate alveolar bone loss, osteoclast formation, periodontal inflammation and pro-inflammatory gene expression	Imipramine inhibited the synergy between metabolic syndrome (MetS) and periodontitis on alveolar bone loss, proposing acid sphingomyelinase (aSMase) as a therapeutic target of periodontitis exacerbated by MetS.
Yamawaki et al., 2022 [74]	Experimental study on rats	Induction of LPS-PG/no depression at t0	Active group treated with imipramine (20 mg/kg) 1 h before LPS-PG (lipopolysaccharide from porphyromonas gingivalis) injection (5 mg/kg).	Cell culture and cell immunoreactivity assay using electrochemiluminescence (ECL) reagent	Imipramine is associated with a reduction in the expression of TNF (tumour necrosis factor) and Il-1 (interleukin 1) in the hippocampus, 24 h after introduction; furthermore, it attenuated microglial-induced neuronal death by inhibiting signaling of an inflammation factor in microglia (NF-κB).

Table 1. *Cont.*

Study	Study Design and Population	Presence of Periodontitis/Depression at t0	Comparison Groups and Pharmacological Administration	Tested Parameters/Analyses Conducted	Outcome
Bhatia et al., 2018 [75]	Observational study on humans	Presence of chronic periodontitis/presence of depression at t0	Group 1 (test): they took a daily dose of 50 mg/day of desvenlafaxine; Group 2 (control group): diagnosed with depression at the first visit who had not started any antidepressant medication.	PI, GI, SBI, BOP, PPD, AL	Patients treated with desvenlafaxine had shallower pocket depth and less bleeding in survey.
Carvalho et al., 2010 [76]	Experimental study on rats	Experimentally induced periodontitis/absence of depression at t0	Group 1: sham-operated (SO); Group 2: experimental periodontitis treated with vehicle; Groups 3 and 4: rats without induced periodontitis treated with 10 or 50 mg/kg of venlafaxine; Groups 5 and 6: rats with induced periodontitis treated orally with venlafaxine 10 or 50 mg/kg.	Bone loss analysed morphometrically and histopathological and immunohistochemical analysis for TNF-α and iNOS	High-dose venlafaxine (50 mg/kg) increased bone loss and worsened the inflammation condition of the tested animals. Furthermore, the drug increased the immunoreactivity of inflammatory biomarkers such as TNF (tumour necrosis factor).
Aguiar et al., 2013 [77]	Experimental study on rats	Experimentally induced periodontitis (before depression)/experimentally induced depression at t0	Groups 1: non-stressed rats; Group 2: non-stressed rats + daily fluoxetine (20 mg/kg) Group C: stressed rats; Group 3: stressed rats + daily fluoxetine (20 mg/kg).	Histological analyses and immunohistochemical staining for IL-1β and IL-6	Animal models with depression and periodontitis had greater bone loss than the non-depressed periodontitis group. Furthermore, fluoxetine reduced levels of bone loss in animal models of induced periodontitis and stress-induced depression.
Bhatia et al., 2015 [78]	Cross- sectional observational study on humans	Periodontitis present/and depression diagnosed at the first visit at t0	Group 1 (test group): periodontal patients taking 20 mg/day of fluoxetine for at least 2 months; Group 2 (control group): periodontal patients who had yet to start antidepressant treatment.	PI, GI, SBI, BOP, PPD, AL	Except plaque index (PI), all parameters were lower in group taking fluoxetine compared to the control group (depressed patients with periodontitis).
Branco-de-Almeida et al., 2012 [79]	Experimental study on rats	Experimentally induced periodontitis/depression absent at t0	Group 1: control rats (without ligation); Group 2: rats with ligation + placebo (saline); Group 3: ligation rats + fluoxetine (20 mg/kg/day).	Bone loss by histometric assessment, expression of IL-1β, COX-2, MMP-9 and iNOS and MMP-9 activity	The periodontitis group and fluoxetine demonstrated less alveolar bone loss at histometric evaluation compared to the group with induced periodontitis alone and placebo. Furthermore, in the fluoxetine group there was a reduced inflammatory expression of IL-1β (interleukin 1-beta) and COX-2 (cyclooxygenase-2).

Table 1. Cont.

Study	Study Design and Population	Presence of Periodontitis/Depression at t0	Comparison Groups and Pharmacological Administration	Tested Parameters/Analyses Conducted	Outcome
Regueira et al., 2017 [80]	Experimental study on rats	Absence of periodontitis/depression at t0	Group 1: sodium chloride administered throughout the pregnancy; Group 2: sodium chloride administered throughout pregnancy and breastfeeding; Group 3: fluoxetine administered throughout the pregnancy; Group 4: fluoxetine administered throughout pregnancy and breastfeeding.	Histometrical, histochemical and immunohistochemical analysis of the maxillary first molar periodontium region of rat pups made under light microscopy; periodontal ligament collagen qualitatively evaluated under a polarizing light microscope	Decreases in osteoblasts, fibroblasts and mercatoblasts were observed, but only in the group in which fluoxetine was taken until the breastfeeding period. However, it is not possible to determine whether this cellular deficiency actually influenced periodontogenesis, as the morphological descriptive analysis did not highlight any alterations or structural elements evident in the periodontal conformation.
Breivik et al., 2006 [81]	Experimental study on rats	Experimentally induced periodontitis (before depression)/experimentally induced depression at t0	Experiment 1: Group 1: mice with periodontitis and induced depression (OB); Group 2: mice with induced periodontitis without depression. Experiment 2: Group 1: OB rats treated with tianeptine; Group 2: OB mice treated with saline; Group 3: control mice.	Radiographic bone loss, analysis of serum corticosterone, tumour necrosis factor TNF-α, IL-10 and TGF-β; RNA isolation in the hippocampus	Depressed mice (OB) had a higher susceptibility to periodontitis than healthy controls without induced depression. Tianeptine treatment of OB rats significantly inhibited periodontal bone loss, normalised behavioural responses, increased TGF-1β levels and abolished the decrease in TNF-α, but did not attenuate the increase in corticosterone response and decreased hippocampal GR expression.
Breivik et al., 2006 [82]	Experimental study on rats	Induced periodontitis/depression absent at t0	Experiment 1: Group 1 (active group): dexamethasone; Group 2 (control group): physiological solution. Experiment 2: Group 1 (active group): 10 mg/kg per day of tianeptine; Group 2 (control group): physiological solution.	Radiographic bone loss, analysis of serum corticosterone, tumour necrosis factor TNF-α, IL-10 and TGF-β; RNA isolation in the hippocampus	Tianeptine-treated group showed significantly reduced periodontal bone loss, increased plasma levels of TNF-α and transforming growth factor-1β; no significant difference was found in corticosterone levels.

Table 1. *Cont.*

Study	Study Design and Population	Presence of Periodontitis/Depression at t0	Comparison Groups and Pharmacological Administration	Tested Parameters/Analyses Conducted	Outcome
Muniz et al., 2018 [83]	Systematic review of 5 experimental studies on rats	Studies involved: Breivick et al., 2006 [81]; Breivick et al., 2006 [82]; Carvalho et al., 2010 [76]; Branco-de-Almeida et al., 2012 [79]; Aguiar et al., 2013 [77];	/	Parameters extracted from each selected study: author, country, number of animals involved, antidepressant used, use of ligature (yes or no), intervention (if any) in the control group, number of days with the ligature placed, number of days the antidepressant was administered, measurement of ABL in each experimental group and additional information.	With the exception of venlafaxine, the antidepressant treatments studied (tianeptine and fluoxetine) can modify the reactivity of the stress response system and modulate susceptibility to periodontitis.

Abbreviations. PPD: Probing pocket depth; CAL: Clinical attachment loss; AL: Attachment loss; BOP: Bleeding on probing; GI: Gingival index; BL: Bone level; PI: Plaque index; SBI: Sulcular bleeding index; DI: Debris index; CI: Calculus index; TNF-α: Tumour necrosis factor; PGE2: Prostaglandin E2; IL: Interleukin; iNOS: Inducible nitric oxide synthase; COX-2: Cyclooxygenase-2; MMP-9: Matrix metallopeptidase 9; TIMP-1: Tissue inhibitor of metalloproteinase 1; TGF-β: Transforming growth factor beta; OPN: Anti-osteopontin antibody; H&E: Haematoxylin plus eosin.

The electronic search yielded 130 results, and 17 articles met the eligibility criteria and were included in this narrative review.

The studies included in the review evaluated the use of several antidepressants, such as amitriptyline (two studies) [69,70], desipramine (one study) [72], imipramine (two studies) [73,74], desvenlafaxine (one study) [75], fluoxetine (six studies) [67,68,77–80], venlafaxine (three studies) [67,68,76] and tianeptine (two studies) [81,82]. One study evaluated several categories of antidepressants, such as selective serotonin reuptake inhibitors (SSRI), serotonin-norepinephrine reuptake inhibitors (SNRI), tricyclic, atypical and monoamine oxidase inhibitors (MAO) [66]; the only included review investigated the effects of fluoxetine, venlafaxine and tianeptine [83].

The antidepressant drug that seems to make periodontal health worse is venlafaxine (in all studies that have analyzed its effects), with an increase in clinical indices such as gingival index, periodontal pocket depth, clinical attachment loss ($p < 0.05$) [67,68] and inflammation and bone loss ($p < 0.001$) [76].

For the two amitriptyline studies, there are two different results: in one study (RCT) where amitriptyline gel or mouthwash was used, there was an improvement in periodontal health and a reduction in the epidemiological indices ($p < 0.001$) analysed (probing depth, attachment level, tooth mobility, plaque index, gingival index and bleeding on probing) [70], while in the second study (in rats), when amitriptyline was administered as a tablet for 4 weeks, a deterioration in periodontal health was noticed, with reduced bone mineral density [71]. Discordant results also emerge from the studies that analysed the effects of fluoxetine: it reduced bone loss and inflammatory parameters, with noted improvements in gingival index, sulcus bleeding index, bleeding on probing, probing depth, attachment level [77–79]; however, other studies have shown a worsening of the epidemiological indices related to periodontal disease [67,68] and a decrease in periodontal cells, although no structural periodontal changes in the analysis were noted [80].

For imipramine, desipramine, desvenlafaxine and tianeptine, there were improvements in periodontal status in all studies.

Table 2 shows a summary of the antidepressant used and its effect on the periodontium.

Table 2. Antidepressants and their effects on the periodontium.

Article	Antidepressant Used	Effects on Periodontium
Hakam et al., 2022 [66]	SSRI (selective serotonin reuptake inhibitors), SNRI (serotonin-norepinephrine reuptake inhibitors), tricyclic, atypical and MAO (monoamine oxidase inhibitors) categories	Antidepressants improve BL and CAL
Bey et al., 2020 [67]	Fluoxetine and Venlafaxine	Fluoxetine and Venlafaxine worsen periodontal health
Majeed et al., 2024 [68]	Fluoxetine and Venlafaxine	Fluoxetine and Venlafaxine worsen periodontal indices
Hasan et al., 2019 [70]	Amitryptiline	Amitryptiline improves periodontal health and periodontal indices
Hassan et al., 2022 [71]	Amitryptiline	Amitryptiline worsens periodontal health
Branco-de-Almeida et al., 2020 [72]	Desipramine	Desipramine reduces alveolar bone loss
Li et al., 2022 [73]	Imipramine	Imipramine improves periodontal health
Yamawaki et al., 2022 [74]	Imipramine	Imipramine inhibits LPS-PG-induced inflammatory responses in microglia and improves periodontal disease-related neural damage
Bhatia et al., 2018 [75]	Desvenlafaxine	Desvenlafaxine improves PPD and BOP
Carvalho et al., 2010 [76]	Venlafaxine	Venlafaxine increases inflammation and bone loss
Aguiar et al., 2013 [77]	Fluoxetine	Fluoxetine reduces bone loss

Table 2. *Cont.*

Article	Antidepressant Used	Effects on Periodontium
Bhatia et al., 2015 [78]	Fluoxetine	Fluoxetine improves GI, SBI, BOP, CAL (bu not plaque index)
Branco-de-Almeida et al., 2012 [79]	Fluoxetine	Fluoxetine reduces inflammation and bone lo
Regueira et al., 2017 [80]	Fluoxetine	Periodontal tissue may be sensitive to fluoxetine, and its interference in reducing periodontal cells depends on exposure tim during lactation
Breivik et al., 2006 [81]	Tianeptine	Tianeptine inhibits bone loss
Breivik et al., 2006 [82]	Tianeptine	Tianeptine inhibits bone loss
Muniz et al., 2018 [83]	Fluoxetine, Tianeptine and Venlafaxine	Only Venlafaxine study was not to able to fi any significant alveolar bone loss reductio while others showed positive effects

Abbreviations. PPD: Probing pocket depth; CAL: Clinical attachment loss; AL: Attachment loss; BOP: Bleeding on probing; GI: Gingival index; BL: Bone level; PI: Plaque index; SBI: Sulcular bleeding index.

Risk of Bias of Studies Included

The evaluation of blinding, randomisation, allocation concealment, outcome data and outcome recording were carried out to assess the bias risk of this review. According to the variable taken into consideration, a green symbol was assigned where the information was complete and accurate; a yellow symbol was allocated where information was missing; and a red symbol was assigned where the information did not meet the requirements. This review has low risk of bias.

Table 3 shows the risk of bias in the main articles examined.

Table 3. Risk of bias of articles [66–68,70–83].

	Adequate Sequence Generated	Allocation Concealment	Blinding	Incomplete Outcome Data	Registration Outcome Data
Hakam et al., 2022 [66]	− (yellow)	− (yellow)	− (red)	✓ (green)	✓ (green)
Bey et al., 2020 [67]	− (yellow)	− (yellow)	− (yellow)	✓ (green)	− (yellow)
Majeed et al., 2024 [68]	− (yellow)	− (yellow)	− (red)	✓ (green)	− (yellow)
Hasan et al., 2019 [70]	− (yellow)	− (yellow)	− (red)	✓ (green)	✓ (green)
Hassan et al., 2022 [71]	✓ (green)	✓ (green)	− (yellow)	✓ (green)	✓ (green)
Branco-de-Almeida et al., 2020 [72]	✓ (green)	✓ (green)	✓ (green)	✓ (green)	✓ (green)
Li et al., 2022 [73]	− (yellow)	− (yellow)	✓ (green)	✓ (green)	− (yellow)
Yamawaki et al., 2022 [74]	− (yellow)	− (yellow)	− (yellow)	✓ (green)	✓ (green)

Table 3. *Cont.*

	Adequate Sequence Generated	Allocation Concealment	Blinding	Incomplete Outcome Data	Registration Outcome Data
atia et al., 2018 [75]	–	–	✓	–	–
Carvalho et al., 2010 [76]	–	–	✓	✓	–
Aguiar et al., 2013 [77]	✓	✓	✓	✓	✓
atia et al., 2015 [78]	–	–	✓	✓	✓
ranco-de-Almeida et al., 2012 [79]	✓	✓	✓	✓	✓
Regueira et al., 2017 [80]	✓	✓	✓	✓	✓
Breivik et al., 2006 [81]	✓	✓	–	✓	–
Breivik et al., 2006 [82]	✓	✓	–	✓	–
Muniz et al., 2018 [83]	–	–	–	✓	–

4. Discussion

Recent studies [32,84] have suggested a strong link between oral health and systemic diseases, one of which is mental health with depression.

The link between periodontal disease and depression can be explained by behavioural, biological and bacteriological factors.

Periodontitis is an inflammatory disease, and inflammatory factors such as IL-1, IL-6 and TNF-α are directly associated with periodontitis [85]. Some of these biomarkers appear to play a central role in regulating the inflammatory process of the immune response and are identified based on the bone destruction that characterises the destructive phase of the disease [86,87]. In particular, IL-1 and TNF are directly involved in osteoclastic resorption [88] by inhibiting osteoblast activity and promoting the release of CSF-1, also known as macrophage colony-stimulating factor [89]. However, a secondary group of cytokines (such as IL-10) have antagonistic and periodontal protective effects [90]. TNF is also involved in the pathogenesis of periodontitis. In fact, high levels of this cytokine up-regulate the expression of RANKL in osteoblasts, T cells and gingival epithelial cells; therefore, it has been hypothesised that it may be associated with the early stage of periodontitis by altering the oral mucosal barrier [91]. These inflammatory factors have also been found in people with depression. In summary, known pro-inflammatory cytokines of the IL-1, IL-6 and TNF families are secreted by periodontal cells and host immune cells after pathological stimulation, which activate and recruit specific immune cell subsets that cause direct tissue damage. Thus, T cells and B cells differentiate into mature T cells or plasma cells under the influence of specific cytokines and further activate or promote other effector cells, such as osteoclasts and neutrophils, which exert pro-inflammatory or anti-inflammatory effects [86–89,92].

In addition to biological factors, there are virological aspects in common between individuals with periodontitis and depression: *Fusobacterium nucleatum* has been identified in the brain tissue of animals with induced periodontitis, suggesting that this may be associated with HPA dysregulation and elevated corticosterone levels [34]. *Porphyromonas gingivalis*, a major pathogen of periodontitis, inoculated into preclinical models every other day for 4 weeks, induced depression-like behaviours [93]. This is followed by changes in the levels of neurotrophic receptors (in rats with both periodontitis and depression) [34]. Also, the presence of stress hormones catecholamine, dopamine and cortisol increased proliferation and growth of *Tannerella forsythia* and *Fusobacterium nucleatum* [94]. Therefore, stress-related adrenal hormones, such as catecholamines, can modulate the growth of some bacterial species, including *Eikenella corrodens, Tannerella forsythia* and *Fusobacterium nucleatum* [94,95], and drive the transition towards dysbiosis [32], a key element in the pathogenesis of periodontal disease [3].

Moreover, there are certain negative habits common to both diseases. Poor oral hygiene, smoking, alcohol consumption and poor or unregulated nutrition remain influential factors in both cases.

The articles analysed in the following review included 17 in vivo studies, which complied with the inclusion criteria, to understand the effects of antidepressant drugs on the periodontium in clinical and preclinical models.

Fluoxetine (an SSRIs) reduced periodontal progression [77], alveolar bone loss and inflammatory responses [79] in rats with induced periodontitis. Furthermore, it appears to influence periodontal genesis in mice without any clinically relevant effects by decreasing the number of periodontal cells [11]. The beneficial effects of fluoxetine could be explained by its ability to reduce pathological inflammatory response and gene transcription when administered in an animal model [60,83]. Intake of tianeptine, imipramine and desipramine is associated with a reduction in the level of alveolar bone loss and periodontal inflammation in mice. These molecules appear to exhibit immunomodulatory effects and can modulate bone remodelling and key inflammatory mediators [72,74,81,82]. Desipramine (belonging to a tricyclic antidepressant) also appears to attenuate alveolar bone loss and modulate gene expression in mice [72].

In light of the results that emerged on animal models, although fluoxetine, imipramine, tianeptine, desvenlafaxine and desipramine appear to have anti-inflammatory and immunomodulatory properties, it is not possible to state with certainty the mechanism of action with which these drugs intervene at the periodontal level [71–73,81,82].

The results of studies performed on clinical models are contradictory. The recent study by Hakam et al. analysed the records of 582 patients divided into those with and without periodontitis [66]. The periodontal parameters of patients taking different classes of antidepressants were compared with those of non-users. Subjects taking antidepressants (especially SSRIs such as fluoxetine or mixed classes) had statistically higher rates of alveolar bone loss and clinical attachment loss than periodontal patients not taking these drugs. Therefore, there are conflicting opinions on the effect of antidepressants on periodontal health: indeed, studies have shown improvements in periodontal and immunological indices with desvenlafaxine and fluoxetine treatment in patients with periodontitis and depression, while others have highlighted how the use of some antidepressants in the presence of periodontitis and depression limits periodontal loss and influences periodontal epidemiological indices [75], such as bleeding on probing and alveolar bone loss [78].

The antidepressant that appears to be more damaging to the periodontium is venlafaxine, which worsens PPD, CAL, GI and DI [67,68] and exacerbates bone loss due to synaptic inhibition of serotonin uptake, which has negative effects on the skeleton [76].

The contrasting results may be due to the different categories of antidepressants used in the studies included in this review: probably the negative or positive effects are linked precisely to the category of the drug and its application.

This review, which would seem to show that there is no effect on periodontal health in patients taking antidepressants (category), shows a strong risk in the studies—animal or human studies, different sample numbers, different antidepressants used and different dosages, different epidemiological indices analysed—these data could confuse the results emerging from this review, but also explain the reason for their diversity.

For future studies, it would be useful to use a uniform sample, with the same degree of periodontitis (even if induced), to which is administered the same type and dosage of antidepressant. In addition, it is possible to make a comparison with an untreated control group or with other groups of patients treated with other antidepressants, in an attempt to highlight the side effects that may arise.

5. Conclusions

Depressive disorders and periodontal disease have been reported to share distinct behavioural, inflammatory and bacterial translocation mechanisms. In particular, the pharmacology of depressive disorders and their association with the course of periodontal disease have been analysed in clinical and preclinical models.

Our analysis suggests that in the presence of comorbidity between periodontitis and depression, pharmacological treatment with SNRIs, SSRIs and mixed antidepressants is associated with an improvement in periodontal parameters (such as probing pocket depth, bleeding on probing, clinical attachment loss and bone loss), with the exception of venlafaxine (with worsening of periodontal indices, including bone loss). Therefore, it is not possible to provide a clear idea of the effect of antidepressants on periodontal health, which depends on their type and dosage.

Healthcare professionals (especially oral and mental health professionals) should assess the adherence to medication in patients with a history of periodontitis and depression.

Pharmacological treatment may modulate and reduce the inflammatory burden in patients diagnosed with both periodontitis and depression. Further studies are needed to analyse the cause-and-effect mechanisms underlying the depression–periodontitis associations and to investigate the anti-inflammatory and immunomodulatory effects of different antidepressants on the periodontium, using a uniform sample of patients with periodontal disease and the same class of antidepressant. These effects have not been well studied.

Author Contributions: Conceptualisation, D.T. and A.B.; methodology, A.C. and C.M.; software, A.S.; validation, A.P., G.L. and A.B.; formal analysis, A.S.; investigation, D.T.; resources, A.B. and C.M.; data curation, S.S.; writing—original draft preparation, A.B. and S.S.; writing—review and editing, A.S.; visualisation, G.L.; supervision, A.S.; project administration, A.B.; funding acquisition, A.C. All authors have read and agreed to the published version of the manuscript.

Funding: This research received no external funding.

Conflicts of Interest: The authors declare no conflicts of interest.

'erences

Chen, M.X.; Zhong, Y.J.; Dong, Q.Q.; Wong, H.M.; Wen, Y.F. Global, regional, and national burden of severe periodontitis, 1990–2019: An analysis of the Global Burden of Disease Study 2019. *J. Clin. Periodontol.* **2021**, *48*, 1165–1188. [CrossRef] [PubMed]

Nazir, M.A. Prevalence of periodontal disease, its association with systemic diseases and prevention. *Int. J. Health Sci.* **2017**, *11*, 72–80.

Kinane, D.F.; Stathopoulou, P.G.; Papapanou, P.N. Periodontal diseases. *Nat. Rev. Dis. Primers* **2017**, *3*, 17038. [CrossRef] [PubMed]

Papapanou, P.N.; Sanz, M.; Buduneli, N.; Dietrich, T.; Feres, M.; Fine, D.H.; Flemmig, T.F.; Garcia, R.; Giannobile, W.V.; Graziani, F.; et al. Periodontitis: Consensus report of workgroup 2 of the 2017 World Workshop on the Classification of Periodontal and Peri-Implant Diseases and Conditions. *J. Periodontol.* **2018**, *89*, S173–S182. [CrossRef] [PubMed]

Lindhe, J.; Lang, N.P. *Clinical Periodontology and Oral Implantology*, 6th ed.; Wiley-Blackwell: Oxford, UK, 2016.

Sabatini, S.; Maiorani, C.; Bassignani, J.; Cotellessa, S.; Di Trani, G.; Fulgenzi, E.; Iacono, R.; Mercogliano, I.; Butera, A. Effectiveness of Ultrasonic and Manual Instrumentation in Nonsurgical Periodontal Therapy: Are Additional Therapies More Effective? A Systematic Review. *Appl. Sci.* **2024**, *14*, 1950. [CrossRef]

Pardo, A.; Butera, A.; Giordano, A.; Gallo, S.; Pascadopoli, M.; Scribante, A.; Albanese, M. Photodynamic Therapy in Non-Surgical Treatment of Periodontitis: A Systematic Review and Meta-Analysis. *Appl. Sci.* **2023**, *13*, 1086. [CrossRef]

Preda, C.; Butera, A.; Pelle, S.; Pautasso, E.; Chiesa, A.; Esposito, F.; Oldoini, G.; Scribante, A.; Genovesi, A.M.; Cosola, S. The Efficacy of Powered Oscillating Heads vs. Powered Sonic Action Heads Toothbrushes to Maintain Periodontal and Peri-Implant Health: A Narrative Review. *Int. J. Environ. Res. Public. Health* **2021**, *18*, 1468. [CrossRef]

9. Wang, C.W. Emerging opportunity to implement host modulation therapy in non-surgical periodontal therapy-The role probiotics and future perspectives. *J. Dent. Sci.* **2024**, *19*, 1305–1306. [CrossRef]
10. Michopoulos, V.; Powers, A.; Gillespie, C.F.; Ressler, K.J.; Jovanovic, T. Inflammation in fear- and anxiety-based disorders: PT GAD, and beyond. *Neuropsychopharmacology* **2017**, *42*, 254–270. [CrossRef]
11. Miller, A.H.; Raison, C.L. The role of inflammation in depression: From evolutionary imperative to modern treatment target. *N Rev. Immunol.* **2016**, *16*, 22–34. [CrossRef]
12. Flux, M.C.; Lowry, C.A. Finding intestinal fortitude: Integrating the microbiome into a holistic view of depression mechanis treatment, and resilience. *Neurobiol. Dis.* **2020**, *135*, 104578. [CrossRef] [PubMed]
13. Raison, C.L.; Miller, A.H. The evolutionary significance of depression in pathogen host defense (PATHOS-D). *Mol. Psychia* **2013**, *18*, 15–37. [CrossRef] [PubMed]
14. Dominy, S.S.; Lynch, C.; Ermini, F.; Benedyk, M.; Marczyk, A.; Konradi, A.; Nguyen, M.; Haditsch, U.; Raha, D.; Griffin, C.; e Porphyromonas gingivalis in Alzheimer's disease brains: Evidence for disease causation and treatment with small-molec inhibitors. *Sci. Adv.* **2019**, *5*, eaau3333. [CrossRef] [PubMed]
15. Parahitiyawa, N.B.; Jin, L.J.; Leung, W.K.; Yam, W.C.; Samaranayake, L.P. Microbiology of odontogenic bacteremia: Beyo endocarditis. *Clin. Microbiol. Rev.* **2009**, *22*, 46–64. [CrossRef] [PubMed]
16. Lockhart, P.B.; Brennan, M.T.; Sasser, H.C.; Fox, P.C.; Paster, B.J.; Bahrani-Mougeot, F.K. Bacteremia associated with toothbrush and dental extraction. *Circulation* **2008**, *117*, 3118–3125. [CrossRef] [PubMed]
17. Frister, A.; Schmidt, C.; Schneble, N.; Brodhun, M.; Gonnert, F.A.; Bauer, M.; Hirsch, E.; Müller, J.P.; Wetzker, R.; Bauer Phosphoinositide 3-kinase γ affects LPS-induced disturbance of blood-brain barrier via lipid kinase-independent control of cA in microglial cells. *Neuromolecular Med.* **2014**, *16*, 704–713. [CrossRef] [PubMed]
18. Kisely, S.; Sawyer, E.; Siskind, D.; Lalloo, R. The oral health of people with anxiety and depressive disorders—A system review and meta-analysis. *J. Affect. Disord.* **2016**, *200*, 119–132. [CrossRef] [PubMed]
19. Cunha, F.A.; Cota, L.O.M.; Cortelli, S.C.; Miranda, T.B.; Neves, F.S.; Cortelli, J.R.; Costa, F.O. Periodontal condition and level bacteria associated with periodontitis in individuals with bipolar affective disorders: A case-control study. *J. Periodontal Res.* **2** *54*, 63–72. [CrossRef] [PubMed]
20. Coelho, J.M.F.; Miranda, S.S.; da Cruz, S.S.; Dos Santos, D.N.; Trindade, S.C.; Cerqueira, E.M.M.; Passos-Soares, J.d.S.; Co M.d.C.N.; Figueiredo, A.C.M.G.; Hintz, A.M.; et al. Common mental disorder is associated with periodontitis. *J. Periodontal* **2020**, *55*, 221–228. [CrossRef]
21. Martínez, M.; Postolache, T.T.; García-Bueno, B.; Leza, J.C.; Figuero, E.; Lowry, C.A.; Malan-Müller, S. The Role of the C Microbiota Related to Periodontal Diseases in Anxiety, Mood and Trauma- and Stress-Related Disorders. *Front. Psychiatry* **2C** *12*, 814177. [CrossRef]
22. Sekhon, S.; Gupta, V. Mood Disorder. [Updated 2023 May 8]. In *StatPearls [Internet]*; StatPearls Publishing: Treasure Island, USA, 2024.
23. Rakofsky, J.; Rapaport, M. Mood Disorders. *Behav. Neurol. Psychiatry* **2018**, *24*, 804–827. [CrossRef] [PubMed]
24. Datta, S.; Suryadevara, U.; Cheong, J. Mood Disorders. *Behav. Neurol. Psychiatry* **2021**, *27*, 1712–1737. [CrossRef]
25. Mitchell, P.B. Bipolar disorder: Defining symptoms and comorbidities. *Lancet* **2016**, *388*, 868–869. [CrossRef] [PubMed]
26. National Collaborating Centre for Mental Health (UK). Bipolar Disorder: The NICE Guideline on the Assessment and Mana ment of Bipolar Disorder in Adults, Children and Young People in Primary and Secondary Care. In *NICE Clinical Guidelines*; T British Psychological Society and The Royal College of Psychiatrists: London, UK, 2014.
27. Liu, Q.; He, H.; Yang, J.; Feng, X.; Zhao, F.; Lyu, J. Changes in the global burden of depression from 1990 to 2017: Findings fr the Global Burden of Disease study. *J. Psychiatr. Res.* **2020**, *126*, 134–140. [CrossRef] [PubMed]
28. Yang, L.; Zhao, Y.; Wang, Y.; Liu, L.; Zhang, X.; Li, B.; Cui, R. The Effects of Psychological Stress on Depression. *C Neuropharmacol.* **2015**, *13*, 494–504. [CrossRef] [PubMed]
29. Jorge, R.E. Mood disorders. In *Handbook of Clinical Neurology*; Elsevier: Amsterdam, The Netherlands, 2015; Volume 128, 613–631.
30. Genco, R.J.; Borgnakke, W.S. Risk factors for periodontal disease. *Periodontology 2000* **2013**, *62*, 59–94. [CrossRef] [PubMed]
31. Klimkiewicz, A.; Klimkiewicz, J.; Jakubczyk, A.; Kieres-Salomonski, I.; Wojnar, M. Comorbidity of alcohol dependence with ot psychiatric disorders. Part I. Epidemiology of dual diagnosis. *Psychiatr. Pol.* **2015**, *49*, 265–275. [CrossRef] [PubMed]
32. Ball, J.; Darby, I. Mental health and periodontal and peri-implant diseases. *Periodontology 2000* **2022**, *90*, 106–124. [CrossR [PubMed]
33. Anttila, S.; Knuuttila, M.; Ylostalo, P.; Joukamaa, M. Symptoms of depression and anxiety in relation to dental health behav and self-perceived dental treatment need. *Eur. J. Oral Sci.* **2016**, *114*, 109–114. [CrossRef]
34. Martinez, M.; Martin-Hernandez, D.; Virto, L.; MacDowell, K.S.; Montero, E.; Gonzalez-Bris, A.; Marin, M.J.; Ambrosio, Herrera, D.; Leza, J.C.; et al. Periodontal diseases and depression: A pre-clinical in vivo study. *J. Clin. Periodontol.* **2021**, 503–527. [CrossRef] [PubMed]
35. Hsu, C.C.; Hsu, Y.C.; Chen, H.J.; Lin, C.C.; Chang, K.H.; Lee, C.Y.; Chong, L.W.; Kao, C.H. Association of Periodontitis a Subsequent Depression: A Nationwide Population-Based Study. *Medicine* **2015**, *94*, e2347. [CrossRef] [PubMed]

Kim, S.R.; Nam, S.H. Comparison of Diagnosed Depression and Self-Reported Depression Symptom as a Risk Factor of Periodontitis: Analysis of 2016–2018 Korean National Health and Nutrition Examination Survey Data. *Int. J. Environ. Res. Public Health* **2021**, *18*, 871. [CrossRef]
Zheng, D.X.; Kang, X.N.; Wang, Y.X.; Huang, Y.N.; Pang, C.F.; Chen, Y.X.; Kuang, Z.L.; Peng, Y. Periodontal disease and emotional disorders: A meta-analysis. *J. Clin. Periodontol.* **2021**, *48*, 180–204. [CrossRef] [PubMed]
Okoro, C.A.; Strine, T.W.; Eke, P.I.; Dhingra, S.S.; Balluz, L.S. The association between depression and anxiety and use of oral health services and tooth loss. *Community Dent. Oral Epidemiol.* **2012**, *40*, 134–144. [CrossRef]
Kassebaum, N.J.; Bernabe, E.; Dahiya, M.; Bhandari, B.; Murray, C.J.; Marcenes, W. Global burden of severe periodontitis in 1990–2010: A systematic review and meta-regression. *J. Dent. Res.* **2014**, *93*, 1045–1053. [CrossRef] [PubMed]
Al-Harthi, L.S.; Cullinan, M.P.; Leichter, J.W.; Thomson, W.M. The impact of periodontitis on oral health-related quality of life: A review of the evidence from observational studies. *Aust. Dent. J.* **2013**, *58*, 274–277. [CrossRef] [PubMed]
Gerritsen, A.E.; Allen, P.F.; Witter, D.J.; Bronkhorst, E.M.; Creugers, N.H. Tooth loss and oral health-related quality of life: A systematic review and meta-analysis. *Health Qual. Life Outcomes* **2012**, *8*, 126. [CrossRef] [PubMed]
Saintrain, M.V.; de Souza, E.H. Impact of tooth loss on the quality of life. *Gerodontology* **2012**, *29*, e632–e636. [CrossRef]
Hohls, J.K.; Konig, H.H.; Quirke, E.; Hajek, A. Anxiety, Depression and Quality of Life-A Systematic Review of Evidence from Longitudinal Observational Studies. *Int. J. Environ. Res. Public Health* **2021**, *18*, 12022. [CrossRef]
Shin, H.S.; Ahn, Y.S.; Lim, D.S. Association Between Chewing Difficulty and Symptoms of Depression in Adults: Results from the Korea National Health and Nutrition Examination Survey. *J. Am. Geriatr. Soc.* **2016**, *64*, e270–e278. [CrossRef]
Sowislo, J.F.; Orth, U. Does low self-esteem predict depression and anxiety? A meta-analysis of longitudinal studies. *Psychol. Bull.* **2013**, *139*, 213–240. [CrossRef] [PubMed]
Dowlati, Y.; Herrmann, N.; Swardfager, W.; Liu, H.; Sham, L.; Reim, E.K.; Lanctot, K.L. A meta-analysis of cytokines in major depression. *Biol. Psychiatry* **2010**, *67*, 446–457. [CrossRef] [PubMed]
Kohler, C.A.; Freitas, T.H.; Maes, M.; de Andrade, N.Q.; Liu, C.S.; Fernandes, B.S.; Stubbs, B.; Solmi, M.; Veronese, N.; Herrmann, N.; et al. Peripheral cytokine and chemokine alterations in depression: A meta-analysis of 82 studies. *Acta Psychiatr. Scand.* **2017**, *135*, 373–387. [CrossRef] [PubMed]
Mac Giollabhui, N.; Ng, T.H.; Ellman, L.M.; Alloy, L.B. The longitudinal associations of inflammatory biomarkers and depression revisited: Systematic review, meta-analysis, and meta-regression. *Mol. Psychiatry* **2021**, *26*, 3302–3314. [CrossRef] [PubMed]
Butera, A.; Maiorani, C.; Gallo, S.; Pascadopoli, M.; Venugopal, A.; Marya, A.; Scribante, A. Evaluation of Adjuvant Systems in Non-Surgical Peri-Implant Treatment: A Literature Review. *Healthcare* **2022**, *10*, 886. [CrossRef]
Dumitrescu, A.L. Depression and Inflammatory Periodontal Disease Considerations-An Interdisciplinary Approach. *Front. Psychol.* **2016**, *7*, 347. [CrossRef]
Butera, A.; Pascadopoli, M.; Nardi, M.G.; Ogliari, C.; Chiesa, A.; Preda, C.; Perego, G.; Scribante, A. Clinical Use of Paraprobiotics for Pregnant Women with Periodontitis: Randomized Clinical Trial. *Dent. J.* **2024**, *12*, 116. [CrossRef] [PubMed]
Neupane, S.P.; Virtej, A.; Myhren, L.E.; Bull, V.H. Biomarkers common for inflammatory periodontal disease and depression: A systematic review. *Brain Behav. Immun. Health* **2022**, *21*, 100450. [CrossRef]
Wang, X.; Tong, Y.; Zhang, J.; Khan, N.; Zhang, K.; Bai, H.; Zhang, Q.; Chen, Y. Neuroinflammation changes with periodontal inflammation status during periodontitis in wild-type mice. *Oral Dis.* **2021**, *27*, 1001–1011. [CrossRef]
Castro, M.M.L.; Ferreira, R.O.; Fagundes, N.C.F.; Almeida, A.; Maia, L.C.; Lima, R.R. Association between Psychological Stress and Periodontitis: A Systematic Review. *Eur. J. Dent.* **2020**, *14*, 171–179. [CrossRef]
Botelho, J.; Machado, V.; Mascarenhas, P.; Rua, J.; Alves, R.; Cavacas, M.A.; Delgado, A.; Joao Mendes, J. Stress, salivary cortisol and periodontitis: A systematic review and meta-analysis of observational studies. *Arch. Oral Biol.* **2018**, *96*, 58–65. [CrossRef] [PubMed]
Biggio, G.; Mostallino, M.C. Stress, cortisol, neuronal plasticity, and depressive disorder. *J. Psychopathol.* **2013**, *19*, 77–83.
DeCarolis, N.A.; Eisch, A.J. Hippocampal neurogenesis as a target for the treatment of mental illness: A critical evaluation. *Neuropharmacology* **2010**, *58*, 884–893. [CrossRef] [PubMed]
Belvederi Murri, M.; Pariante, C.; Mondelli, V.; Masotti, M.; Atti, A.R.; Mellacqua, Z.; Antonioli, M.; Ghio, L.; Menchetti, M.; Zanetidou, S.; et al. HPA axis and aging in depression: Systematic review and meta-analysis. *Psychoneuroendocrinology* **2014**, *41*, 46–62. [CrossRef] [PubMed]
Nascimento, G.G.; Gastal, M.T.; Leite, F.R.M.; Quevedo, L.A.; Peres, K.G.; Peres, M.A.; Horta, B.L.; Barros, F.C.; Demarco, F.F. Is there an association between depression and periodontitis? A birth cohort study. *J. Clin. Periodontol.* **2019**, *46*, 31–39. [CrossRef] [PubMed]
Bansal, T.; Pandey, A.D.D.; Asthana, A.K. C-Reactive Protein (CRP) and its Association with Periodontal Disease: A Brief Review. *J. Clin. Diagn. Res.* **2014**, *8*, ZE21–ZE24.
Jiang, H.; Zhang, Y.; Xiong, X.; Harville, E.W.; O, K.; Qian, X. Salivary and serum inflammatory mediators among pre-conception women with periodontal disease. *BMC Oral Health* **2016**, *16*, 131. [CrossRef]
Wang, I.C.; Askar, H.; Ghassib, I.; Wang, C.W.; Wang, H.L. Association between periodontitis and systemic medication intake: A case-control study. *J. Periodontol.* **2020**, *91*, 1245–1255. [CrossRef]
Hashioka, S.; McGeer, P.L.; Monji, A.; Kanba, S. Anti-inflammatory effects of antidepressants: Possibilities for preventives against Alzheimer's disease. *Cent. Nerv. Syst. Agents Med. Chem.* **2009**, *9*, 12–19. [CrossRef]

64. Martino, M.; Rocchi, G.; Escelsior, A.; Fornaro, M. Immunomodulation Mechanism of Antidepressants: Interactions betw Serotonin/Norepinephrine Balance and Th1/Th2 Balance. *Curr. Neuropharmacol.* **2012**, *10*, 97–123. [CrossRef]
65. Tynan, R.J.; Weidenhofer, J.; Hinwood, M.; Cairns, M.J.; Day, T.A.; Walker, F.R. A comparative examination of the a inflammatory effects of SSRI and SNRI antidepressants on LPS stimulated microglia. *Brain Behav. Immun.* **2012**, *26*, 469– [CrossRef] [PubMed]
66. Hakam, A.E.; Duarte, P.M.; Mbadu, M.P.; Aukhil, I.; da Silva, H.D.P.; Chang, J. Association of different antidepressant clas with clinical attachment level and alveolar bone loss in patients with periodontitis: A retrospective study. *J. Periodontal Res.* **2** *57*, 75–84. [CrossRef] [PubMed]
67. Bey, A.; Ahmad, S.S.; Azmi, S.A.; Ahmed, S. Effect of antidepressants on various periodontal parameters: A case-control stud *Indian Soc. Periodontol.* **2020**, *24*, 122–126. [CrossRef] [PubMed]
68. Majeed, R.; Sathi, K.V.; Patil, R.S.; Singh, N.; Duseja, S.; Kondreddy, K. Association of the Antidepressants and the Periodo Status: An Original Research. *J. Pharm. Bioallied Sci.* **2024**, *16*, S215–S218. [CrossRef] [PubMed]
69. Page, M.J.; McKenzie, J.E.; Bossuyt, P.M.; Boutron, I.; Hoffmann, T.C.; Mulrow, C.D.; Shamseer, L.; Tetzlaff, J.M.; Akl, E Brennan, S.E.; et al. The PRISMA 2020 statement: An updated guideline for reporting systematic reviews. *BMJ* **2021**, *372*, 1 [CrossRef] [PubMed]
70. Hasan, F.; Ikram, R.; Simjee, S.U.; Iftakhar, K.; Asadullah, K. Effects of 1% amitriptyline gel and mouthwash in patients w periodontal diseases via local drug delivery system: A randomized control clinical trial. *Pak. J. Pharm. Sci.* **2019**, *32*, 1855–1 [PubMed]
71. Hassan, R.; Ahmed, N.F.; Hussein, S.I. Histological, immunohistochemical and radiographic evaluation of Amitripty administration on the periodontium of albino rats (An experimental study). *Saudi Dent. J.* **2022**, *34*, 449–457. [CrossRef] [PubM
72. Branco-de-Almeida, L.S.; Franco, G.C.; Castro, M.L.; Vieira, M.S.; Galvão-Moreira, L.V.; Cortelli, S.C.; Anbinder, A.L.; Kawai Rosalen, P.L. Protective effects of desipramine on alveolar bone in experimental periodontitis. *J. Periodontol.* **2020**, *91*, 1694–1 [CrossRef]
73. Li, Y.; Lu, Z.; Zhang, L.; Kirkwood, C.L.; Kirkwood, K.L.; Lopes-Virella, M.F.; Huang, Y. Inhibition of acid sphingomyelinase imipramine abolishes the synergy between metabolic syndrome and periodontitis on alveolar bone loss. *J. Periodontal Res.* **2** *57*, 173–185. [CrossRef]
74. Yamawaki, Y.; So, H.; Oue, K.; Asano, S.; Furusho, H.; Miyauchi, M.; Tanimoto, K.; Kanematsu, T. Imipramine preve Porphyromonas gingivalis lipopolysaccharide-induced microglial neurotoxicity. *Biochem. Biophys. Res. Commun.* **2022**, *634*, 92- [CrossRef]
75. Bhatia, A.; Sharma, R.K.; Tewari, S.; Narula, S.C.; Khurana, H. Periodontal status in chronic periodontitis depressed patients desvenlafaxine: An observational study. *J. Indian Soc. Periodontol.* **2018**, *22*, 442–446. [CrossRef] [PubMed]
76. Carvalho, R.S.; de Souza, C.M.; Neves, J.C.; Holanda-Pinto, S.A.; Pinto, L.M.; Brito, G.A.; de Andrade, G.M. Effect of venlafax on bone loss associated with ligature-induced periodontitis in Wistar rats. *J. Negat. Results Biomed.* **2010**, *9*, 3. [CrossRef] [PubM
77. Aguiar, J.C.A.; Gomes, E.P.P.; Fonseca-Silva, T.; Velloso, N.A.; Vieira, L.T.; Fernandes, M.F.; Santos, S.H.S.; Neto, J.F.R.; De-Pa A.M.B.; Guimarães, A.L.S. Fluoxetine reduces periodontal disease progression in a conditioned fear stress model in rats *Periodontal Res.* **2013**, *48*, 632–637. [CrossRef] [PubMed]
78. Bhatia, A.; Sharma, R.K.; Tewari, S.; Khurana, H.; Narula, S.C. Effect of Fluoxetine on Periodontal Status in Patients W Depression: A Cross-Sectional Observational Study. *J. Periodontol.* **2015**, *86*, 927–935. [CrossRef] [PubMed]
79. Branco-De-Almeida, L.S.; Franco, G.C.; Castro, M.L.; dos Santos, J.G.; Anbinder, A.L.; Cortelli, S.C.; Kajiya, M.; Kawai, T.; Rosa P.L. Fluoxetine inhibits inflammatory response and bone loss in a rat model of ligature-induced periodontitis. *J. Periodontol.* **2** *83*, 664–671. [CrossRef] [PubMed]
80. Regueira, L.S.; Marcelos, P.G.; Santiago-Jaegger, I.M.; Perez, D.E.; Evêncio, J.; Neto Baratella-Evêncio, L. Fluoxetine effe on periodontogenesis: Histomorphometrical and immunohistochemical analyses in rats. *J. Appl. Oral Sci.* **2017**, *25*, 159–1 [CrossRef] [PubMed]
81. Breivik, T.; Gundersen, Y.; Myhrer, T.; Fonnum, F.; Osmundsen, H.; Murison, R.; Gjermo, P.; Von Hörsten, S.; Opstad, Enhanced susceptibility to periodontitis in an animal model of depression: Reversed by chronic treatment with the anti-depress tianeptine. *J. Clin. Periodontol.* **2006**, *33*, 469–477. [CrossRef] [PubMed]
82. Breivik, T.; Gundersen, Y.; Osmundsen, H.; Fonnum, F.; Opstad, P.K. Neonatal dexamethasone and chronic tianeptine treatm inhibit ligature-induced periodontitis in adult rats. *J. Periodontal Res.* **2006**, *41*, 23–32. [CrossRef]
83. Muniz, F.W.M.G.; Melo, I.M.; Rösing, C.K.; Andrade, G.M.; Martins, R.S.; Moreira, M.M.S.M.; Carvalho, R.D.S. Use of antidep sive agents as a possibility in the management of periodontal diseases: A systematic review of experimental studies. *J. Inves Clin. Dent.* **2018**, *9*, e12291. [CrossRef]
84. Palomer, T.; Ramírez, V.; Ortuño, D. Correction: Relationship between oral health and depression: Data from the National Hea Survey 2016–2017. *BMC Oral Health* **2024**, *24*, 399. [CrossRef]
85. Cecoro, G.; Annunziata, M.; Iuorio, M.T.; Nastri, L.; Guida, L. Periodontitis, Low-Grade Inflammation and Systemic Health Scoping Review. *Medicina* **2020**, *56*, 272. [CrossRef]
86. de Molon, R.S.; Park, C.H.; Jin, Q.; Sugai, J.; Cirelli, J.A. Characterization of ligature-induced experimental periodontitis. *Micr Res. Tech.* **2018**, *81*, 1412–1421. [CrossRef] [PubMed]

Plemmenos, G.; Evangeliou, E.; Polizogopoulos, N.; Chalazias, A.; Deligianni, M.; Piperi, C. Central Regulatory Role of Cytokines in Periodontitis and Targeting Options. *Curr. Med. Chem.* **2021**, *28*, 3032–3058. [CrossRef]
Hienz, S.A.; Paliwal, S.; Ivanovski, S. Mechanisms of Bone Resorption in Periodontitis. *J. Immunol. Res.* **2015**, 615486. [CrossRef] [PubMed]
Tsurukai, T.; Udagawa, N.; Matsuzaki, K.; Takahashi, N.; Suda, T. Roles of macrophage-colony stimulating factor and osteoclast differentiation factor in osteoclastogenesis. *J. Bone Miner. Metab.* **2020**, *18*, 177–184. [CrossRef] [PubMed]
Garlet, G.P. Destructive and protective roles of cytokines in periodontitis: A re-appraisal from host defense and tissue destruction viewpoints. *J. Dent. Res.* **2010**, *89*, 1349–1363. [CrossRef]
Pan, W.; Wang, Q.; Chen, Q. The cytokine network involved in the host immune response to periodontitis. *Int. J. Oral Sci.* **2019**, *11*, 30. [CrossRef]
Harsanyi, S.; Kupcova, I.; Danisovic, L.; Klein, M. Selected Biomarkers of Depression: What Are the Effects of Cytokines and Inflammation? *Int. J. Mol. Sci.* **2022**, *24*, 578. [CrossRef] [PubMed]
Wang, Y.X.; Kang, X.N.; Cao, Y.; Zheng, D.X.; Lu, Y.M.; Pang, C.F.; Wang, Z.; Cheng, B.; Peng, Y. Porphyromonas gingivalis induces depression via downregulating p75NTR-mediated BDNF maturation in astrocytes. *Brain Behav. Immun.* **2019**, *81*, 523–534. [CrossRef]
Jentsch, H.F.; Marz, D.; Kruger, M. The effects of stress hormones on growth of selected periodontitis related bacteria. *Anaerobe* **2013**, *24*, 49–54. [CrossRef]
Roberts, A.; Matthews, J.B.; Socransky, S.S.; Freestone, P.P.; Williams, P.H.; Chapple, I.L. Stress and the periodontal diseases: Effects of catecholamines on the growth of periodontal bacteria in vitro. *Oral Microbiol. Immunol.* **2002**, *17*, 296–303. [CrossRef] [PubMed]

Journal of
Clinical Medicine

MDPI

Review

Minimally Invasive Surgical Techniques for Periodontal Regeneration: Preserving the Entire Papilla Without Dissection—A Narrative Review

Sylwia Jakubowska * and Bartłomiej Górski

Department of Periodontology and Oral Mucosa Diseases, Medical University of Warsaw, Binieckiego 6 St., 02-097 Warsaw, Poland; bgorski@wum.edu.pl
* Correspondence: sylwiajakubowska999@interia.pl

Abstract: Background: The aim of the present narrative review is to synthesize the available scientific evidence on the minimally invasive surgical techniques for periodontal regeneration preserving the entire papilla without dissection. Surgical treatment of intrabony defects may result in compromising the integrity of the interdental tissues and subsequent papilla loss. Therefore, it is indicated to investigate the approaches avoiding papillary incision over the osseous defect, thus optimizing wound healing conditions. **Methods:** Authors performed a search of literature via electronic databases such as PubMed, Web of Science, Cochrane, and Scopus, and extended by manual searching with a stop date of February 2025. Based on inclusion criteria only randomized clinical trials (RCT), cohort studies, case–control studies, and case series were included, and 106 records were initially identified. Various aspects of described novel approaches preserving the entire papilla were finally discussed. **Results:** A total of 12 studies were evaluated. There is a significant lack of randomized controlled clinical trials on minimally invasive techniques without incision in the papilla. However, numerous modifications of existing techniques have emerged, mainly in the form of case series and case reports with short-term data. Among them, some authors stated that the entire papilla preservation approaches may facilitate early soft tissue healing, reduce papilla trauma and the risk of gingival recession, minimize procedure time, improve flap stability, and alleviate discomfort and side effects, while others reported similar outcomes to conventional approaches and emphasize the need for further comparative clinical trials. **Conclusions:** Preserving papilla integrity and the soft tissue profile is essential for minimizing complications, especially in the esthetic zone. Within the limitations of this narrative review, presented findings emphasize the effectiveness of entire papilla preservation techniques in preventing post-surgery tissue loss compared to conventional incisions and flaps. Randomized controlled trials with longer follow-up periods and larger sample sizes are necessary to validate the efficacy of these approaches in comparison to established papilla preservation techniques.

Keywords: periodontal regeneration; intrabony defects; entire papilla preservation; interdental papilla; periodontics; soft tissue surgery

1. Introduction

Periodontitis is a persistent inflammatory condition of multifactorial origin, characterized by the gradual degradation of the periodontium. The associated alveolar bone loss may manifest in distinct morphological patterns—horizontal, angular, or vertical—frequently leading to the development of intrabony periodontal defects. These osseous defects are considered critical indicators of disease severity and progression, and they commonly necessitate regenerative periodontal interventions to restore lost tissue architecture and function [1–3]. After initial periodontal therapy, the persistence of pathological pockets with intrabony bone loss patterns is considered a significant risk factor for continued disease progression. These sites frequently require further surgical management to achieve favorable clinical results [2–7]. Extensive scientific evidence supports the effectiveness of periodontal reconstructive surgery in managing teeth with deep periodontal pockets and pronounced clinical attachment loss, contributing to sustained functional stability [8,9]. Although contemporary minimally invasive techniques for the treatment of intrabony defects have shown substantial success in reducing probing depths and improving clinical attachment levels, multiple studies have noted a consistent occurrence of marginal soft tissue contraction following surgery. Furthermore, despite overall favorable clinical outcomes, complete resolution of the intrabony defect is often not achieved [10–12]. In the majority of conventional minimally invasive periodontal regenerative techniques, the defect is accessed via incisions made in the marginal gingiva. However, this approach may present notable challenges, especially in cases where the incision is positioned at the base of the interdental papilla directly above the defect. The challenging anatomical features of the interdental area, combined with the specific morphology of intrabony defects, may predispose these sites to early wound dehiscence. Such complications heighten the risk of surgical site exposure, creating favorable conditions for bacterial contamination and the development of an inflammatory infiltrate, which are predisposing factors that may significantly compromise the success of the regenerative procedure [12,13]. Conventional marginal surgical techniques, characterized by sulcular incisions and the elevation of papillary and marginal soft tissues, are linked to an elevated risk of both horizontal and vertical tissue collapse. Functional forces and micromovements generated during mastication and routine oral hygiene can jeopardize clot stability at the root surface, potentially undermining the regenerative outcome. Additionally, the inherent difficulty in securing stable adaptation of marginal tissues to the root surface may contribute to esthetic concerns, such as postoperative soft tissue recession and irregular gingival contours [12,14]. Gingival recession (REC) often increases after surgical treatment of intraosseous defects, which is an undesirable outcome commonly linked to the selected flap design. Since gingival recession significantly affects oral health-related quality of life, it is highly recommended to adopt simplified surgical methods that reduce postoperative REC while maximizing clinical results [15]. Key components of contemporary minimally invasive surgical approaches include the utilization of magnification for enhanced visualization, limited flap extension and reflection to reduce tissue trauma, and conservation of the papilla and surrounding supracrestal tissues, supported by the application of scrupulous suturing. To minimize complications and enhance the outcome of PPT [16], MIST [17], M-MIST [18], and SFA [19], several innovative minimally invasive surgical procedures have been developed over the last years to preserve the entire papilla without dissection. This review summarizes records on Entire Papilla Preservation Technique (EPPT), Non-Incised Papillae Surgical Approach (NIPSA), the apically incised coronally advanced surgical technique (AICAST), Vestibular Incision Subperiosteal Tunnel Access (VISTA), and periodontal endoscopy-aided non-incisional regeneration technique (NIT), which are all periodontal regeneration techniques in the treatment of intrabony defects that avoid the traumatic incisions in at the papilla base. The principles are to maintain the integrity of the vascular supply, support optimal healing and reduce the risk of tissue necrosis. These approaches minimize surgical trauma, lower the likelihood of gingival recession or scarring, and preserve the natural gingival contour—key factors for achieving favorable esthetic outcomes. Additionally, they enhance soft tissue stability around grafts or biomaterials and contribute to improved patient comfort and faster recovery, making them highly valuable in minimally invasive periodontal surgery. Preventing complications in the esthetic region relies heavily on protecting the shape and integrity of the soft tissues between the teeth [20]. Therefore, it is indicated to investigate the approaches avoiding papillary incision over the osseous defect, thus optimizing wound healing conditions and advancing further than traditional PPT and MIST to reduce trauma. The aim of the present narrative review is to synthesize the available scientific evidence on the novel surgical techniques for periodontal regeneration preserving the entire papilla without dissection.

2. Materials and Methods

Search strategy and data extraction: an electronic search of the literature was conducted in February 2024. Four databases—PubMed/Medline, Web of Science, Cochrane, and Scopus—were screened for relevant articles. Prior to the screening process, the first 50 titles and abstracts retrieved by the electronic literature search were used for calibration of the two reviewers (S.J and B.G) with an independent supervising researcher (B.G). Agreement between reviewers was assessed using the kappa statistic. Consequently, titles and abstracts were independently screened by two reviewers (S.J and B.G). Authors obtained full texts of studies that potentially met the inclusion criteria and evaluated them for possible inclusion. Disagreement between the reviewers was discussed with an independent supervising researcher.

The first reviewer managed the article selection process by importing all records from the databases into Mendeley Reference Manager, where duplicates were removed and the articles were screened. The search strategy was adapted to each specific database and utilized Boolean operators to refine the results. The search was conducted using the following strategy: {(intervention) AND (outcome). (Intervention: [MeSH Terms] periodontal regeneration OR intrabony defects OR gingival recession OR clinical attachment level OR probing depth) AND (outcomes: [MeSH Terms] papilla preservation techniques OR minimally invasive surgery OR entire papilla preservation technique OR non-incised papillae surgical approach OR Soft tissue surgery)}.

The eligibility criteria for this narrative review were structured according to the PICOS framework: P (Population): studies on humans diagnosed with (a) periodontitis, (b) with the evidence of at least one deep intrabony defect, (c) in good general health, (d) with full-mouth plaque score (FMPS) and full-mouth bleeding score $\leq 20\%$.

I (Intervention): surgical techniques preserving the entire papilla.

C (Comparison): (a) papilla preservation techniques (PPTs), (b) MIST, (c) M-MIST.

O (outcome measures): average change in PPD, CAL, REC, periodontal tissue stability.

S (Study design): randomized clinical trials (RCT), case series, case–control studies, cohort studies. Only articles published in English were considered eligible.

The following were excluded: abstract-only publications, both narrative and systematic reviews, studies involving antimicrobial interventions, and animal or in vitro studies.

Data from the selected studies were extracted, organized into evidence tables, and visualized through figures such as flowcharts. The general findings were then synthesized in a narrative manner.

The risk of bias of included randomized clinical trials was assessed with The Cochrane Risk of Bias 2 tool for randomized trials (RoB2). The NIH Quality Assessment Tool for Case Series Studies was used to evaluate remaining 9 case series.

3. Results

A total of 106 articles were retrieved from the database searches [Figure 1]. Duplicates and studies that did not meet the predefined search criteria were subsequently eliminated. After abstracts revision, 68 studies were discarded. Following full-text evaluation, 12 studies focusing on the implementation and effectiveness of the novel surgical techniques for periodontal regeneration preserving the entire papilla without dissection were evaluated [21–32]. The main objectives of the chosen studies and summary of reported results are depicted in Table 1 (clinical relevance) and Table 2 (clinical outcomes). Included reports of non-incised entire papilla preservation techniques applications and their clinical relevance were finally discussed. Three RCTs [22,25,28] demonstrated an unclear risk of bias. Detailed risk of bias assessment is demonstrated in Figure 2. Six case series present good quality ratings [26,27,29–32], and three series present fair quality ratings [21,23,24]. A detailed assessment is depicted in Figure 3. A short summary of included approaches is depicted in Figure 4.

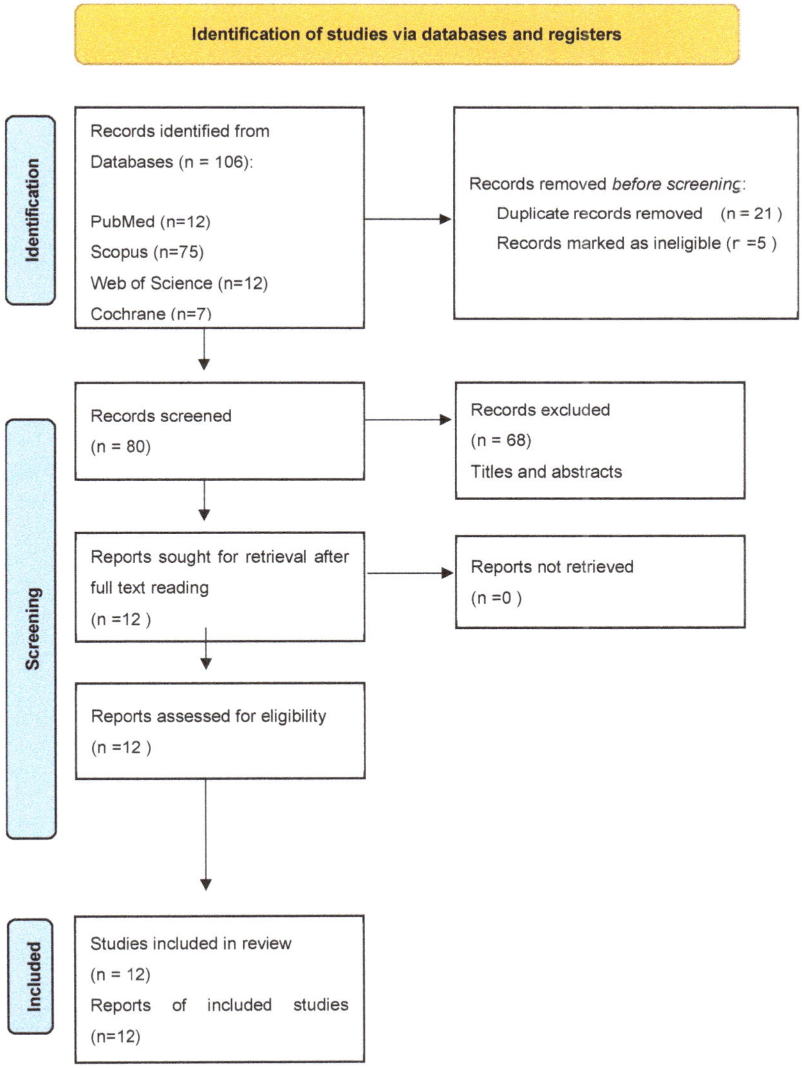

Figure 1. Flow chart of the selection process.

Table 1. Main characteristics of the selected studies and summary of objectives and clinical relevance.

Author/Year	Title	Type of Article	Objectives	Clinical Relevance
Sanz et al., 2024 [21]	"Entire papilla preservation technique for treatment of periodontal intrabony defects: a series of cases."	Prospective case series	To evaluate the use of EPPT without biomaterials for periodontal intrabony defect regeneration, assessing clinical and CBCT-based radiographic outcomes, as well as postoperative complications.	Study demonstrates that the EPPT improves key clinical parameters (PD reduction, CAL gain) without grafts. CBCT enabled precise defect assessment and confirmed post-treatment bone formation, supporting the EPPT as a regenerative, minimally invasive, and cost-effective approach.
Kobe et al., 2024 [22]	"Prehydrated collagenated cortico-cancellous heterologous bone gel and papillae tunneling for isolated intrabony defects: 12-month noninferiority trial."	Randomized, controlled clinical trial	To determine how prehydrated collagenated xenogenic bone gel and a collagenated cortico-cancellous heterologous bone mixture together with EPP or NIPSA are effective in periodontal regenerative procedures.	Results indicate that prehydrated collagen cortico-cancellous bone gel combined with papilla-preserving procedures (EPP or NIPSA) produces similar reductions in PD and clinical attachment gain, with only minor gingival recession compared to conventional slowly resorbable solid particulate bone graft substitutes.
Górski et al., 2023 [23]	"Entire Papilla Preservation Technique with Enamel Matrix Proteins and Allogenic Bone Substitute for the Treatment of Isolated Intrabony Defects: A Prospective Case Series."	Prospective case series	To evaluate clinical and radiographic outcomes of a modified EPPT with extended buccal flap elevation, combined with EMD and radiation-sterilized allogenic grafts for treating isolated intrabony defects.	Study suggests that the modified EPPT may benefit isolated intrabony defects. However, results are based on a single treatment concept without a control group and influenced by variables like SCTG. These results should be considered pilot data, and further trials are needed to evaluate each component's role. Given similar results to established methods, justifying combination therapy remains challenging.

Table 1. *Cont.*

Author/Year	Title	Type of Article	Objectives	Clinical Relevance
Pohl et al., 2023 [24]	"VISTA Approach in Conjunction with Enamel Matrix Derivative, Corticocancellous Bone, and Connective Tissue Graft for Periodontal Defect Surgery: A Case Series."	Prospective case series	To describe the VISTA approach with CCTB (cortico-cancellous tuberosity bone) grafting, debridement, EMD application, and CTG for periodontal regeneration and soft tissue maintenance in the anterior region.	Results suggest that the VISTA approach with EMD, CCTB, and CTG is a promising technique for regenerating periodontal defects with intact lingual bone.
Moreno Rodríguez et al., 2022 [25]	"Apical approach in periodontal reconstructive surgery with enamel matrix derivate and enamel matrix derivate plus bone substitutes: a randomized, controlled clinical trial."	Randomized controlled clinical trial	To assess whether the effectiveness of the non-incised papillae surgical approach (NIPSA) could be impacted by additional use of bone substitutes (BS) and enamel matrix derivative (EMD). Report describes deep, isolated, non-containing defects combining intrabony and supra-alveolar components.	Regardless of whether bone substitutes were used, the NIPSA technique demonstrated significantly improved clinical outcomes along with effective preservation of soft tissue integrity. The use of bone substitutes may promote interproximal soft tissue gain.
Calzavara et al., 2021 [26]	"The apically incised coronally advanced surgical technique (AICAST) for periodontal regeneration in isolated defects: a case series."	Retrospective case series	To report the performance of AICAST (the apically incised coronally advanced surgical technique) in treating non-containing periodontal intrabony defects.	AICAST represents a recent treatment approach. Although study is based on a single treatment approach, preliminary outcomes present favorable clinical attachment gains and preservation of the soft tissues with eventual reduction in the associated gingival recessions.

Table 1. *Cont.*

Author/Year	Title	Type of Article	Objectives	Clinical Relevance
Aslan et al., 2021 [27]	"Reconstructive surgical treatment of isolated deep intrabony defects with guided tissue regeneration using entire papilla preservation technique: A prospective case series."	Prospective case series	To evaluate how effective is the entire papilla preservation (EPP) in combination with native collagen membrane and bone grafting materials in periodontal regeneration.	Presented technique, which avoids incision of the interdental papilla associated with the defect, appears promising for ensuring optimal biomaterial protection and healing conditions, even when a collagen barrier is used.
Aslan et al., 2020 [28]	"Clinical outcomes of the entire papilla preservation technique with and without biomaterials in the treatment of isolated intrabony defects: A randomized controlled clinical trial."	Randomized controlled clinical trial	To evaluate and compare the clinical effectiveness of the entire papilla preservation technique (EPP), both as a standalone approach and in combination with enamel matrix derivatives and bovine-derived bone substitutes (EPP + EMD + BS), in the treatment of isolated interdental intrabony periodontal defects	The use of the EPP, both with and without adjunctive regenerative biomaterials, led to significant CAL gains and probing depth PD reductions, with minimal gingival recession. The adjunctive use of regenerative biomaterials did not yield additional clinical benefits over EPP alone
Moreno Rodríguez et al., 2019 [29]	"Supra-alveolar attachment gain in the treatment of combined intra-suprabony periodontal defects by non-incised papillae surgical approach."	Prospective cohort study	To evaluate the clinical applicability of NIPSA in managing both intrabony and supra-alveolar components of periodontal defect.	Principal findings show that NIPSA improved clinical outcomes, including the supra-alveolar component, reducing soft tissue collapse risk. NIPSA may be a promising approach in periodontal reconstructive surgery, enhancing esthetic outcomes through optimal supra-alveolar tissue stability.

Table 1. *Cont.*

Author/Year	Title	Type of Article	Objectives	Clinical Relevance
Moreno Rodríguez et al., 2019 [30]	"Periodontal reconstructive surgery of deep intraosseous defects using an apical approach. Non-incised papillae surgical approach (NIPSA): A retrospective cohort study."	Retrospective cohort study	To compare a minimally invasive surgical technique (MIST) and a non-incised papilla surgical approach (NIPSA) in periodontal reconstructive surgery of deep intraosseous defects.	NIPSA showed significant soft tissue preservation. NIPSA may represent a promising papillae preservation technique in the treatment of intraosseous periodontal defects.
Aslan et al., 2017 [31]	"Entire papilla preservation technique in the regenerative treatment of deep intrabony defects: 1-Year results."	Prospective case series	To report the clinical outcomes and potential benefits of a surgical "tunnel-like" approach in managing deep, isolated intrabony lesions.	Presented technique reduces wound failure risk, particularly in early healing, preventing biomaterial exposure, stabilizing blood clots in deep intrabony defects, and improving clinical outcomes.
Shi et al., 2023 [32]	"A novel periodontal endoscopy-aided non-incisional periodontal regeneration technique in the treatment of intrabony defects: a retrospective cohort study."	Retrospective cohort study	To explore the feasibility of periodontal endoscopy-aided NIT in comparison with periodontal endoscopy-aided SRP (PSRP).	By eliminating flap elevation, PE-aided NIT preserves an optimal periodontal microenvironment for regeneration, making it a potential alternative technique for treating intrabony defects.

Table 2. Tabular presentation of quantitative clinical outcomes.

Author/Year	Defects (n), Diagnostic Criteria for Defects	Follow-Up	Smoking, Mean Age	Type of Procedure	Outcomes	CAL (mm) Mean ± SD	PD (mm) Mean ± SD	REC/GMP (mm) Mean ± SD
Sanz et al., 2024 [21]	6, PD ≥ 6 mm with CAL ≥ 6 mm, ≥3 mm in depth with at least two bony walls	6 months	No, 48 ± 13.07 years	EPPT	Average change in PD, CAL, GMP, PP, PW, KTW	3.67 ± 1.03 ($p < 0.05$)	4.00 ± 0.63 ($p < 0.05$)	0.33 ± 0.52

Table 2. *Cont.*

Author/Year	Defects (n), Diagnostic Criteria for Defects	Follow-Up	Smoking, Mean Age	Type of Procedure	Outcomes	CAL (mm) Mean ± SD	PD (mm) Mean ± SD	REC/GMP (mm) Mean ± SD
Kobe et al., 2024 [22]	20, periodontitis stage III/IV, at least one deep isolated 2/3-wall intraosseous defect, (PD) ≥ 5 mm and (CAL) ≥ 6 mm	12 months	4 smokers, 16 non-smokers, 53 ± 9 years	Control: collagenous corticocellular xenogeneic bone graft + EPPT/NIPSA Test: prehydrated collagen-containing corticocellular heterologous bone gel + EPPT/NIPSA	Average change in CAL, REC, PD, and TP in mm.	Control: −3.70 ± 1.83 Test: −3.60 ± 1.51	Control: −3.90 ± 1.66 Test: −3.50 ± 0.97	Control: 0.20 ± 0.79 Test: −0.10 ± 0.99
Górski et al., 2023 [23]	18, Stage III periodontitis, one-wall/two-wall/three-wall, PD ≥ 5 mm, CAL ≥ 6 mm, DD ≥ 3 mm	6 months	No, 42.61 ± 6.94 years	Control: Modified EPPT + EMD + allogeneic bone graft Test: Modified EPPT + EMD + allogeneic bone graft + SCTG	Average change in PD, CAL, REC, KTW, DD, FMPS, FMBS	Control: −4.87 ± 1.36 mm ($p < 0.0001$) Test: −4.66 ± 1.98	Control: −4.33 ± 1.25 mm ($p < 0.0001$) Test: −4.67 ± 2.08	Control: −0.03 ± 0.48 Test: −0.5 ± 0.5
Pohl et al., 2023 [24]	6, Three-wall/two-wall, CAL ≥ 6 mm	Average 30 months	No, 37–54 years	VISTA + CTG + CCTB	PPD, CAL, REC, PT	Initial: 8.5 ± 0.83 Post: 2.7 ± 0.52	Initial: 8.2 ± 0.75 Post: 2.7 ± 0.52	Initial: 0.3 ± 0.52 Post: 0
Moreno Rodríguez et al., 2022 [25]	24, periodontitis stage III and IV, grade A, PD > 6 mm and extension of the intrabony defect > 3 mm, 1 and/or 2 walls	12 months	No, Control: 46.50 ± 10.47 years Test: 50.33 ± 9.02 years	Control: NIPSA + EMD Test: NIPSA + EMD + BS	Average change in BOP, PPD, CAL, REC, PT, KTW, SUPRA-AG	Control: 8.33 ± 2.74 Test: 7.08 ± 2.68	Control: 8.25 ± 2.70 Test: 6.83 ± 0.81	Control: − 0.25 ± 0.45 (increased) Test: − 0.17 ± 0.58 (increased)

Table 2. Cont.

Author/Year	Defects (n), Diagnostic Criteria for Defects	Follow-Up	Smoking, Mean Age	Type of Procedure	Outcomes	CAL (mm) Mean ± SD	PD (mm) Mean ± SD	REC/GMP (mm) Mean ± SD
Calzavara et al., 2021 [26]	9, periodontitis stage III/IV, 1 or 2 walls, residual PPD ≥ 6 mm and intrabony component ≥ 3 mm	18 months (7 cases) 5 years (2 cases)	No	AICAST + EMD + bovine bone-derived xenograft	Average change in PPD, CAL, REC	18 months follow up cases: 5.66 ± 0.73 5-years follow up cases: 7.42 ± 4.12	18 months follow up cases: 6.81 ± 2.19 5-years follow up cases: 8.58 ± 1.53	18 months follow up cases: 1.14 ± 2.01 5-years follow up cases: 1.16 ± 2.59
Aslan et al., 2021 [27]	15, Periodontitis stage III/IV, 1 or 2 wall, (PD) ≥ 6 mm, (CAL) ≥ 6 mm and at least 4 mm intrabony component in the interdental area	12 months	No, 47.73 ± 12.18	EPPT + deproteinized bovine-derived bone substitute + collagen barrier	Average change in PPD, CAL, REC	5.86 ± 1.28 ($p < 0.0001$)	6.1 ± 1.47 ($p < 0.0001$)	0.23 ± 0.62 (increased)
Aslan et al., 2020 [28]	30, isolated intrabony defect (PD) ≥ 7 mm, (CAL) ≥ 8 mm and an intrabony component ≥ 4 mm measured radiographically	12 months	No, 43.93 ± 12.85 years	Control: EPPT Test: EPPT + EMD + bovine-derived bone substitutes (BS)	Average change in PPD, CAL, REC	Control: 5.83 ± 1.12 Test: 6.3 ± 2.5	Control: 6.2 ± 1.33 Test: 6.5 ± 2.65	Control: −0.36 ± 0.54 (increased) Test: −0.2 ± 0.25 (increased)
Moreno Rodríguez et al., 2019 [29]	20, (PD) > 5 mm, and an intrabony component ≥ 4 mm	12 months	5 smokers and 7 former smokers, 30–60 years	NIPSA + EMD + deproteinized bovine bone xenograft	Average change in PPD, CAL, REC, TP, KTW, SUPRA-AG	5.9 ± 2.38 (<0.001)	5.6 ± 2.48 (<0.001)	0.25 ± 0.44

Table 2. *Cont.*

Author/Year	Defects (n), Diagnostic Criteria for Defects	Follow-Up	Smoking, Mean Age	Type of Procedure	Outcomes	CAL (mm) Mean ± SD	PD (mm) Mean ± SD	REC/GMP (mm) Mean ± SD
Moreno Rodríguez et al., 2019 [30]	30, (PD) > 5 mm, intrabony defect > 3 mm, intrabony defect configuration including a 1 and/or 2-wall involving the buccal wall	12 months	14 smokers, 16 non-smokers, 44.36 ± 5.9 years	Control: MIST + EMD + de-proteinized bovine bone xenograft Test: NIPSA + EMD + de-proteinized bovine bone xenograft	Average change in PPD, CAL, REC, TP, KTW,	MIST: 3.6 ± 1.40 $p < 0.001$ NIPSA: 5.33 ± 2.47 $p < 0.001$	MIST: 4.33 ± 1.45 $p < 0.001$ NIPSA: 5.53 ± 2.56 $p < 0.001$	MIST: −0.73 ± 0.88 (increased) NIPSA: −0.20 ± 0.41 (increased)
Aslan et al., 2017 [31]	12, isolated two- or three-wall intrabony defect with (PD) ≥ 7 mm, (CAL) ≥ 7 mm and at least 4 mm intrabony component	12 months	No, 42.6 ± 13.1 years	EPPT + EMD + de-proteinized porcine-derived bone substitute	Average change in PPD, CAL, REC	6.83 ± 2.51 $p < 0.001$	7 ± 2.8 $p < 0.001$	0.16 ± 0.38
Shi et al., 2023 [32]	117, stage III/IV periodontitis, at least one tooth with probing depth (PD) ≥ 5 mm and bleeding on probing, at least one intrabony defect with the depth ≥ 3 mm	12 months	No, NIT: 21 subjects (32.67 ± 5.83 years) PSRP: 21 subjects (35.76 ± 9.63 years)	Control: periodontal endoscopy- aided SRP (PSRP) Test: periodontal endoscopy-aided non-incisional regeneration technique (NIT)	Average change in PPD, CAL, REC, IBD	PSRP: −2.38 ± 1.60 NIT: −3.62 ± 2.70	PSRP: −3.07 ± 1.66 NIT: −4.14 ± 2.16	PSRP: 0.70 ± 1.15 (decreased) NIT: 0.71 ± 0.90

Author/Year	Adequate Sequence Generation?	Allocation Concealment?	Blinding?	Incomplete Outcome Data Addressed?	Free of Selective Reporting?	Free of Other Bias?
Kobe et al., 2024	Yes	Yes	Yes	Yes	Yes	Unclear
Moreno Rodríguez et al., 2022	Yes	Yes	Yes	Yes	Yes	Unclear
Aslan et al.,2020	Yes	Yes	Yes	Yes	Yes	Unclear

Figure 2. Summary of risk of bias of three included RCTs (ROB 2) [22,25,28].

thor/Year	Q1	Q2	Q3	Q4	Q5	Q6	Q7	Q8	Q9
nz et al., 2024	Yes	Yes	CD	NA	Yes	Yes	No	Yes	Yes
rski et al., 2023	Yes	Yes	CD	NA	Yes	Yes	No	Yes	Yes
hl et al., 2023	Yes	Yes	CD	NA	Yes	Yes	Yes	No	Yes
lzavara et al., 2021	Yes	Yes	CD	NA	Yes	Yes	Yes	Yes	Yes
slan et al., 2021	Yes	Yes	CD	Yes	Yes	Yes	Yes	Yes	Yes
oreno Rodríguez et , 2019	Yes	Yes	CD	Yes	Yes	Yes	Yes	Yes	Yes
oreno Rodríguez et , 2019	Yes	Yes	CD	NA	Yes	Yes	Yes	Yes	Yes
slan et al., 2017	Yes	Yes	CD	Yes	Yes	Yes	Yes	Yes	Yes
i et al., 2023	Yes	Yes	CD	NA	Yes	Yes	Yes	Yes	Yes

Figure 3. Summary of The NIH Quality Assessment Tool for Case Series Studies [21,23,24,26,27,29–32].

It is important to note that this review included different biomaterials, which were primarily used in two- and three-walled intrabony defects treated with various non-incision entire papilla preservation techniques.

Although levels of evidence are important in clinical and research decision-making, it is also essential to carefully evaluate the strengths and weaknesses of each individual study. In this review, only three randomized controlled trials and nine case series were included. Case series are limited by small sample sizes and the absence of control groups, which increases the risk of bias. Therefore, conclusions drawn from such studies should be interpreted with caution.

The clinical effectiveness of periodontal regeneration procedures may be reduced in high-risk populations, such as heavy smokers or individuals with inadequate oral hygiene. It is important to note that the majority of the studies included in this review involved only non-smokers or participants who had quit smoking at least one year prior to enrollment. Only RCT by Kobe et al. [22] and prospective case series by Calzavara et al. [26] allowed for inclusion patients smoking less than 10 cigarettes per day. They constituted

4 out of 20 patients in the Kobe et al. [22] trial and an unknown number in the Calzavara et al. [26] series.

Entire papilla preservation technique EPPT	A buccal intracrevicular incision combined with a single short vertical releasing incision is made, followed by the creation of an interdental tunnel beneath the papilla to access the defect.
Non incised papilla surgical approach NIPSA	A buccal horizontal incision is made apical to the periodontal defect, and the flap is elevated in a coronal direction, providing access to the defect while preserving the integrity of the marginal tissues.
Vestibular incision subperiosteal tunnel access VISTA	A vertical vestibular incision was made near the defect, followed by subperiosteal tunneling to adjacent teeth and papillae using elevators. The tunnels from the vestibular and sulcular approaches were connected, allowing coronal advancement of the buccal soft tissue.
Apically Incised coronally advanced surgical technique AICAST	A horizontal incision was made in the vestibular mucosa, at least 10 mm apical to the gingival margin, and extended mesiodistally to include the affected tooth and its two neighbors. From this incision, a full-thickness mucoperiosteal flap was elevated coronally up to the gingival margins of the involved teeth.
Endoscopy-aided non-incisional regeneration technique NIT	Granulation tissue was gently removed using a mini curette under endoscopic visualization. Bio-Oss Collagen was carefully inserted into the bone defects with the help of a gingival retractor, ensuring precise placement without extensive tissue reflection.

Figure 4. Short summary of included approaches.

Only one prospective case series by Sanz et al. [21] did not report the additional use of bone substitute materials or bone grafts in the surgical procedure. The EMD (Emdogain®; Straumann, Basel, Switzerland) was not reported in this series either. Moreno-Roudrigez et al. [25,30], Calzavara et al. [26], Shi et al. [32], and Aslan et al. [27,28,31] used deproteinized bovine-derived bone substitute (BS, Cerabone, Botiss Biomaterials GmbH, Berlin, Germany or Bio-Oss/Bio-Oss Collagen, Geistlich Biomaterials, Zurich, Switzerland), while Kobe et al. [22] reported that in the experimental group, a prehydrated collagen-containing corticocellular heterologous bone gel (OsteoBiol® Gel, Tecnoss, Torino, Italy) was applied, and in the control group patient's blood-soaked collagenous corticocellular xenogeneic bone graft (OsteoBiol® Gen-Os, Tecnoss, Torino, Italy) was utilized. Meanwhile, Górski et al. [23] applied frozen, radiation-sterilized, allogeneic bone granules consisting of cortical and cancellous bone. Pohl et al. [24] were the first to use corticocancellous tuberosity bone (CCTB) for periodontal regeneration.

While the beneficial effects of EMD and its capacity to enhance regeneration have been widely recorded, two studies did not mention the additional use of amelogenins [21,22].

There was notable heterogeneity in the follow-up periods among the included studies. Two studies reported outcomes at 6 months [21,23], seven studies had a 12-month follow-up [22,25,27,28,30–32], and only two studies extended beyond 12 months [24,26]. Of these, one study reported long-term results for two cases with a follow-up of 5 years, highlighting the limited availability of long-term data in this area.

According to Aimetti et al. [6], two criteria for probing depth (PD)—$\leq$3 mm and $\leq$4 mm—were assessed among studies. Each included study report a mean PD $\leq$ 4 mm at the follow-up for the treated sites, but not every study recorded the PD $\leq$ 3 mm after the observation period. In one RCT [25], both groups accomplished the residual PD < 5 mm (NIPSA EMD 2.50 $\pm$ 0.67 mm; NIPSA EMD + BS 2.67 $\pm$ 0.78 mm). The residual probing depth was 2 mm in 58.33% of cases treated with NIPSA EMD and in 50% of cases treated with NIPSA EMD + BS. A residual probing depth of 4 mm was observed in one case within the NIPSA EMD group and in two cases within the NIPSA EMD + BS group. In RTC using the EPPT [28] both groups showed a significant decrease in PD in the first years post-op. No significant inter-group differences were found ($p = 0.866$). In the EPP EMD + BS group, 33% of defects (n = 5) exhibited a residual probing depth of 2 mm, 53% (n = 8) had 3 mm, and 14% (n = 2) presented with a depth of 4 mm or more.

Among the EPP group, 20% of defects (n = 3) had a residual PD of 2 mm, 60% (n = 9) measured 3 mm, and another 20% (n = 3) had depths $\geq$ 4 mm. Some studies presented only mean PD difference values without percentage of reached pocket resolutions. In studies that did not use bone substitutes, the residual PD was 2.67 $\pm$ 1.03 mm (EPPT) and 2.59 $\pm$ 0.92 mm (AICAST) accordingly [21,26]. Meanwhile, cases series using the EPPT with BS and a collagen barrier membrane [27] reported residual PD 2.93 $\pm$ 0.59 mm after 1 year and a case series using the EPPT with BS recorded PD 2.67 $\pm$ 0.78 after 1 year [31].

Q1: Was the study question or objective clearly stated?, Q2: Was study population clearly and fully described, including case definition?, Q3: Were cases consecutive?, Q4: Were subjects comparable?, Q5: Was intervention clearly described?, Q6: Were outcome measures clearly defined, valid, reliable, and implemented consistently across all study participants?, Q7: Was length of follow-up adequate?, Q8: Were statistical methods well-described?, Q9: Were results well-described?, Good: Met 7–9 criteria, Fair: Met 4–6 criteria, Poor: Met 0–3 criteria. NA = not applicable, NIH = National Institutes of Health, NR = not reported.

In 2017, Aslan [31] published the first report on the tunnel-like surgical technique (EPPT) as 1 year follow-up of a prospective case series. The application of this technique supports the use of amelogenins and grafting materials. Three years later, an RCT was published by the same authors, Aslan et al. [28], where they combined the EPPT with biomaterials (EMD + BS). The outcomes were comparable to established methods, and it was documented that the use of the EPP, regardless of the use of adjunctive regenerative biomaterials, led to significant CAL gains and probing depth PD reductions, with minimal gingival recession. Moreover, authors concluded that the adjunctive use of regenerative biomaterials did not yield additional clinical benefits over EPP alone. In 2021, Aslan et al. [27] investigated another configuration of the EPPT in combination with GTR using native collagen membrane and bone grafting materials. According to the results, the technique may potentially provide effective protection for the biomaterial and optimal conditions for healing, even with the presence of a collagen barrier. The following authors went further to investigate the possibilities of the EPPT, and in 2023, Gorski et al. [23] proposed the modification to the original method design. In their modification, the buccal flap is extended mesiodistally in order to reduce flap tension and to enhance surgical access to a one-wall defect. Furthermore, the vertical releasing incision is lengthened as necessary to improve visualization. The findings of this study indicate that the modified EPPT, combined with EMD and allogenic bone grafting, may be considered as a potential treatment modality for intrabony defects. Follow-up of this case series demonstrated statistically significant and sustained clinical improvements over a 3-year period. The most recent prospective case series published by Sanz et al. in 2024 [21] evaluated the use of the EPPT without biomaterials for periodontal intrabony defect regeneration, assessing clinical and CBCT-based radiographic outcomes, as well as postoperative complications.

NIPSA was first proposed in 2018 (Moreno Rodriguez & Caffesse, 2018) [33]. One year later, the results of a prospective cohort study were published by the same authors [29]. It revealed that PD decrease was 5.53 ± 2.56 mm and CAL gain was 5.33 ± 2.47 mm. Moreover, the early wound healing index after one week was 1.5 ± 0.7, but recession increased by 0.20 ± 0.41 mm. The keratinized tissue width remained unchanged. In 2019, in the retrospective cohort study by Moreno Rodríguez et al. [30], the minimally invasive surgical technique (MIST) was compared with a non-incised papilla surgical approach (NIPSA). No significant differences between the two techniques were shown regarding PD reduction. However, authors report that after 1 year, the NIPSA group presented favorable, significant CAL gain ($p < 0.05$. It is suggested that a different soft tissue response (REC, TP, KT) is related to the approach used. The NIPSA design seems to minimize surgical trauma of tissues resulting in REC increase by only 0.2 ± 0.41 mm, while MIST resulted in the 0.73 ± 0.88 mm increase. Three years later, Moreno-Rodriguez et al. [25] presented an RCT in which they evaluate how non-incised papillae surgical approach (NIPSA) can be influenced by enamel matrix derivate (EMD) and bone substitutes (BS) in resolving combined non-contained periodontal defects with intrabony and supra-alveolar components. BoP was negative in all cases at the 1-year follow-up. Both groups demonstrated notable improvements, with substantial reductions in probing depth (NIPSA + EMD: 8.25 ± 2.70 mm; NIPSA + EMD + BS: 6.83 ± 0.81 mm) and gains in clinical attachment level (NIPSA + EMD: 8.33 ± 2.74 mm; NIPSA + EMD + BS: 7.08 ± 2.68 mm), all statistically significant ($p < 0.001$). However, no meaningful differences were detected in the inter-group comparison ($p > 0.05$). Soft tissue integrity was maintained in both groups, with no statistically significant differences observed between them (recession: NIPSA + EMD 0.25 ± 0.45 mm vs. NIPSA + EMD + BS 0.17 ± 0.58 mm, $p > 0.05$; keratinized tissue width: 0.00 ± 0.43 mm vs. 0.08 ± 0.67 mm, $p > 0.05$). Interestingly, although both groups exhibited improvements in papillary height, statistical significance was reached only in the NIPSA + EMD + BS group (0.45 ± 0.52 mm; $p < 0.05$), while the NIPSA + EMD group recorded a non-significant gain (0.33 ± 0.49 mm; $p > 0.05$).

Recently, in 2024, an RCT by Kobe et al. [22] was published, in which both papillae tunneling techniques (PTT), EPPT and NIPSA, were utilized in the treatment. Authors implemented prehydrated collagenated xenogenic bone gel in one group and collagenated cortico-cancellous heterologous bone mixture in the second group adjunctive to non-incised papilla preservation techniques. In this regard, incisors and canines were treated with NIPSA (n = 11) (Aslan et al., 2017) [31], whereas EPP was used with premolars or molars (n = 9). The authors noted that both surgical modalities ensured complete wound closure during the early healing phase and prevented biomaterial exposure in both the test and control groups.

In 2023, Pohl et al. [24] described a prospective case series using the VISTA approach with cortico-cancellous tuberosity bone grafting, debridement, EMD application, and CTG for periodontal regeneration. The authors used a single vertical incision just adjacent to the defect for gaining access and sulcular approach for root scaling. Visualization of the treated area was reported to be sufficient. The probing pocket depth improved from 8.2 ± 0.75 mm initially to 2.7 ± 0.52 mm at follow-up, clinical attachment level changed from 8.5 ± 0.83 mm initially to 2.7 ± 0.52 mm at follow-up, and gingival recession of 1 mm at two sites was corrected. The papillae remained stable across all sites, maintaining an average distance of 4.8 mm from the incisal edge to the papilla tip. Another innovative surgical design for preserving the entire papilla whilst avoiding dissection is the apically incised coronally advanced surgical technique (AICAST) proposed by Calzavara et al. in 2021 [26]. The case series presents the modification to surgical approach to reconstruct the interdental papilla by an apical incision in the lining mucosa described by Azzi et al. [34]. The modification facilitates the coronal advancement of both the gingival margin and the interdental papilla. In four out of nine cases where a buccal gingival recession was preoperatively present, a ctg was applied. CAL gains ≥ 6 mm were achieved in eight out of nine treated sites (88.9%), and PPD ≤ 3 mm was detected in all cases. Moreover, cases treated with an additional use of CTG resulted in a non-statistically significantly higher recession reduction and lower PPD reduction than the cases treated without the adjunctive use of ctg.

In 2023, a new non-incisional periodontal regeneration technique was proposed by Shi et al. [32]. In a retrospective cohort study, the authors analyzed the periodontal endoscopy-aided non-incisional regeneration technique (NIT) for the management of intrabony defects. In NIT, full access to the defect was achieved using periodontal endoscopy instead of flap elevation. Bone substitutes were then placed into the thoroughly debrided defect under endoscopic guidance. The NIT method was proposed as a further effort to reduce the invasiveness of periodontal regeneration surgery. The study aimed to explore the feasibility of periodontal endoscopy-aided NIT and to compare its effectiveness with periodontal endoscopy-aided SRP (PSRP). After 1 year, significant improvements in probing depth (PD), clinical attachment level gain (CAL), intrabony defect (IBD) depth, and gingival recession (GR) were demonstrated in both groups. Changes in these parameters between baseline and 1 year were statistically significant in both the NIT and PSRP groups ($p < 0.001$). Interestingly, CAL improved more in the NIT than the PSRP ($p = 0.012$). Regarding the changes in the GR no inter-group differences were noted ($p = 0.232$).

4. Discussion

This review was focused on the clinical outcomes of the novel surgical techniques for periodontal regeneration preserving the entire papilla without dissection. Maintaining papilla integrity and the soft tissue profile has tremendous value in periodontal regenerative surgery, especially in the esthetic area. The findings of this study are analyzed in comparison to the existing literature on the pre-established regenerative approaches, of which the core is to preserve the papilla and minimize the invasiveness of surgery. The recent EFP S3-Level Clinical Practice Guideline advocates for the use of specific flap designs that prioritize the preservation of interdental soft tissues, such as papilla preservation flaps [4,5]. In certain cases, minimizing flap elevation is also recommended to enhance wound stability and reduce patient morbidity [4]. Clinical outcomes of each included study showed a beneficial result in terms of average change in CAL, PD, and differences in REC during the follow-up. In a majority of studies, a positive change in CAL and PD exhibited a statistically significant value [21,23,27,29–31].

Conventional periodontal surgery frequently results in postoperative gingival recession, characterized by a concave contour at the coronal portion of the papilla. This morphology tends to promote plaque accumulation and persistent soft tissue inflammation. Additionally, the interdental papilla faces challenges in tissue regeneration due to its limited blood supply and the difficulty in achieving tension-free wound closure during the early healing phase. Research has demonstrated that guided tissue regeneration surgery (GTRS) is often associated with wound dehiscence and barrier membrane exposure, complications that compromise the stability and integration of bone graft materials, particularly in the interdental region. A recent systematic review and meta-analysis by Nibali et al. [35] concluded that guided tissue regeneration (GTR) offered additional benefits over open flap debridement (OFD), with gains of 1.15 mm in clinical attachment level (CAL-G) and 1.24 mm in probing pocket depth reduction (PPD-R) at 12 months. Furthermore, the incorporation of deproteinized bovine bone mineral (DBBM) further enhanced GTR outcomes, resulting in a CAL gain of 1.5 mm and a PPD reduction of 1.13 mm. Interestingly, the analysis also indicated that papillary preservation flaps led to improved clinical outcomes compared to conventional access flaps. This finding may suggest that, when performing regenerative procedures to treat intrabony defects, papillary preservation techniques should be considered the surgical approach of choice. [7]. With the development of new regenerative materials, such as enamel matrix derivatives, the use of barrier membranes is no longer essential for achieving successful outcomes. Papilla preservation flap techniques have progressed over time, beginning with traditional approaches and later advancing to the modified PPT (Checchi et al., 2009) [36], followed by the simplified PPT by Di Tullio et al. in 2013 [37]. In these techniques, the incision for the papilla preservation technique (PPT) is made at the papillary base. In spite of offering a reduction in papilla trauma compared to traditional methods, these methods still require mesio-distal dissection through the papilla. As a result, biomaterials placed beneath the incision line remain vulnerable to exposure. After one year, the SPPF with EMD showed significantly greater PD reduction (3.4 ± 0.7 mm), CAL gain (2.8 ± 0.8 mm), and less GR increase (0.6 ± 0.4 mm) compared to the non-EMD group (PD: 2.2 ± 0.8 mm; CAL: 1.0 ± 0.6 mm; GR: 1.2 ± 0.7 mm) ($p < 0.001$). The minimally invasive surgical technique (MIST), introduced by Cortellini et al. in combination with the use of an enamel matrix derivative (EMD), was developed to minimize both the mesio-distal extension and the corono-apical reflection of the flap. This approach aims to reduce surgical trauma while enhancing flap stability [17]. At 1-year follow-up, authors reported a significant clinical attachment level gain of 4.9 ± 1.7 mm ($p < 0.0001$) in comparison to the baseline and an increase in gingival recession of 0.4 ± 0.7 mm.

The single-flap approach (SFA) was introduced by Trombelli et al. in 2009 [19,38]. The SFA involves flap elevation on only one side (buccal or oral), preserving the opposite side. PD reduced from 9.0 ± 2.8 mm to 3.8 ± 1.5 mm, while GR increased slightly from 2.2 ± 1.9 mm to 2.6 ± 1.3 mm post-surgery. The Single Flap Approach (SFA) has shown promising results in minimizing postoperative gingival recession (REC), with six out of seven prospective clinical studies reporting mean REC changes of less than 1 mm at six months following surgery. Moreover, compared to papilla preservation techniques, SFA was associated with a lower occurrence of postoperative REC in both conservative and regenerative treatments of intraosseous defects [39].

While previous surgical techniques have significantly minimized trauma to the interdental papilla, they still fail to fully preserve its vascular supply. In cases involving isolated and deep intrabony defects, the use of suboptimal flap designs may markedly compromise the efficacy of regenerative treatment.

In the EPP technique [31], the initial surgical step involves making a vertical incision at the buccal line angle of the affected tooth, located distal to the osseous defect, along with an intrasulcular incision directed toward the defect. This design allows entry to the bony lesion through a tunneled approach. The papilla is elevated as a full-thickness flap, while preserving its natural, uninterrupted blood supply. This ensures optimal vascular perfusion, which helps reduce the risk of wound exposure. The authors reported that all sites healed without complications in the early stage, and at 1-year follow-up, all sites maintained a primary wound closure. EPP without the addition of biomaterials resulted in CAL gain of 5.83 ± 1.12 mm, PD reduction of 6.2 ± 1.33 mm, and gingival margin reduction of 0.36 ± 0.54 mm. According to Górski et al., modification to the EPPT maintained significant improvements from baseline at the 3-years follow-up. The authors reported significant reductions in PPD (7.03 ± 1.61 to 3.33 ± 0.89 mm, $p < 0.0001$), CAL improvement (to 3.08 ± 1.16 mm, $p < 0.001$), and DD decrease (4.59 ± 1.24 to 0.38 ± 0.31 mm, $p < 0.001$), while changes in gingival recession and keratinized tissue were not statistically significant [40].

The Non-Incised Papillae Surgical Approach (NIPSA) is founded on the principle of performing a single horizontal incision on the buccal mucosa, positioned as apically as possible relative to both the periodontal defect and the marginal soft tissues [29,30,33]. This technique entails the elevation of a coronally advanced mucoperiosteal flap, which allows apical access to the defect while maintaining the integrity of the marginal tissues. The preserved marginal tissue acts as a protective covering over the interproximal defect, supposedly helping to maintain soft tissue architecture and prevent papillary collapse. While the supraperiosteal gingival vessels neighboring the mucogingival junction are transected, the continuity of the non-incised gingival vasculature with the periodontal ligament is preserved, along with a strong lingual blood supply. This preservation of vascular integrity may provide an advantage over traditional extended flap techniques by ensuring enhanced perfusion to the surgical site [29,30].

The clinical outcomes reported in the case series by Calzavara et al. [26] utilizing the AICAST flap design are comparable to those reported in clinical trials using the MIST, M-MIST, SFA, and EPPT. However, the AICAST suggests additional suprabony clinical attachment gains in comparison to forementioned papilla preservation techniques. According to Calzavara et al. [26], the AICAST demonstrates positive performance in treating deep isolated intrabony lesions and the long-term maintenance of this outcomes. In study by Calzavara et al. [26], after the surgery, healing was 100% uneventful, and primary closure was achieved in all cases. At the last follow-up (5 years), PPD reduced by 6.05 ± 1.76 mm, and CAL gained 7.20 ± 2.13 mm (both $p < 0.01$), while the REC reduction of 1.15 ± 1.97 mm was not significant. The authors' proposed modification enables the gingival margin and interdental papilla to be advanced coronally, creating an additional vertical space. When this space is filled with a scaffold, it has the potential to extend the attachment gain vertically, including the suprabony component of the defect. Furthermore, this coronal repositioning may correct existing gingival recessions and deficiencies in the interdental papillae, therefore enhancing the esthetic results. It has to be highlighted that this was the first publication of this technique, and the results have to be interpreted with caution. In order to minimize the post-operative gingival recession and patient discomfort, Shi et al. [32] performed a retrospective analysis after 1 year where 21 subjects were treated with non-incisional regeneration technique (NIT) and 21 subjects underwent periodontal endoscopy-aided scaling and root planning (PSRP). Based on the hypothesis that the stability of blood clot can improve without open flap, this study presents a promising approach for enhanced healing by creating an optimal periodontal microenviorment. Both groups showed significant improvements in PD, CAL, and IBD, along with an increase in gingival recession over the follow-up period. The NIT group demonstrated significantly greater CAL gains compared to PSRP ($p = 0.012$). In NIT-treated sites, 32.7% achieved ≥5 mm CAL gain, and 52.7% showed ≥4 mm PD reduction. The average CAL gain of 3.62 ± 2.70 mm in the NIT group aligns with outcomes reported in other studies using GTR or EMD-based regenerative therapies. The periodontal endoscopic system allows for direct visualization of subgingival biofilms, root surfaces, and calculus within periodontal pockets. Through real-time, magnified imaging, it enables clinicians to perform precise and targeted debridement of subgingival deposits, potentially making periodontal therapy less invasive. While traditionally used to improve the effectiveness of scaling and root planing (SRP) by allowing accurate removal of biofilms and calculus, its capacity to visually access the walls of intrabony defects also highlights its potential in regenerative procedures—specifically by facilitating defect debridement without the need for flap elevation [41]. The studies included in the presented review are characterized by keeping the flap as short as possible, with minimal exposure to the residual bone crest reaching a stable primary wound closure to seal the regenerated region and permitting an incident-free healing phase. Clinical outcomes are comparable to pre-established papilla preservation techniques in terms of clinical attachment gain and periodontal depth reduction. However, the majority of the presented studies report minimal post-operative gingival recession, maintenance, or even coronal advancement of the gingival margin, suggesting that the approaches may also enhance the esthetic outcomes. On the other hand, Rasperini et al. [42] suggest that the combination of conventional papilla preservation techniques with connective tissue grafts and coronal flap advancement can promote intrabony defect regeneration while simultaneously achieving interproximal root coverage and papilla reconstruction.

Several key factors must be taken into account when interpreting scientific data on techniques preserving entire papilla.

Establishing a threshold for pocket resolution is essential, as the chosen cut-off values influence how treatment success is defined. According to Aimetti et al. [6], two criteria for probing depth (PD)—≤3 mm and ≤4 mm—were considered in the results. A PD of ≤3 mm reflects the physiological depth of a healthy gingival sulcus, aligning with the ultimate goal of periodontal regeneration—to restore lost attachment. In contrast, a PD of ≤4 mm is often used to indicate periodontal stability in successfully treated patients, particularly when there are no sites with PD > 4 mm or PD = 4 mm with bleeding on probing [4,5]. Aimetti et al. [6] support the declining use of non-resorbable membranes in the last decade, likely due to their association with a high rate of complications and the requirement for a second surgical procedure for membrane removal. However, they also state that the probability of pocket resolution was higher for regenerative procedures than PPTs in meta-analysis for both thresholds of treatment outcomes, but there was a heterogeneity in surgical techniques used. They also state that greater weighted mean reductions in probing depth (PD) and gains in clinical attachment level (CAL) were observed in intrabony defects treated with enamel matrix derivative (EMD) combined with biomaterials or non-resorbable membranes, compared to other regenerative approaches. Additionally, papilla preservation techniques (PPTs) used alone were less effective than guided tissue regeneration (GTR) in achieving PD reduction and CAL gain, as shown in the pairwise meta-analyses. Therefore, authors of this review emphasize the need for randomized controlled trials comparing the use of EPPT without papilla dissection in conjunction with regenerative procedures to determine their superiority or inferiority.

The techniques have certain limitations and drawbacks, which the authors acknowledge and are aware of. The EPPT, NIPSA, and VISTA approaches would not be appropriate if the defect involved the lingual bone crest. The AICAST was reported specifically for only one or two-wall defects with a missing buccal bone on a single rooted teeth. VISTA was advised for use in the anterior region, whereas EPP was not preferred for this area due to the potential for visible scarring along the vertical incision line. EPPT was also not suggested for a narrow interproximal space, because of an increased risk of rupturing the fragile papilla [20]. The disadvantage of NIPSA is the risk of cutting-off the blood supply through a horizontal incision. Suturing in the EPP technique was the simplest, requiring only interrupted sutures, whereas NIPSA and VISTA necessitated more advanced methods such as horizontal mattress and sling sutures. In the NIT [32], case selection is a critical issue. The use of endoscopic instruments may be limited by narrow pocket openings, furcation morphology, or restricted mouth opening. In thin-scalloped biotypes, there is a risk of gingival stripping. Root anomalies like enamel pearls or palatal grooves can hinder NIT application.

A follow-up period of more than 12 months is preferred in periodontal regeneration studies because it allows for the evaluation of long-term stability, true tissue regeneration, and the detection of any delayed complications or relapse. It provides more reliable and clinically meaningful evidence compared to shorter-term follow-up. However, there is a heterogeneity among the included records and only two studies presented follow up period exceeding 12 months [24,26].

Most of the studies were prospective, retrospective and nonrandomized, and there was majority of small sample case series, insufficient to fully detail the procedures. One has to keep in mind that three RCTs and three case series presented an unclear or fair risk of bias, while six case series were assessed good quality, which could also influence the overall summary.

More robust evidence could be gained from randomized clinical trials and multicenter studies. There is a need for large, prospective, and well-designed research in this area. Lastly, the limitations inherent to the design of this narrative review, including a higher degree of bias, should be taken into account before drawing conclusions [43].

5. Conclusions

Within the limitations of this narrative review, it cannot be conclusively determined whether entire papilla preservation techniques that avoid papilla base dissection represent a viable or superior therapeutic approach for the regenerative treatment of intrabony defects. Clinical results of the analyzed studies seem to be comparable to those achieved with conventional papilla preservation techniques. Some findings also report the effectiveness in preventing post-surgery papilla loss, emphasizing the importance of selecting the appropriate technique based on the defect area and patient esthetics. Therefore, the authors indicate a possible area of interest and research for the future on innovative treatment modalities further reducing invasiveness of periodontal regenerative surgical procedures.

Funding: This research received no external funding.

Conflicts of Interest: The authors declare no conflicts of interest.

Abbreviations

BD	Base of the Defect
CAL	Clinical Attachment Level
CAL-G	Clinical Attachment Level Gain
CEJ	Cementoenamel Junction
DBBM	Deproteinized Bovine Bone Mineral
DD	Radiographic Defect Depth
FMBS	Full-Mouth Bleeding Score
FMPS	Full-Mouth Plaque Score

GTR	Guided Tissue Regeneration
MPPT	Modified Papilla Preservation Technique
n	Number of Defects
OFD	Open-Flap Debridement
PPD	Probing Pocket Depth
PPD-R	Probing Pocket Depth Reduction
RCT	Randomized Controlled Trial
SD	Standard Deviation
PPT	Papilla Preservation Technique
EPPT	Entire Papilla Preservation Technique
MIST	Minimally Invasive Surgical Technique
M-MIST	Modified Minimally Invasive Surgical Technique
NIPSA	Non-Incised Papillae Surgical Approach
SRP	Scaling and Root Planing
NIT	Non-Incisional Regeneration Technique
PESRP	Periodontal Endoscopy-Aided Scaling and Root Planning
SFA	Single-Flap Approach
IBD	Intra-Bony Defect

References

1. Cui, Y.; Mai, Y.; Liu, X.; Mu, H. Clinical benefits of autologous platelet concentrate in periodontal intrabony defects: A netw meta-analysis of randomized controlled trials. *Eur. J. Oral Sci.* **2024**, *132*, e12978. [CrossRef] [PubMed]
2. Górski, B.; Brodzikowska, A.; Nijakowski, K.; Sanz, M. Guided Tissue Regeneration of Periodontal Infrabony Defects with Fro Radiation-Sterilized Allogenic Bone Graft Versus Deproteinized Bovine Bone Mineral: 5-Year Outcomes of RCT. *J. Funct. Biom* **2025**, *16*, 95. [CrossRef] [PubMed]
3. Papapanou, P.N.; Wennströmm, J.L. The angular bony defect as indicator of further alveolar bone loss. *J. Clin. Periodontol.* **1** *18*, 317–322. [CrossRef]
4. Sanz, M.; Herrera, D.; Kebschull, M.; Chapple, I.; Jepsen, S.; Beglundh, T.; Sculean, A.; Tonetti, M.S. EFP Workshop Participa and Methodological Consultants. Treatment of stage I-III periodontitis-The EFP S3 level clinical practice guideline. *J. C Periodontol.* **2020**, *47* (Suppl. S22), 4–60. [CrossRef] [PubMed]
5. Herrera, D.; Sanz, M.; Kebschull, M.; Jepsen, S.; Sculean, A.; Berglundh, T.; Papapanou, P.N.; Chapple, I.; Tonetti, M.S. E Workshop Participants and Methodological Consultant. Treatment of stage IV periodontitis: The EFP S3 level clinical prac guideline. *J. Clin. Periodontol.* **2022**, *49* (Suppl. S24), 4–71. [CrossRef]
6. Aimetti, M.; Fratini, A.; Manavella, V.; Giraudi, M.; Citterio, F.; Ferrarotti, F.; Mariani, G.M.; Cairo, F.; Baima, G.; Roman Pocket resolution in regenerative treatment of intrabony defects with papilla preservation techniques: A systematic review a meta-analysis of randomized clinical trials. *J. Clin. Periodontol.* **2021**, *48*, 843–858. [CrossRef]
7. Jepsen, K.; Sculean, A.; Jepsen, S. Complications and treatment errors related to regenerative periodontal surgery. *Periodor 2000* **2023**, *92*, 120–134. [CrossRef]
8. Kazarian, E.; Inozemtseva, K.; Lebedeva, E. A Novel 3D Tunneling (3DT) Surgical Technique for the Treatment of Gingi Recessions with Reconstruction of the Deficient Interdental Papilla and Interproximal Attachment Regeneration: A Case Se *Int. J. Periodontics Restor. Dent.* **2025**, *45*, 31–45. [CrossRef]
9. Prato, G.P.; Cortellini, P. Thirty-year stability after regeneration of a deep intrabony defect: A case report. *J. Clin. Periodontol.* **2** *43*, 857–862. [CrossRef]
10. Cortellini, P.; Tonetti, M.S. Clinical and radiographic outcomes of the modified minimally invasive surgical technique w and without regenerative materials: A randomized-controlled trial in intra-bony defects. *J. Clin. Periodontol.* **2011**, *38*, 365– [CrossRef]
11. Trombelli, L.; Simonelli, A.; Minenna, L.; Vecchiatini, R.; Farina, R. Simplified procedures to treat periodontal intraosseous def in esthetic areas. *Periodontology 2000* **2018**, *77*, 93–110. [CrossRef] [PubMed]
12. Pardo-Zamora, G.; Moreno-Rodríguez, J.A.; Ortiz-Ruíz, A.J. Non-Incised Papilla Surgical Approach and Leukocyte Platelet-R Fibrin in Periodontal Reconstruction of Deep Intrabony Defects: A Case Series. *Int. J. Environ. Res. Public Health* **2021**, *18*, 2 [CrossRef] [PubMed]
13. Farina, R.; Simonelli, A.; Rizzi, A.; Pramstraller, M.; Cucchi, A.; Trombelli, L. Early postoperative healing following buccal sin flap approach to access intraosseous periodontal defects. *Clin. Oral Investig.* **2012**, *17*, 1573–1583. [CrossRef]

Burkhardt, R.; Magaz, V.R.; Hämmerle, C.H.; Lang, N.P. Interposition of a connective tissue graft or a collagen matrix to enhance wound stability—An experimental study in dogs. *J. Clin. Periodontol.* **2016**, *43*, 366–373. [CrossRef]

Trombelli, L.; Simonelli, A.; Minenna, L.; Rasperini, G.; Farina, R. Effect of a Connective Tissue Graft in Combination with a Single Flap Approach in the Regenerative Treatment of Intraosseous Defects. *J. Periodontol.* **2017**, *88*, 348–356. [CrossRef] [PubMed]

Takei, H.H.; Han, T.J.; Carranza, F.A.; Jr Kenney, E.B.; Lekovic, V. Flap technique for periodontal bone implants. Papilla preservation technique. *J. Periodontol.* **1985**, *56*, 204–210. [CrossRef]

Cortellini, P.; Tonetti, M.S. A minimally invasive surgical technique with an enamel matrix derivative in the regenerative treatment of intra-bony defects: A novel approach to limit morbidity. *J. Clin. Periodontol.* **2007**, *34*, 87–93. [CrossRef]

Cortellini, P.; Tonetti, M.S. Improved wound stability with a modified minimally invasive surgical technique in the regenerative treatment of isolated interdental intrabony defects. *J. Clin. Periodontol.* **2009**, *36*, 157–163. [CrossRef]

Trombelli, L.; Simonelli, A.; Pramstraller, M.; Wikesjö, U.M.E.; Farina, R. Single flap approach with and without guided tissue regeneration and a hydroxyapatite biomaterial in the management of intraosseous periodontal defects. *J. Periodontol.* **2010**, *81*, 1256–1263. [CrossRef]

Pei, X. New surgery approaches preserving entire papilla to treat isolated interdental intrabony defects: A narrative review. *Clin. Exp. Dent. Res.* **2021**, *7*, 719–725. [CrossRef]

Sanz, A.; Anwandter, A.; Novoa, F.; Messina, M.; Valdés, M. Entire papilla preservation technique for treatment of periodontal intrabony defects: A series of cases. *Quintessence Int.* **2024**, *55*, 202–211. [CrossRef] [PubMed]

Kobe, T.; Povšič, K.; Gašperšič, R. Prehydrated collagenated cortico-cancellous heterologous bone gel and papillae tunneling for isolated intrabony defects: 12-month noninferiority trial. *Clin. Exp. Dent. Res.* **2024**, *10*, e853. [CrossRef]

Górski, B.; Kowalski, J.; Wyrębek, B. Entire Papilla Preservation Technique with Enamel Matrix Proteins and Allogenic Bone Substitute for the Treatment of Isolated Intrabony Defects: A Prospective Case Series. *Int. J. Periodontics Restor. Dent.* **2023**, *43*, 387–397. [CrossRef]

Pohl, S.; Buljan, M. VISTA Approach in Conjunction with Enamel Matrix Derivative, Corticocancellous Bone, and Connective Tissue Graft for Periodontal Defect Surgery: A Case Series. *Int. J. Periodontics Restor. Dent.* **2023**, *43*, 715–723. [CrossRef]

Moreno Rodríguez, J.A.; Ortiz Ruiz, A.J. Apical approach in periodontal reconstructive surgery with enamel matrix derivate and enamel matrix derivate plus bone substitutes: A randomized, controlled clinical trial. *Clin. Oral Investig.* **2022**, *26*, 2793–2805. [CrossRef]

Calzavara, D.; Morante, S.; Sanz, J.; Noguerol, F.; Gonzalez, J.; Romandini, M.; Sanz, M. The apically incised coronally advanced surgical technique (AICAST) for periodontal regeneration in isolated defects: A case series. *Quintessence Int.* **2021**, *53*, 24–34. [CrossRef] [PubMed]

Aslan, S.; Buduneli, N.; Cortellini, P. Reconstructive surgical treatment of isolated deep intrabony defects with guided tissue regeneration using entire papilla preservation technique: A prospective case series. *J. Periodontol.* **2021**, *92*, 488–495. [CrossRef]

Aslan, S.; Buduneli, N.; Cortellini, P. Clinical outcomes of the entire papilla preservation technique with and without biomaterials in the treatment of isolated intrabony defects: A randomized controlled clinical trial. *J. Clin. Periodontol.* **2020**, *47*, 470–478. [CrossRef] [PubMed]

Moreno Rodríguez, J.A.; Ortiz Ruiz, A.J.; Caffesse, R.G. Supra-alveolar attachment gain in the treatment of combined intra-suprabony periodontal defects by non-incised papillae surgical approach. *J. Clin. Periodontol.* **2019**, *46*, 927–936. [CrossRef]

Moreno Rodríguez, J.A.; Ortiz Ruiz, A.J.; Caffesse, R.G. Periodontal reconstructive surgery of deep intraosseous defects using an apical approach. Non-incised papillae surgical approach (NIPSA): A retrospective cohort study. *J. Periodontol.* **2019**, *90*, 454–464. [CrossRef]

Aslan, S.; Buduneli, N.; Cortellini, P. Entire papilla preservation technique in the regenerative treatment of deep intrabony defects: 1-Year results. *J. Clin. Periodontol.* **2017**, *44*, 926–932. [CrossRef]

Shi, J.; Wang, J.; Yang, Z.; Li, J.; Lei, L.; Li, H. A novel periodontal endoscopy-aided non-incisional periodontal regeneration technique in the treatment of intrabony defects: A retrospective cohort study. *BMC Oral Health* **2023**, *23*, 962. [CrossRef]

Moreno Rodriguez, J.A.; Caffesse, R.G. Nonincised Papillae Surgical Approach (NIPSA) in Periodontal Regeneration: Preliminary Results of a Case Series. *Int. J. Periodontics Restor. Dent.* **2018**, *38*, s105–s111. [CrossRef] [PubMed]

Azzi, R.; Takei, H.H.; Etienne, D.; Carranza, F.A. Root coverage and papilla reconstruction using autogenous osseous and connective tissue grafts. *Int. J. Periodontics Restor. Dent.* **2001**, *21*, 141–147.

Nibali, L.; Koidou, V.P.; Nieri, M.; Barbato, L.; Pagliaro, U.; Cairo, F. Regenerative surgery versus access flap for the treatment of intra- bony periodontal defects: A systematic review and meta-analysis. *J. Clin. Periodontol.* **2020**, *47* (Suppl. S22), 320–351. [CrossRef] [PubMed]

Checchi, L.; Montevecchi, M.; Checchi, V.; Bonetti, G.A. A modified papilla preservation technique, 22 years later. *Quintessence Int.* **2009**, *40*, 303–311. [PubMed]

37. Di Tullio, M.; Femminella, B.; Pilloni, A.; Romano, L.; D'Arcangelo, C.; De Ninis, P.; Paolantonio, M. Treatment of supra-alveo type defects by a simplified papilla preservation technique for access flap surgery with or without enamel matrix proteins *Periodontol.* **2013**, *84*, 1100–1110. [CrossRef]
38. Trombelli, L.; Simonelli, A.; Schincaglia, G.P.; Cucchi, A.; Farina, R. Single-flap approach for surgical debridement of de intraosseous defects: A randomized controlled trial. *J. Periodontol.* **2012**, *3*, 27–35. [CrossRef]
39. Schincaglia, G.P.; Hebert, E.; Farina, R.; Simonelli, A.; Trombelli, L. Single versus Double Flap Approach in periodon regenerative procedures. *J. Clin. Periodontol.* **2015**, *42*, 557–566. [CrossRef]
40. Górski, B.; Jakubowska, S.; Wyrębek, B. Entire Papilla Preservation Technique with Enamel Matrix Proteins and Allogenic Bo Substitutes for the Treatment of Isolated Intrabony Defects: A 3-Year Follow-Up of a Prospective Case Series. *J. Clin. Med.* **20** *14*, 2374. [CrossRef]
41. Jakubowska, S.; Górski, B. Periodontal Endoscopy for Mechanical Debridement in the Non-Surgical Management of F Implantitis: A Narrative Review. *J. Clin. Med.* **2025**, *14*, 346. [CrossRef] [PubMed]
42. Rasperini, G.; Tavelli, L.; Barootchi, S.; McGuire, M.K.; Zucchelli, G.; Pagni, G.; Stefanini, M.; Wang, H.L.; Giannobile, W Interproximal attachment gain: The challenge of periodontal regeneration. *J. Periodontol.* **2021**, *92*, 931–946. [CrossRef] [PubMe
43. Green, B.N.; Johnson, C.D.; Adams, A. Writing narrative literature reviews for peer-reviewed journals: Secrets of the trade *Chiropr. Med.* **2006**, *5*, 101–117. [CrossRef] [PubMed]

Journal of
Clinical Medicine

MDPI

e Report

ntire Papilla Preservation Technique with Enamel Matrix roteins and Allogenic Bone Substitutes for the Treatment of olated Intrabony Defects: A 3-Year Follow-Up of a Prospective ase Series

·tłomiej Górski *, Sylwia Jakubowska and Beata Wyrębek

Department of Periodontology and Oral Mucosa Diseases, Medical University of Warsaw, Binieckiego 6 St., 02-097 Warsaw, Poland; sylwiajakubowska999@interia.pl (S.J.); beatawyrebek@gmail.com (B.W.)
* Correspondence: bgorski@wum.edu.pl

Abstract: Background: This study aimed to assess the effectiveness of a modified entire papilla preservation technique (MEPPT) for treating isolated intrabony defects in patients with stage III periodontitis. **Material and Methods**: Fifteen patients with 15 interdental intrabony defects were treated with a MEPPT using enamel matrix derivative and allogenic bone. Their probing pocket depth (PPD), clinical attachment level (CAL), gingival recession (GR), keratinized tissue width (KTW), defect depth (DD), full-mouth plaque score (FMPS), full mouth bleeding score (FMBS), radiographic images (radiographic angles, BF and LDF) and intrasurgical parameters were assessed at baseline and 3 years postsurgery. Standardized measurements were taken to evaluate the defect characteristics and treatment outcomes. **Results**: At 3 years, significant improvements from baseline were maintained. Probing pocket depth (PPD) decreased from 7.03 ± 1.61 mm to 3.33 ± 0.89 mm ($p < 0.0001$), clinical attachment level (CAL) improved to 3.08 ± 1.16 mm ($p < 0.001$) and defect depth (DD) decreased from 4.59 ± 1.24 mm to 0.38 ± 0.31 mm ($p < 0.001$). The changes in gingival recession and keratinized tissue were not statistically significant. The results demonstrate sustained clinical stability over a 3-year period. **Conclusions**: Within the limitations of this study, the findings suggest that the modified entire papilla preservation technique (MEPPT) in conjunction with enamel matrix proteins and allogenic bone grafting is an effective approach for the treatment of intrabony defects, leading to statistically significant and sustained clinical improvements over a 3-year period. The study protocol was registered in ClinicalTrials.gov ID NCT05029089.

Keywords: modified entire papilla preservation technique; intrabony defect; periodontitis; enamel matrix protein; allogenic bone

1. Introduction

Currently, the professional mechanical debridement of subgingival plaque using ultrasonic devices and/or hand instruments constitutes a fundamental phase of periodontal therapy. In the majority of cases, non-surgical periodontal treatment effectively maintains periodontal health, reducing the need for surgical intervention [1]. While non-surgical periodontal therapy generally leads to a reduction in pocket depth, in specific clinical scenarios, such as deep vertical bone loss, complete pocket closure may not be attainable [2]. Residual pockets (≥6 mm) associated with intrabony defects constitute a risk factor for periodontitis progression and require surgical therapy [3]. Various regenerative biomaterials and flap designs are employed in periodontal surgery to improve periodontal regeneration [4–10]. Barrier membranes, either alone or in combination with allogeneic or xenogenic bone substitutes, have been utilized to enhance clot stabilization and provide osteoconductive support for bone regeneration [4]. However, the presence of a membrane may lead to postoperative flap dehiscence, biomaterial exposure and delayed healing [5]. To decrease early wound healing complications, the application of enamel matrix derivative (EMD, Emdogain, Straumann) was implemented to stimulate osteoinduction and regenerate the periodontal ligament and cementum [6].

Several surgical techniques have been developed to enhance periodontal regeneration and to minimize invasiveness in the surgical area. In recent years, the treatment of intrabony defects has increasingly favored minimally invasive surgical techniques aimed at preserving the interdental papilla. In 1985, Takei et al. introduced the papilla preservation technique [7], later modified by Cortellini et al. [8,9,11], with the aim of favoring wound healing, diminishing the risk of flap dehiscence in the interdental area and preserving the soft tissues. The incision at the base of the interdental papilla provides a sufficient view of intrabony defects, although it compromises the vascular integrity of the interdental tissues. Consequently, postsurgical recession, dental hypersensitivity and esthetic problems may occur. In 2017, Aslan et al. [12,13] introduced the entire papilla preservation technique (EPPT). This technique is based on preserving the integrity of the defect-associated interdental papilla through a tunnel-like incision. Therefore, the papilla remains fully supplied by its native, continuous vascular network, effectively preventing wound exposure. Maintaining the papilla intact creates a sealed gingival chamber that stabilizes the blood clot, preserves vascular supply, promotes angiogenesis and enhances the wound healing process. In this technique, vertical incisions are performed, and a full-thickness flap is raised around the tunneled defect-associated papilla. This technique provides significant improvements in clinical outcomes [14]. It was proposed for the treatment of isolated deep and wide intrabony defects that did not involve lingual sites. However, in cases where a higher risk of tearing the interdental papilla occurs, such as for a thin phenotype, narrow interdental space, or fragile interdental papilla with the presence of a crater, the modification of the EPPT offers advantages. This modification involves extending the buccal flap mesiodistally to expose the cortical bone of adjacent teeth, thereby enhancing access to the surgical site, providing less tension on the flap while still preserving the papilla. Additionally, to improve visualization and access to a single-wall intrabony defect, the vertical releasing incision is lengthened as needed. Therefore, the aim of this study was to evaluate the clinical and radiographic outcomes of a modified EPPT (EPPT with the elevation of the larger buccal flap) in combination with EMD and radiation-sterilized, allogeneic bone substitution in the treatment of isolated intrabony defects.

2. Materials and Methods

Participants: Patients diagnosed with stage III periodontitis at the Department of Periodontology of the Medical University of Warsaw who fulfilled the inclusion criteria were included. Non-surgical periodontal treatment was conducted and reevaluated after 3 months. The patients were informed of the procedure, potential risks and the benefits of their participation in the study. All signed consent forms. Inclusion criteria: 1. diagnosis of stage III periodontitis [15]; 2. no systemic diseases; 3. no use of medications affecting the periodontal status; 4. non-smokers; 5. neither pregnant nor lactating; 6. presence of at least one tooth with PPD $\geq$ 6 mm, CAL $\geq$ 5 mm and bone defect depth (5DD) $\geq$ 3 mm as detected in periapical radiographs; 7. full-mouth plaque score (FMPS) $\leq$ 20% and full-mouth bleeding score (FMBS) $\leq$ 20%; 8. tooth has to be vital or properly treated; 9. no furcation involvement.

Study Design: The clinical measurements were taken by the same experienced examiner. FMPS was calculated as the percentage of tooth surfaces that exhibited plaque [16] and FMBS as the percentage of periodontal pockets that bled from the bottom 15 s after careful probing [17]. The clinical parameters were registered with a millimeter periodontal probe (15 mm University of North Carolina (UNC) probe, Hu-Friedy, Chicago, IL, USA) as follows: 1. PPD as the distance from the gingival margin to the base of the periodontal pocket at six points per tooth (i.e., distobuccal, buccal, mesiobuccal, distolingual, lingual and mesiolingual); 2. CAL as the distance from the cemento-enamel junction (CEJ) to the base of the periodontal pocket at six points per tooth; 3. gingival recession (GR) as the distance from the CEJ to the gingival margin at the mid-buccal point of the tooth; 4. keratinized tissue width (KTW) as the distance from the gingival margin to the mucogingival junction at the mid-buccal point of the tooth after staining with an iodine solution. The clinical measurements were taken immediately before and 3 years after periodontal surgery.

The following intrasurgery measurements were recorded upon the completion of debridement during surgery: (1) defect depth as the distance between the bottom of the defect and the most coronal point of the bony walls surrounding the defect; (2) defect width as the distance from the most coronal point of the bony walls surrounding the defect to the root surface; (3) the number of remaining walls of the defect (defects were classified as one-wall, two-wall and three-wall defects).

Radiographic measurements: Standardized digital periapical radiographs were collected from each patient with film holders and a paralleling technique using an X-ray unit operating at 70 kV, 4 mA and a 0.1 s exposure time prior to surgery and 3 years postoperatively. The radiographs were analyzed using Planmeca Romexis Viewer software (Planmeca, Helsinki, Finland). Anatomic landmarks, which included the CEJ, alveolar crest (AC) and base of the defect (BD), were selected on the radiographs. Two auxiliary lines were drawn, the first in the tooth axis (AUX1) and the second line (AUX2) from the AC, perpendicular to AUX1. Defect depth (DD) was measured as the distance from the spot where AUX2 crossed the CEJ-BD line to the base of the defect. The radiographic defect angle was calculated between the intersection of the CEJ-BD line of the tooth and the delimitation of the wall of the defect [18]. During the follow-up analysis, the radiographic bone-fill (BF) was quantified utilizing the Planmeca Romexis Viewer software program as the percentage of bone-fill, depicting the change in bone level as compared to the preset landmarks and initial radiograph. Linear radiographic measurements were taken of the present landmarks using the Planmeca Romexis Viewer software program, which provides a computerized ruler, and were compared with the initial situation.

Surgical Procedures: All surgical procedures were performed by one surgeon (BG) using surgical loupes (×3.3). The anesthetic of choice was 4% articaine hydrochloride with adrenaline (1:100,000) (Ubistesin Forte 1.7 mL, 3-M ESPE, Saint Paul, MN, USA) based on its reported superiority over local anesthetic agents in oral surgical procedures [19,20]. After local anesthesia, a buccal intra-crevicular incision of the defect-associated tooth and the adjacent tooth was performed. Subsequently, a short buccal vertical incision positioned contralaterally to the intrabony defect was extended beyond the mucogingival line. A buccal full-thickness flap was elevated, extending from the vertical incision to the defect-associated papilla and to the contralateral site of the whole width of the adjacent tooth. The interdental papilla was carefully elevated in a full-thickness manner to the coronal edge of the lingual bone crest. The intrabony defect was meticulously debrided and the roots were carefully planned. The surgical area was rinsed with sterile saline and the exposed root surfaces were conditioned for 2 min with 24% Ethylenediaminetetraacetic acid (EDTA) (PrefGel®, Straumann, Basel, Switzerland) and then thoroughly rinsed with sterile saline. Subsequently, enamel matrix derivative (EMD) (Emdogain, Straumann) was applied on the exposed and air-dried root surface. In the next step, EMD mixed with frozen, radiation-sterilized, allogenic bone granules consisting of cortical and cancellous bone prepared by the Department of Transplantology and Central Tissue Bank, Medical University of Warsaw, was placed into the defect [21]. The suturing approach consisted of a single sling suture (Seralon 6/0 12 mm 3/8) at the buccal site of the adjacent tooth and simple sutures in vertical incisions (Seralon 7/0 10 mm 3/8).

Postsurgical Care: The patients received postoperative instructions and were asked to avoid brushing, flossing and chewing in the treated area for 2 weeks. Patients were advised to rinse their mouth with 0.12% chlorhexidine three times a day for 4 weeks. At week 2, the sutures were removed and patients resumed careful brushing with a soft toothbrush. The patients were placed on a 2-week recall system for 3 months and every 2 months for 6 months [22].

Schematic illustrations of the described technique are presented in Figure 1, whereas Figure 2 shows one representative case clinically and radiographically at the baseline, at the time of the surgery and subsequently after 6 months and 3 years.

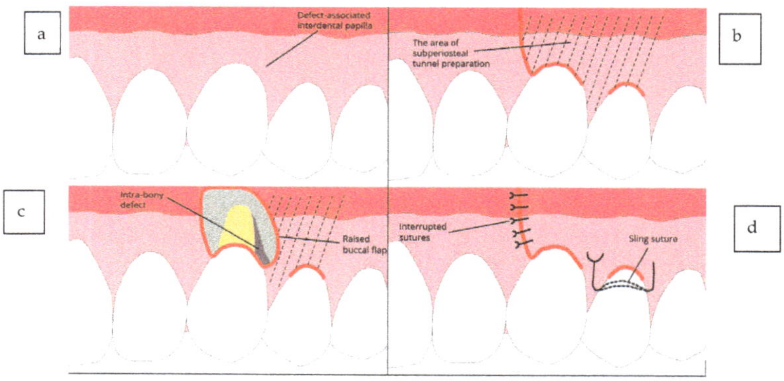

Figure 1. Diagrams illustrating the EPPT. (**a**) Intrabony defect affecting the maxillary left canine. (**b**) Flap design with a single vertical incision on the buccal side along with two sulcular incisions. (**c**) Elevation of the buccal flap. (**d**) Primary closure of the vertical incision using simple interrupted sutures and a sling suture at the neighboring tooth.

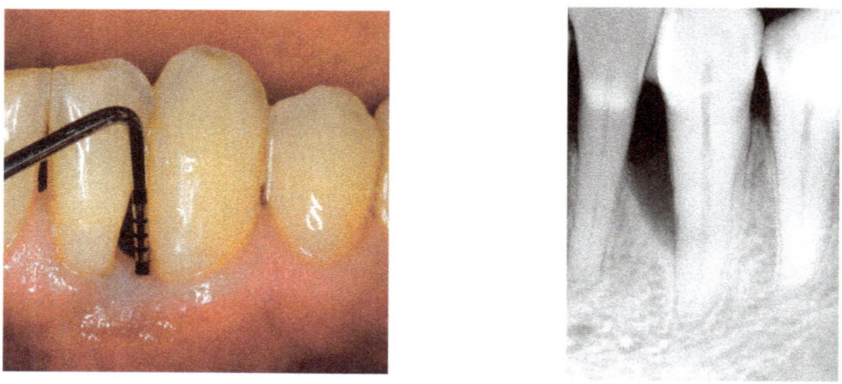

(**a**) (**b**)

Figure 2. *Cont.*

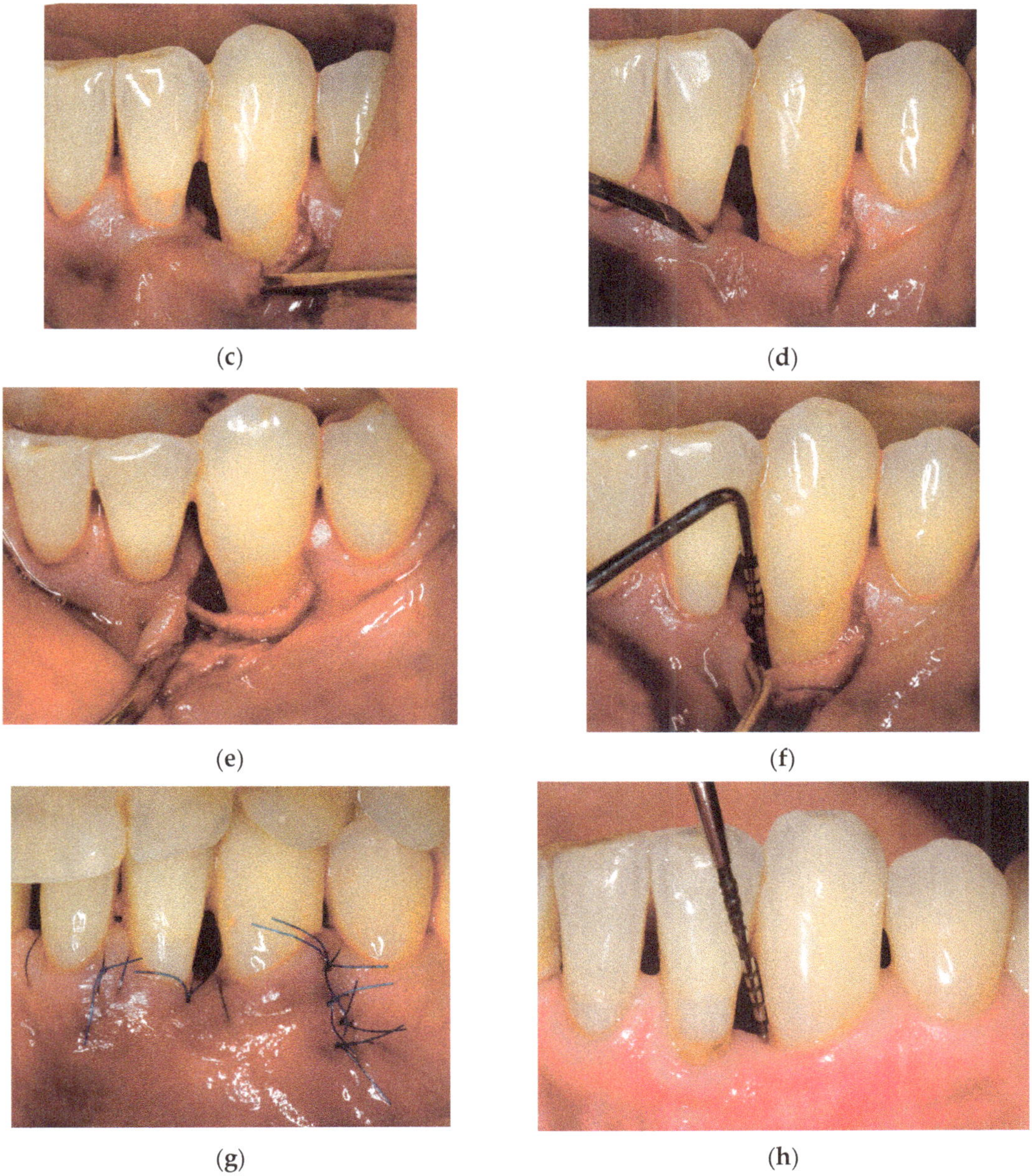

Figure 2. *Cont.*

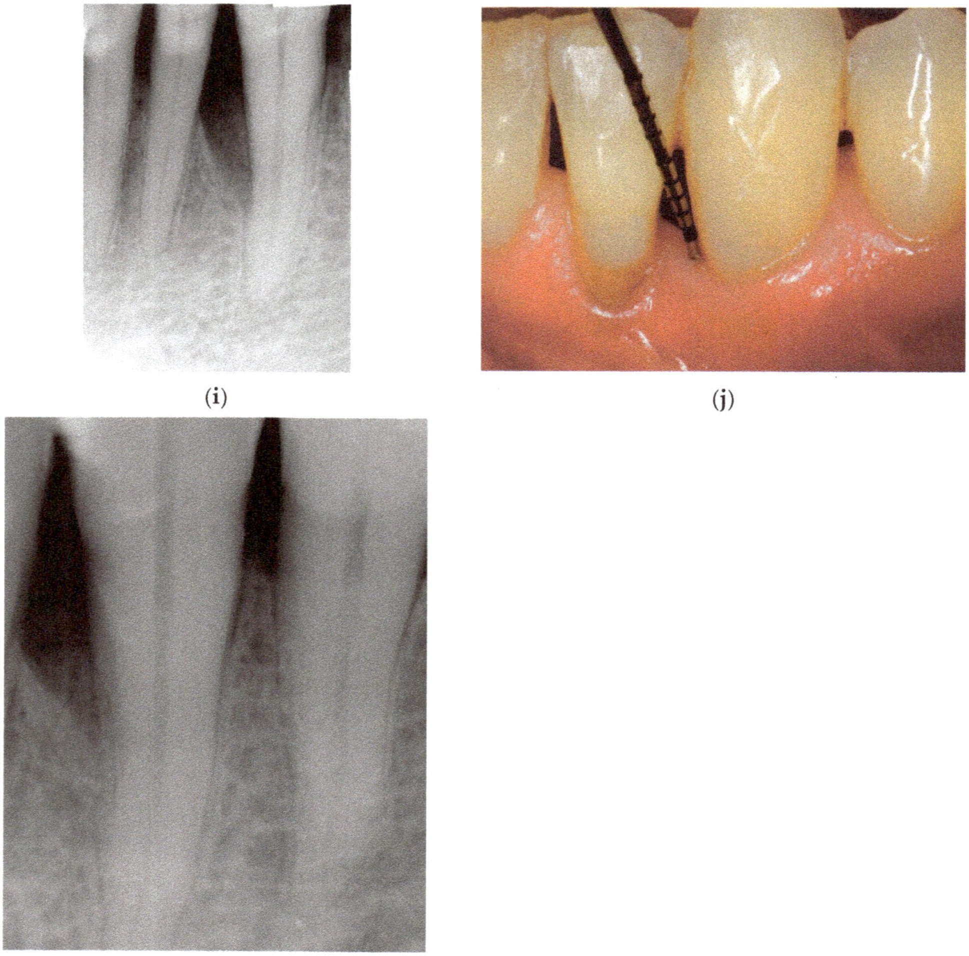

(**i**) (**j**) (**k**)

Figure 2. Representative case 1. (**a**) Baseline radiographic view. (**b**) Baseline clinical measurements. (**c**) A single vertical incision was made at the distal aspect of the mandibular left canine. (**d**) The flap was elevated, and the interdental tunnel was created by carefully dissecting beneath the papilla adjacent to the defect. (**e**,**f**) A clinical view of the intrabony defect after debridement. (**g**) the primary closure of the surgical area with interrupted sutures over the vertical incision and single sling suture. (**h**,**i**) Clinical and radiographic views at 6 months postsurgery. (**j**,**k**) Clinical and radiographic views 3 years after the surgery.

3. Results

3.1. Statistical Analysis

All data were collected and analyzed at the Department of Periodontology, Medical University of Warsaw. Data analysis was conducted using a statistical software package (Statistica 13). Each patient contributed only one intrabony defect to the study. The variables PD, CAL, GR, KTA and DD were expressed in millimeters, and FMPS and FMBS were expressed in percentages, while the radiographic angles were reported in degrees. The mean and standard deviation (SD) was calculated for each parameter. The assumption of normal distribution was checked for all parameters by means of the Shapiro–Wilk test. The intra-group analyses for the variables FMPS, FMBS, PD, CAL, GR, KTW and DD were carried out using a paired *t*-test or Wilcoxon signed-rank test accordingly. Each comparison was tested separately and refers to specific time points (e.g., baseline vs. 6 months (P1), 6 months vs. 3 years (P2) and baseline vs. 3 years (P3)). A statistically significant difference was set at p-value < 0.05 and should be interpreted for specific intervals during this study.

3.2. Results

Fifteen patients (eight women and seven men) with an average age of 42.61 ± 6.94 years, ranging from 30 to 57 years, were included in this study, with each contributing one intrabony defect. The baseline defect characteristics are summarized in Table 1. At 6 months and at 3 years, all patients with one intrabony defect each were available for the analysis. All patients completed the study without any dropouts. During the follow-up, no adverse events were recorded, and no teeth were lost.

At the initial assessment, the average FMPS and FMBS values remained below 15%, reflecting a high standard of oral hygiene and minimal residual infection. Among the 15 identified intrabony defects, the majority were located in esthetically significant areas, including 3 in the incisors, 7 in the canines, 6 in the premolars and 2 in the molars. The defects were classified into three categories: four presented as one-wall defects, seven as two-wall and seven as three-wall. At baseline, the mean FMPS and mean FMBS values were below 15%, indicating good oral hygiene and low levels of residual infection. Healing after the surgery was uneventful in all patients. Complete gingival wound closure was accomplished for all defect sites. All participants completed the 6-month follow-up. The mean FMPS and FMBS values did not change significantly from baseline. The following changes in the assessed variables were observed: a PPD reduction of 4.33 ± 1.25 mm ($p < 0.0001$), CAL gain of 4.87 ± 1.36 mm ($p < 0.0001$) and DD reduction of 4.27 ± 1.19 mm ($p < 0.0001$) (Table 1). The changes in GR and KTW between baseline and after 6 months were not statistically significant. No formation of scar tissue was detected.

At the secondary assessment 3 years postsurgery, the results were the following. All patients exhibited changes in FMPS and FMBS over time. FMPS increased from approximately 11.93% at baseline to 14.13% at 6 months and further to 22.67% at 3 years. FMBS followed a similar trend, increasing continuously from 11.07% to 13.07% at 6 months and reaching 18.75 at 3 years. (Table 1). These differences over time were statistically significant ($p < 0.05$) for both P2 and P3. In terms of changes in PPD, a significant reduction in PPD was observed at 6 months and 3 years in both groups ($p < 0.05$). PPD decreased from 7.03 ± 1.61 mm at baseline to 2.70 ± 0.70 mm at 6 months and then increased to 3.33 ± 0.89 mm at 3 years. The differences between the time points were statistically significant ($p < 0.0001$ for both P1 and P3). CAL decreased from approx. 7.60 ± 1.92 mm at baseline to 2.73 ± 1.44 mm at 6 months and then to 3.08 ± 1.16 mm at 3 years. The changes between these time points were statistically significant ($p < 0.001$ for both P1 and P3). Significant changes in DD were observed for intervals P1 and P3 ($p < 0.05$). DD decreased from 4.59± 1.24 mm at baseline to 0.32 ± 0.35 mm at 6 months and then increased to 0.38 ± 0.31 mm at 3 years. The reductions were statistically significant between two of the points ($p < 0.001$ for both comparisons from baseline). Significant changes in BF% and LDF were shown over time ($p < 0.05$). BF% decreased from approximately 92.48% at 6 months to 92.00% at 3 years. LDF followed a similar trend, decreasing from approximately 4.325 mm at 6 months to 4.10 mm at 3 years. The minor decreases in both parameters were statistically significant for LDF ($p = 0.0236$) and not significant for BF ($p = 0.1332$). The changes in GR and KTW between 6 months and 3 years were not statistically significant.

Table 1. Baseline parameters and 6-month post-treatment clinical outcomes.

Variables	Baseline (Mean ± SD)	95% CI	6 Months (Mean ± SD)	95% CI	3 Years (Mean ± SD)	95% CI	Baseline-6 Months (Mean ± SD)	95% CI	P1	6 Months–3 Years (Mean ± SD)	95% CI	P2	Baseline-3 Years (Mean ± SD)	95% CI	P3
Tooth type, *n*															
Incisor	3														
Canine	7														
Premolar	3														
Molar	2														
Tooth position, *n*															
Maxilla	7														
Mandible	8														
FMPS, %	11.93 ± 4.08	9.67, 14.19	14.13 ± 3.81	12.02, 16.25	22.67 ± 9.31	6.59, 15.80	+2.20 ± 3.36	−4.06, −0.34	0.0487	8.42 ± 9.12	−14.21, −2.62	0.0085	10.58 ± 7.70	−15.48, −5.69	0.0006
FMBS, %	11.07 ± 5.12	8.23, 13.90	13.07 ± 4.01	10.85, 15.29	18.75 ± 4.77	3.38, 8.10	+2.00 ± 3.16	−3.75, −0.25	0.1113	6.08 ± 4.21	−8.76, −3.41	0.0004	8.00 ± 4.77	−11.51, −4.49	0.0004
PPD, mm	7.03 ± 1.61	6.14, 7.92	2.70 ± 0.70	2.31, 3.09	3.33 ± 0.89	0.63, 1.51	−4.33 ± 1.25	3.64, 5.02	<0.0001	0.58 ± 0.79	−1.09, −0.08	0.0271	−3.63 ± 1.75	2.52, 7.73	<0.0001
CAL, mm	7.60 ± 1.92	6.54, 8.66	2.73 ± 1.44	1.94, 3.53	3.08 ± 1.16	0.82, 1.98	−4.87 ± 1.36	4.12, 5.62	<0.0001	0.25 ± 1.14	−0.97, 0.47	0.4627	−4.42 ± 1.73	3.32, 5.52	<0.0001
GR, mm	0.67 ± 0.82	0.21, 1.12	0.63 ± 0.85	0.16, 1.11	0.33 ± 0.65	0.46, 1.11	−0.03 ± 0.48	−0.23, 0.30	0.9905	0.17 ± 0.94	−0.76, 0.43	0.5505	0.08 ± 0.90	−0.66, 0.49	0.7545
KTW, mm	3.27 ± 1.16	2.62, 3.91	3.17 ± 1.19	2.51, 3.83	3.50 ± 1.09	0.77, 1.85	+0.10 ± 0.28	−0.06, 0.26	0.9339	−0.08 ± 0.29	-	-	−0.08 ± 0.29	−0.10, 0.27	0.3388
Intrabony depth, mm	5.37 ± 1.86	4.34, 6.39													
Intrabony width, mm	2.33 ± 0.84	1.87, 2.80													
Main defect configuration, *n*															
One-wall	4														
Two-wall	7														
Three-wall	7														
DD, mm	4.59 ± 1.24	3.90, 5.27	0.32 ± 0.35	0.12, 0.52	0.38 ± 0.31	0.22, 0.52	−4.27 ± 1.19	3.61, 4.93	<0.0001	0.09 ± 0.25	0.25, 0.07	0.2308	−4.18 ± 1.15	3.45, 4.92	<0.0001
Radiographic angle, degrees	32.99 ± 8.28	28.41, 37.58													
LDF, mm			4.325 ± 1.147	3.60, 5.04	4.10 ± 1.28	0.90, 2.17				−0.28 ± 0.37	0.05, 0.52	0.0236			
BF, %			92.48 ± 7.83	86.74, 98.22	92.00 ± 5.95	4.21, 10.10				−2.00 ± 4.27	−0.72, 4.72	0.1332			

CAL = clinical attachment level; DD = radiographic defect depth; FMBS = full-mouth bleeding score; FMPS = full-mouth plaque score; GR = gingival recession; KTW = keratinized tissue width; PPD = probing pocket depth. In the Difference column (mean ± SD), growth is indicated with a "+" symbol, and loss is indicated with a "−" symbol.

4. Discussion

Maintaining papilla integrity and the soft tissue profile has tremendous value in periodontal regenerative surgery, especially in the esthetic area. In the presented results, the modified EPPT significantly reduced PPD, improved CAL and decreased DD. No statistically significant differences were observed in regard to GR and KTW. Modification included extending the buccal flap elevation mesiodistally to expose the cortical bone around the defect at the adjacent tooth to enable better access to the surgical area. Moreover, trauma to the interdental papilla was minimized, indicating that the described technique was minimally invasive. This technique is especially valuable in cases of a narrow interdental space, a thin periodontal phenotype, a reduced papilla, or extensive bone loss. The findings of this study are analyzed in comparison with the existing literature on the EPPT introduced by Aslan et al. [13,14,23] and our previous research, which included a 6-month follow-up assessment [24]. The prospective case series by Aslan et al. in 2021 [23] reported that the EPPT with a combination of EMD and deproteinized bovine bone mineral resulted in a statistically significant PPD reduction and CAL gain, as well as a negligible GR increase. A gain in clinical attachment level (CAL) may be achieved through the preservation of the integrity of the papilla, which enables space and stability for the blood clot. The healing phase was uneventful in all cases, and primary wound closure was obtained in all cases. The data from this research points towards the conclusion that the EPPT with a collagen barrier and bone substitutes facilitated uninterrupted wound healing. This finding provides strong evidence for the high potential of this distinct flap design to enhance wound stability and healing, even in the presence of a collagen membrane [23]. Authors in the literature suggest that the proper indication for the EPPT is a 2-wall intrabony defect with a missing buccal wall and a relatively well-preserved lingual wall [12–14,23]. In our study, the majority of the defects were 2-wall and 3-wall; however, by using our modification of the EPTT and extending the flap mesiodistally, access was enhanced even for two single-wall intrabony defects. Moreover, to optimize access and improve the visualization of a single-wall intrabony defect, the length of the vertical releasing incision can be extended. Furthermore, a significant radiographic improvement was achieved, as indicated by the defect fill and bone defect depth (DD). The bone grafts used in this study were radiation-sterilized with a dose of 35 kGy in an accelerator with the use of a high-speed electron beam [21]. Radiation-sterilized deep-frozen bone allografts demonstrate osteoinductive properties and are removed faster than lyophilized irradiated bone [25]. Various allogeneic bone substitutes have demonstrated the ability to promote the regeneration of intrabony defects [24–26]. For instance, Majzoub et al. [27] reported a mean clinical attachment level (CAL) gain of 3.55 $\pm$ 1.85 mm and a probing pocket depth (PPD) reduction of 3.87 $\pm$ 1.87 mm one year after guided tissue regeneration (GTR) using either freeze-dried or solvent-dehydrated bone allografts. The meta-analysis by Trombelli et al. suggests that the combination of enamel matrix derivative (EMD) and bone grafting may be advantageous in the treatment of unsupported deep bone defects [28]. However, a multi-center randomized controlled clinical trial by Tonetti et al. indicated that when combined with a minimally invasive flap, EMD showed a 269% higher success rate in achieving a $\geq$3 mm CAL gain in 3-wall defects with papilla preservation flaps compared to 1-wall defects [29]. Postoperative gingival recession is an adverse outcome of surgical intervention for intrabony defects and may be associated with the morphological characteristics of bone dehiscence. By preserving the volume of intact supracrestal soft tissues through the avoidance of papilla incision, as demonstrated in the presented technique, postsurgical flap shrinkage is effectively minimized. This is particularly crucial in esthetic regions, where minimizing postsurgical gingival recession is essential, as esthetic preservation represents a key objective of surgical periodontal therapy [30]. In a meta-analysis of randomized controlled trials by Graziani et al., it was mentioned that flap surgeries for intrabony defect treatment are associated with an average increase in recession depth of 1.15 mm at 1 year postsurgery [31]. Moreover, according to Vandana et al., regions with a thin gingival biotype or reduced keratinized tissue exhibit lower resistance to recession following surgical trauma [32]. Even though microsurgical techniques are recommended for their ability to enhance visualization of the surgical field and to allow atraumatic flap manipulation, according to Rasperini et al., gingival recession and increased recession depth following periodontal regeneration remain a relatively common occurrence [33]. In the present study, there was not only a lack of an increase in gingival recession after surgical therapy but there was also a slight improvement in gingival recession reduction and an increase in keratinized tissue width observed; however, these changes did not reach statistical significance. In recent years, many authors have contributed to the development of a technique for periodontal regeneration that aims to maintain intact or even coronally advance the gingival margin, such as the "soft tissue wall technique" proposed by Rasperini et al. [34], the "entire papilla preservation" technique by Aslan et al. [12], modified vestibular incision subperiosteal tunnel access (M- VISTA) [35] and the "non-incised papillae surgical approach" (NIPSA) [36]. In order to improve root coverage in intrabony defect treatment, techniques based on connective tissue grafts (CTGs) have been suggested [37]. Nevertheless, there is a considerable paucity of well-conducted randomized controlled trials (RCTs) in the literature to objectively compare and assess the reported techniques. No conclusive evidence supports the superiority of one method over another. Therefore, further comparative studies involving the EPPT and the presented MEPPT are essential to elucidate their true benefits and their relevance to established approaches. To consider treatment outcomes, Trombelli et al. [38] proposed a suitable endpoint for implementing the treat-to-target approach in studies assessing the effectiveness of active periodontal therapy. The authors defined the targeted endpoint as a postsurgery PD $\leq$ 4 mm in the short-term. A recent systemic review and meta-analysis by Aimetti et al. [39] reported that GTR compared to PPTs achieved a higher probability of pocket resolution. However, the use of non-resorbable membranes over the past years has been declining due to their high complication rates. Therefore, studies tend to corroborate that newer, minimally invasive techniques may enhance wound stability due to reduced flap extension and minimal interdental tissue elevation, thereby raising doubts about the added value of incorporating supportive biomaterials for regeneration [40]. Justification for the modified EPPT therapy may be challenging if comparable outcomes can be achieved using standard techniques. In the systematic review and meta-analysis by Pasqualini et al. [41], the authors investigated clinical periodontal parameters (PPD, CAL and gingival recession) after treatment using the Minimally Invasive Surgical Technique (MIST), Modified Minimally Invasive Surgical Technique (M-MIST) and/or any technique for papilla preservation, such as Entire Papilla Preservation (EPP), the modified-papilla preservation technique (M-PPT) or the simplified-papilla preservation technique (SPPT). Their conclusions indicated that MIST, M-MIST and papilla preservation techniques demonstrate significant efficacy in improving periodontal conditions in intrabony defect sites while maintaining minimal patient morbidity. However, modifications to the entire papilla preservation technique could offer advantages in the surgical management of certain isolated intrabony defects in terms of flap design, wound healing, better visualization, minimal morbidity and similar, satisfactory clinical results at the same time. One of the main surgical challenges is to achieve sufficient access and visibility of the intraosseous defect to perform precise instrumentation while minimizing trauma to the interproximal papilla. At the same time, the use of magnification and microsurgical instruments plays a crucial role in addressing these difficulties. Any minimally invasive regenerative procedure is a technique-sensitive approach, and any damage to the papilla resulting from a suboptimal surgical technique may negatively affect regenerative outcomes. The findings of this study indicate that the modified EPPT, combined with EMD and allogenic bone grafting, is an effective approach for treating intrabony defects, demonstrating statistically significant and sustained clinical improvements over a 3-year period. However, it is important to note that the outcomes are derived from a single treatment modality without a control group, limiting the ability to draw definitive conclusions about the proposed approach and its superiority over previously established techniques. Further follow-up clinical trials are necessary to determine the contribution of each component utilized in the presented procedure to the overall results and to validate the presented findings.

5. Conclusions

Within the limitation of this case series, it can be concluded that the proposed modification of the entire papilla preservation technique might be beneficial in the surgical treatment of isolated intrabony defects. Although the findings are encouraging, further research involving larger cohorts and more diverse patient populations is necessary to confirm the long-term clinical efficacy of the modified EPPT.

6. Study Limitations

A limitation of this study is the sample population recruited for the trial, as it was selected based on strict eligibility criteria. However, it is important to note that a significant proportion of patients with severe periodontitis are smokers and may also present with systemic comorbidities such as diabetes. Therefore, further research involving a more diverse patient population is required to establish the efficacy and reliability of the modified entire papilla preservation technique (M-EPPT) as a regenerative approach for the treatment of periodontitis.

Author Contributions: All authors contributed to the study's conception and design. All authors have read and agreed to the published version of the manuscript.

Funding: This research received no external funding.

Institutional Review Board Statement: This study was carried out in accordance with the Helsinki Declaration of 1975, as revised in Tokyo in 2004 after approval of the study design by the Bioethics Committee (KB/118/2021, 2021-07-30).

Informed Consent Statement: Written informed consent was obtained from the patients.

Data Availability Statement: The corresponding author will share the data upon request due to legal and ethical reasons.

Conflicts of Interest: The authors declare no conflicts of interest.

Abbreviations

FMPS%	Full-mouth plaque score
FMBS%	Full-mouth bleeding score
PPD, mm	Probing pocket depth (measured in millimeters)
CAL, mm	Clinical attachment level (measured in millimeters)
GR, mm	Gingival recession (measured in millimeters)
KTW, mm	Keratinized tissue width (measured in millimeters)
DD, mm	Radiographic defect depth (measured in millimeters)
LDF, mm	Linear defect fill
BF, %	Bone-fill percentage

References

1. Lang, N.P.; Salvi, G.E.; Sculean, A. Nonsurgical Therapy for Teeth and Implants—When and Why? *Periodontology 2000* **2019**, 15–21. [PubMed]
2. Tomasi, C.; Leyland, A.H.; Wennstrom, J.L. Factors Influencing the Outcome of Non-Surgical Periodontal Treatment: A Multile Approach. *J. Clin. Periodontol.* **2007**, *34*, 682–690.
3. Matuliene, G.; Pjetursson, B.E.; Salvi, G.E.; Schmidlin, K.; Brägger, U.; Zwahlen, M.; Lang, N.P. Influence of Residual Pock on Progression of Periodontitis and Tooth Loss: Results After 11Years of Maintenance. *J. Clin. Periodontol.* **2008**, *35*, 685–6 [CrossRef]
4. Cortellini, P.; Tonetti, M.S. Clinical concepts for regenerative therapy in intrabony defects. *Periodontology 2000* **2015**, *68*, 282–3 [PubMed]
5. Trombelli, L.; Kim, C.K.; Zimmerman, G.J.; Wikesjo, U.M. Retrospective analysis of factors related to clinical outcome of guid tissue regeneration procedures in intrabony defects. *J. Clin. Periodontol.* **1997**, *24*, 366–371. [CrossRef] [PubMed]
6. Sanz, M.; Tonetti, M.S.; Zabalegui, I.; Sicilia, A.; Blanco, J.; Rebelo, H.; Rasperini, G.; Merli, M.; Cortellini, P.; Suvan, J.E. Treatm of intrabony defects with enamel matrix proteins or barrier membranes: Results from a multicenter practice-based clinical t *J. Periodontol.* **2004**, *75*, 726–733.
7. Takei, H.H.; Han, T.; Carranza, F.A., Jr.; Kenney, E.B.; Lekovic, V. Flap technique for periodontal bone implants. Papi preservation technique. *J. Periodontol.* **1985**, *56*, 204–210. [CrossRef]
8. Cortellini, P.; Pini-Prato, G.; Tonetti, M.S. The modified papilla preservation technique. A new surgical approach for interproxi regenerative procedures. *J. Periodontol.* **1995**, *66*, 261–266.
9. Cortellini, P.; Pini-Prato, G.; Tonetti, M.S. The simplified papilla preservation flap. A novel surgical approach for the managem of soft tissues in regenerative procedures. *Int. J. Periodontics Restor. Dent.* **1999**, *19*, 589–599.
10. Trombelli, L.; Farina, R.; Franceschetti, G.; Calura, G. Single-flap approach with buccal access in periodontal reconstruct procedures. *J. Periodontol.* **2009**, *80*, 353–360. [CrossRef]
11. Cortellini, P.; Tonetti, M.S. Improved wound stability with a modified minimally invasive surgical technique in the regenerat treatment of isolated interdental intrabony defects. *J. Clin. Periodontol.* **2009**, *36*, 157–163. [CrossRef]
12. Aslan, S.; Buduneli, N.; Cortellini, P. Entire papilla preservation technique: A novel surgical approach for regenerative treatm of deep and wide intrabony defects. *Int. J. Restor. Periodontics Restor. Dent.* **2017**, *37*, 227–233. [CrossRef] [PubMed]
13. Aslan, S.; Buduneli, N.; Cortellini, P. Entire papilla preservation technique in the regenerative treatment of deep intrabony defe 1-year results. *J. Clin. Periodontol.* **2017**, *44*, 926–932. [CrossRef]
14. Aslan, S.; Buduneli, N.; Cortellini, P. Clinical outcomes of the entire papilla preservation technique with and without biomateri in the treatment of isolated intrabony defects: A randomized controlled clinical trial. *J. Clin. Periodontol.* **2020**, *47*, 470–4 [CrossRef] [PubMed]
15. Tonetti, M.S.; Greenwell, H.; Kornman, K.S. Staging and grading of periodontitis: Framework and proposal of a new classificati and case definition. *J. Clin. Periodontol.* **2018**, *45* (Suppl. S20), S149–S161. [CrossRef]
16. O'Leary, T.J.; Drake, R.B.; Naylor, J.E. The plaque control record. *J. Periodontol.* **1972**, *43*, 38–46. [CrossRef] [PubMed]
17. Cortellini, P.; Pini-Prato, G.; Tonetti, M.S. Periodontal regeneration of human infrabony defects I. Clinical measures. *J. Periodon* **1995**, *64*, 254–260. [CrossRef]
18. Eickholz, P.; Hörr, T.; Klein, F.; Hassfeld, S.; Kim, T.S. Radiographic parameters for prognosis of periodontal healing of infrab defects. Two different definitions of defect depth. *J. Periodontol.* **2004**, *75*, 399–407. [CrossRef]
19. Krishna, S.; Bhaskaran, R.; Kumar, S.P.; Krishnan, M. Comparison of the Efficacy Between Articaine and Lignocaine in multaneous Bilateral Orthodontic Maxillary Premolar Extractions: A Split-Mouth Comparative Study. *Cureus* **2023**, *6*. [CrossRef]
20. Martin, E.; Nimmo, A.; Lee, A.; Jennings, E. Articaine in dentistry: An overview of the evidence and meta-analysis of the lat randomized controlled trials on articaine safety and efficacy compared to lidocaine for routine dental treatment. *BDJ Open* **20** *7*, 27. [CrossRef]
21. Krasny, K.; Kamiński, A.; Krasny, M.; Czech, T.; Wojtowicz, A. Preparation of allogeneic bone for alveolar ridge augmenta *Cell Tissue Bank* **2017**, *18*, 313–321. [PubMed]
22. Revill, S.I.; Robinson, J.O.; Rosen, M.; Hogg, M.I. The reliability of a linear analogue for evaluating pain. *Anaesthesia* **1976**, 1191–1198. [PubMed]
23. Aslan, S.; Buduneli, N.; Cortellini, P. Reconstructive surgical treatment of isolated deep intrabony defects with guided tiss regeneration using entire papilla preservation technique: A prospective case series. *J. Periodontol.* **2021**, *92*, 488–495. [CrossR [PubMed]
24. Górski, B.; Kowalski, J.; Wyrębek, B. Entire Papilla Preservation Technique with Enamel Matrix Proteins and Allogenic Bo Substitute for the Treatment of Isolated Intrabony Defects: A Prospective Case Series. *Int. J. Periodontics Restor. Dent.* **2023**, 387–397.

Dziedzic-Gocławska, A.; Ostrowski, K.; Stachowicz, W.; Michalik, J.; Grzesik, W. Effect of radiation sterilization on the osteoinductive properties and the rate of remodelling of bone implants preserved by lyophilization and deep-freezing. *Clin. Orthop.* **1991**, *272*, 30–37.
Kao, R.T.; Nares, S.; Reynolds, M.A. Periodontal regeneration—Intrabony defects: A systematic review from the AAP Regeneration Workshop. *J. Periodontol.* **2015**, *86* (Suppl. S2), 77–104. [CrossRef]
Majzoub, J.; Barootchi, S.; Tavelli, L.; Wang, C.-W.; Chan, H.-L.; Wang, H.-L. Guided tissue regeneration combined with bone allograft in intrabony defects: Clinical outcomes and assessment of prognostic factors. *J. Periodontol.* **2020**, *91*, 746–755.
Trombelli, L.; Simonelli, A.; Quaranta, A.; Tu, Y.K.; Li, H.; Agusto, M.; Jiao, X.; Farina, R. Effect of flap design for enamel matrix derivative application in intraosseous defects. *JDR Clin. Transl. Res.* **2021**, *16*, 184–194.
Tonetti, M.S.; Lang, N.P.; Cortellini, P.; Suvan, J.E.; Adriaens, P.; Dubravec, D.; Fonzar, A.; Fourmousis, I.; Mayfield, L.; Rossi, R.; et al. Enamel matrix proteins in the regenerative therapy of deep intrabony defects. A multi-center randomized controlled clinical trial. *J. Clin. Periodontol.* **2002**, *29*, 317–325.
Farina, R.; Simonelli, A.; Minenna, L.; Rasperini, G.; Schincaglia, G.P.; Tomasi, C.; Trombelli, L. Change in the gingival margin profile after the single flap approach in periodontal intraosseous defects. *J. Periodontol.* **2015**, *86*, 1038–1046.
Graziani, F.; Gennai, S.; Cei, S.; Cairo, F.; Baggiani, A.; Miccoli, M.; Gabriele, M.; Tonetti, M. Clinical performance of access flap surgery in the treatment of the intrabony defect. A systematic review and meta-analysis of randomized clinical trials. *J. Clin. Periodontol.* **2012**, *39*, 145–156. [CrossRef] [PubMed]
Vandana, K.L.; Gupta, I. The relation of gingival thickness to dynamics of gingival margin position pre- and post-surgically. *J. Indian Soc. Periodontol.* **2016**, *20*, 167–173.
Rasperini, G.; Tavelli, L.; Barootchi, S.; McGuire, M.K.; Zucchelli, G.; Pagni, G.; Stefanini, M.; Wang, H.L.; Giannobile, W.V. Interproximal attachment gain: The challenge of periodontal regeneration. *J. Periodontol.* **2021**, *92*, 931–946.
Rasperini, G.; Acunzo, R.; Barnett, A.; Pagni, G. The soft tissue wall technique for the regenerative treatment of non-contained infrabony defects: A case series. *Int. J. Periodontics Restor. Dent.* **2013**, *33*, e79–e87.
Najafi, B.; Kheirieh, P.; Torabi, A.; Cappetta, E.G. Periodontal Regenerative treatment of intrabony defects in the esthetic zone using Modified Vestibular Incision Subperiosteal Tunnel Access (M-VISTA). *Int. J. Periodontics Restor. Dent.* **2018**, *38*, e9–e16.
Moreno Rodriguez, J.A.; Ortiz Ruiz, A.J.; Caffesse, R.G. Periodontal reconstructive surgery of deep intraosseous defects using an apical approach. Non-incised papillae surgical approach (NIPSA): A retrospective cohort study. *J. Periodontol.* **2019**, *90*, 454–464.
Zucchelli, G.; Mounssif, I.; Marzadori, M.; Mazzotti, C.; Felice, P.; Stefanini, M. Connective tissue graft wall technique and enamel matrix derivative for the treatment of infrabony defects: Case reports. *Int. J. Periodontics Restor. Dent.* **2017**, *37*, 673–681.
Trombelli, L.; Farina, R.; Vecchiatini, R.; Maietti, E.; Simonelli, A. A simplified composite outcome measure to assess the effect of periodontal regenerative treatment in intraosseous defects. *J. Periodontol.* **2020**, *91*, 723–731.
Aimetti, M.; Fratini, A.; Manavella, V.; Giraudi, M.; Citterio, F.; Ferrarotti, F.; Mariani, G.M.; Cairo, F.; Baima, G.; Romano, F. Pocket resolution in regenerative treatment of intrabony defects with papilla preservation techniques: A systematic review and meta-analysis of randomized clinical trials. *J. Clin. Periodontol.* **2021**, *48*, 843–858.
Cortellini, P.; Cortellini, S.; Bonaccini, D.; Tonetti, M.S. Modified minimally invasive surgical technique in human intrabony defects with or without regenerative materials-10-year follow-up of a randomized clinical trial: Tooth retention, periodontitis recurrence, and costs. *J. Clin. Periodontol.* **2022**, *49*, 528–536.
Pasqualini, E.; Castro, F.; Curado, D.; Martelete, A.; Heboyan, A.; Saleh, M.H.; Fernandes, J.C.H.; Fernandes, G.V.O. Minimally invasive periodontal regeneration with the buccal approach: A systematic review and meta-analysis of clinical studies. *Evid.-Based Dent.* **2024**, *25*, 54. [CrossRef] [PubMed]

Journal of
Clinical Medicine

MDPI

Article

Associations Between Glycemic Control, Self-Reported Gingival Bleeding and Lifestyle Factors in Hospitalized Diabetic Patients

Aida Meto [1,2,3,*], Adora Shpati [1], Adela Alushi [1], Tommaso Filippini [4,*], Alba Kamberi [1], Agron Meto [1] and Adem Alushi [5]

1 Department of Dentistry, Faculty of Dental Sciences, University of Aldent, 1007 Tirana, Albania; adorashpati@yahoo.com (A.S.); adela.alushi@ual.edu.al (A.A.); albakamberi@hotmail.com (A.K.); agron.meto@ual.edu.al (A.M.)
2 Department of Surgery, Medicine, Dentistry and Morphological Sciences with Interest in Transplant, Oncology and Regenerative Medicine, University of Modena and Reggio Emilia, 41125 Modena, Italy
3 Department of Dental Research Cell, Dr. D.Y. Patil Dental College and Hospital, Dr. D.Y. Patil Vidyapeeth, Pimpri, Pune 411018, Maharashtra, India
4 Department of Biomedical, Metabolic and Neural Sciences, University of Modena and Reggio Emilia, 41125 Modena, Italy
5 Department of Dental Therapy, Faculty of Dental Medicine, University of Medicine, 1005 Tirana, Albania; adem.alushi@umed.edu.al
* Correspondence: aida.meto@ual.edu.al or aidameto@yahoo.com (A.M.); tommaso.filippini@unimore.it (T.F.)

Abstract: Background/Objectives: Diabetes mellitus is associated with significant health complications, including challenges in periodontal health. Gingival inflammation is especially common among diabetic patients and can significantly impact overall diabetes management. This study aims to investigate the correlation between glycosylated hemoglobin (HbA1c) levels, an established marker of glycemic control, and gingival inflammation using the Quantitative Gingival Bleeding Index (QGBI) among hospitalized diabetic patients, thereby placing the question within a broader clinical context. **Methods**: The study enrolled 671 hospitalized patients with diabetes complications at "Mother Theresa University Hospital" in Tirana, AL, USA. Glycemic control was assessed through glycosylated hemoglobin (HbA1c) levels, and gingival health was evaluated using the Quantitative Gingival Bleeding Index (QGBI). Behavioral variables were also documented, including smoking habits and routine oral care practices. Spearman's correlation coefficient (r_s) was applied to determine the relationship between HbA1c levels and QGBI scores. **Results**: Our findings revealed a strong positive correlation between glycemic control (HbA1c) and gingival inflammation (QGBI) among the participants (Spearman's coefficient $r_s = 0.868$, $p < 0.001$). Additionally, significant positive associations were observed between behavioral factors, such as smoking habits and regular oral care practices, further underscoring their role in periodontal health in diabetic patients. **Conclusions**: The study highlights a significant positive relationship between poor glycemic control and increased gingival inflammation, emphasizing the importance of periodontal health in the comprehensive management of diabetes mellitus. Our results support integrating periodontal evaluation and management into standard diabetes care, which could improve patient outcomes and overall well-being.

Keywords: diabetes mellitus; HbA1c levels; Quantitative Gingival Bleeding Index; gingival health; oral health; dental care; hospitalized patients

1. Introduction

Diabetes mellitus is a long-term metabolic condition characterized by persistent hyperglycemia due to reduced insulin production, insulin resistance, or both. It affects millions worldwide and is a public health concern, contributing to significant morbidity and mortality [1]. Type 1 diabetes is caused by the autoimmune destruction of pancreatic β-cells and requires lifelong insulin therapy. Type 2 diabetes, on the other hand, is mainly linked to insulin resistance and progressive β-cell dysfunction, often associated with lifestyle factors like obesity, high-fat diets, and physical inactivity [2–4]. As illustrated in Figure 1, periodontal inflammation in diabetic patients is interconnected with systemic complications, including cardiovascular, renal, and ocular effects, and is influenced by both behavioral and biological risk factors.

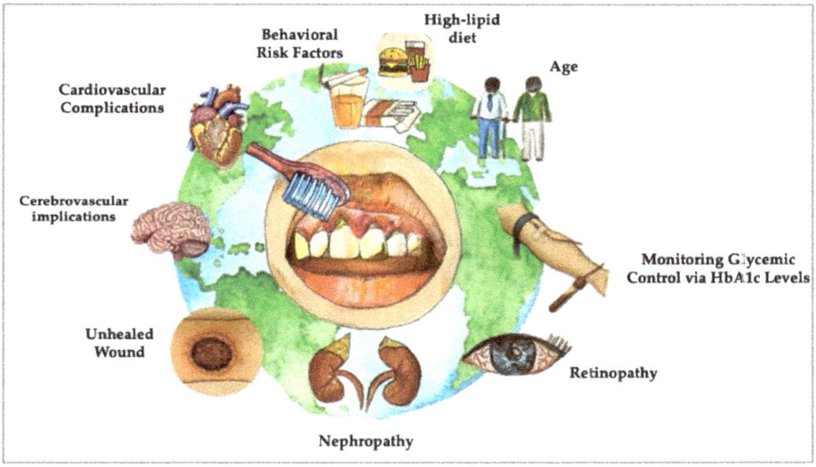

Figure 1. This illustration depicts the multisystemic impact of periodontal inflammation in individuals with diabetes mellitus. A clinical representation of gingival bleeding and inflammation at the center highlights active periodontal disease. Around the central illustration are depicted several complications associated with diabetes, along with key contributing factors. Cardiovascular and cerebrovascular implications are shown, reflecting the increased risk of heart disease and stroke associated with chronic inflammation and poor glycemic control. An unhealed wound reflects the reduced healing capacity often seen in diabetes. Nephropathy and retinopathy represent microvascular damage affecting the kidneys and eyes, respectively. A blood draw highlights the importance of monitoring glycemic control through HbA1c levels. Behavioral risk factors such as smoking and alcohol use, a high-lipid diet, and aging are identified as contributors to disease progression. A world map in the background underscores the global relevance of these interrelated health challenges and the potential of integrating oral health assessments into comprehensive diabetes care. Illustration by Nensi Kallfani.

Glycated hemoglobin (HbA1c) is a widely recognized biomarker for long-term glycemic control, reflecting average blood glucose levels over the past two to three months [5,6]. Higher HbA1c levels are associated with an increased risk of both microvascular (retinopathy, nephropathy, and neuropathy) and macrovascular (cardiovascular disease, stroke, and peripheral artery disease) complications [7–10]. The growing prevalence of diabetes, projected to increase from 536.6 million in 2021 to nearly 783.2 million by 2045, highlights the urgent need for more effective management strategies to reduce associated complications [11,12].

One often-overlooked complication of diabetes is its impact on gingival health. Diabetes and periodontal disease have a well-documented bidirectional relationship, where poor glycemic control worsens periodontal inflammation and untreated periodontal disease further impairs glucose regulation [13,14]. Chronic hyperglycemia contributes to increased inflammation and impaired wound healing, making individuals with diabetes more susceptible to gingival bleeding and periodontitis [15,16].

The Quantitative Gingival Bleeding Index (QGBI) objectively measures gingival inflammation by quantifying bleeding during brushing [17]. Compared to traditional bleeding indices that only show whether bleeding is present or not, QGBI provides a graded measure of bleeding severity, giving better insight into the progression of periodontal disease [18,19]. Given the increased susceptibility of diabetic patients to oral inflammation, QGBI may serve as an important tool for monitoring gingival health and its potential impact on glycemic control [20–22]. In Albania, patients are not regularly monitored through laboratory examinations, often due to the associated costs. To address this gap, we considered evaluating an index (QGBI) that patients can assess at home, enabling them to recognize early warning signs and obtain timely consultation with a specialist.

This study aims to investigate the correlation between HbA1c levels and the QGBI in hospitalized diabetic patients, providing insight into the relationship between glycemic control and gingival health. Furthermore, we examined the impact of lifestyle factors, including smoking habits and the frequency of dental check-ups, on gingival bleeding severity. By understanding these associations, our findings may contribute to a more integrated diabetes management approach, emphasizing both systemic and oral health.

2. Methods

2.1. Study Population

This cross-sectional study enrolled patients with diabetes at Mother Teresa University Hospital in Tirana, AL, USA, between May and December 2023. This care facility serves a diverse patient population from various regions of Albania, requiring specialized services provided exclusively by the country's sole tertiary health center. The center delivers advanced, multidisciplinary care aimed at addressing major complications linked to diabetes. The total number of patients participating in our study was 671, which included 388 (57.8%) male patients and 283 (42.2%) female patients.

Inclusion Criteria: Hospitalized patients aged 16 to 85 years with a diagnosis of type 1 or type 2 diabetes mellitus were included, as individuals in this age range can manage their condition and provide reliable self-reported information.

Exclusion Criteria: Participants with thyroid disorders were excluded due to their potential impact on HbA1c levels, which could confound the study's assessment of diabetes-related glycemic control. Similarly, individuals with anemia or chronic renal failure, altered liver function, and splenomegaly were excluded, as both conditions may influence HbA1c test results. To isolate the effects of smoking on periodontal health and diabetes management, participants with a history of alcohol consumption were also excluded. Additional exclusions were patients with other metabolic or systemic conditions, those on medication affecting gingival bleeding, individuals with peripheral diabetic neuropathy, edentulous patients unable to undergo QGBI assessment, and those who declined to participate. Participants were given clear, standardized instructions before data collection to ensure consistent and reliable QGBI measurements. All assessments followed a validated protocol to keep patient-reported bleeding severity data uniform. These well-defined procedures helped recruit a similar group of participants, improving the accuracy and reliability of the study results.

2.2. Data Collection

Medical records were reviewed to determine each patient's type of diabetes, and HbA1c levels were measured using standardized laboratory tests. We conducted a structured interview to collect detailed information on participants' behavioral patterns, including smoking habits, oral care habits, hypertension, and awareness of the connection between diabetes and gingival health. Gingival health was assessed using the QGBI, a validated tool for evaluating gingival bleeding based on patient-reported outcomes through a structured questionnaire. Rather than a simple self-assessment, patients reported the severity of their gingival bleeding, which the interviewer interpreted and scored according to the QGBI criteria. Patients were asked to describe their bleeding experience during toothbrushing, and their responses were categorized and scored based on the QGBI criteria outlined in Table 1.

Table 1. QGBI scores.

Score	Description
0	No bleeding during brushing, with bristles completely free of blood stains.
1	Slight bleeding during brushing, with blood visible only on the bristle tips.
2	Moderate bleeding during brushing, with blood staining about half the length of the toothbrush bristles from the tip downward.
3	Severe bleeding during brushing, with blood covering the full length of all bristles and the brush head.

2.3. Statistical Analysis

The data was initially coded in MS Excel, double-checked for accuracy, and subsequently imported into Stata software (StataNow/MP 18.5, StataCorp LCC, College Station, TX, USA, 2023). The Shapiro–Wilk test was used to evaluate the data's conformity to a normal distribution. Descriptive statistics were reported, including absolute and relative frequencies, as well as median and interquartile range (IQR) for continuous variables that showed a non-normal distribution. The relationship between glycemic control (measured by HbA1c levels) and gingival bleeding severity (measured by QGBI) was assessed using Spearman's correlation coefficient (r_s).

We used multivariable linear regression analysis to examine the associations between patients' characteristics and QGBI scores, adjusting for all relevant factors and potential confounders, including HbA1c levels, sex, age, smoking status, hypertension, oral care habits, and awareness of the diabetes gingival health link. Since age and HbA1c were non-normally distributed, they were log-transformed to perform the analysis. Results were reported as linear regression coefficients (r_c) with 95% confidence intervals (CI). We also evaluated the risk of moderate to severe gingival bleeding (QGBI scores ≥ 2) based on patient characteristics by calculating odds ratios (OR) with corresponding 95% confidence intervals (CI).

2.4. Ethics

Ethical approval for the study (Protocol no. 144/23) was obtained from the Institutional Review Board of the University of Aldent before data collection. Informed consent was secured from all participants, ensuring their voluntary participation. Appropriate measures were taken to ensure participant confidentiality and anonymity, maintaining the highest standards of privacy. No identifying information was recorded through the questionnaires, and responses were securely stored in a password-protected file. To prevent identification through indirect identifiers or combined information, additional precautions were implemented to keep all patient data secure and fully de-identified throughout the research process.

3. Results

Patient characteristics are presented in Table 2. A total of 671 patients (388 males and 283 females) were enrolled, with a median age of 56 years (IQR: 31–79). Smokers and non-smokers were nearly equally represented in the study population. Type 2 diabetes was the most frequent diagnosis, with a median HbA1c of 7.9% (IQR: 7.1–9.4). The majority of patients (73.2%) did not attend regular oral check-ups, while 17.3% reported annual visits and 9.5% visited the dentist twice a year.

Table 2. Characteristics of study participants (n = 671). Values are reported as numbers (N) and percentages (%) unless otherwise specified. IQR: interquartile range.

Characteristics	N (%)
Sex	
Male	388 (57.8)
Female	283 (42.2)
Age	
Median (IQR)	56 (31–79)
<18 years	15 (2.2)
18–30 years	148 (22.1)
31–64 years	235 (35.0)
65–79 years	128 (19.1)
≥80 years	145 (21.6)
Diabetes type	
Type 1	89 (13.3)
Type 2	582 (86.7)
HbA1c	
Median (IQR)	7.9 (7.1–9.4)
HbA1c ≤ 7.0%	160 (23.8)
HbA1c > 7.0%	512 (76.2)
Hypertension	
Patients with hypertension	256 (38.2)
Patients without hypertension	415 (61.8)
Smoking habits	
Non-smokers	320 (47.7)
Smokers	351 (52.3)
Routine oral check-up	
Not regularly	491 (73.2)
Once a year	116 (17.3)
Twice a year	64 (9.5)
Awareness of the relation between diabetes and gingival health	
No	657 (97.9)
Yes	14 (2.1)
Quantitative Gingival Bleeding Index	
Normal (Score = 0)	16 (2.4)
Mild inflammation with no bleeding (Score = 1)	184 (27.4)
Moderate inflammation and bleeding on probing (Score = 2)	285 (42.5)
Severe inflammation and tendency of spontaneous bleeding (Score = 3)	186 (27.7)

The awareness of the link between diabetes and gingival health was generally very low, with only about 2% of patients reporting knowledge of this relationship. QGBI scores indicated mild to severe gingival bleeding in the vast majority of patients.

The analysis showed a strong association between smoking and poor oral care habits, with smokers being more likely than non-smokers to skip regular dental check-ups (Table 3).

Table 3. Relation between routine oral care frequency and smoking habits.

	Non-Regularly	Once a Year	Twice a Year
	N (%)	N (%)	N (%)
Smoking habits			
Non-Smokers	179 (36.5)	86 (74.1)	55 (35.9)
Smokers	312 (63.5)	30 (25.9)	9 (14.1)

The distribution of patient characteristics by QGBI scores showed a positive association with age (Table 4). An increasing proportion of smokers was also observed with higher QGBI scores, particularly in cases of moderate to severe gingival bleeding.

Table 4. Distribution of patients' characteristics according to QGBI scores.

	QGBI = 0	QGBI = 1	QGBI = 2	QGBI = 3
Age categories				
<18 years	0 (0.0)	12 (6.5)	3 (1.1)	0 (0)
18–30 years	6 (37.5)	84 (45.7)	53 (18.6)	5 (2.7)
31–64 years	9 (56.3)	75 (40.8)	137 (48.1)	14 (7.5)
65–79 years	1 (6.2)	10 (5.4)	46 (16.1)	71 (38.2)
≥80 years	0 (0)	3 (1.6)	46 (16.1)	96 (51.6)
Smoking habits				
Non-smokers	12 (75.0)	150 (81.5)	102 (35.8)	56 (30.1)
Smokers	4 (25.0)	34 (18.5)	183 (64.2)	130 (69.9)
Hypertension				
No	11 (68.8)	119 (64.8)	171 (60.0)	114 (61.3)
Yes	5 (31.2)	65 (35.3)	114 (40.0)	72 (38.7)
Routine oral check-up				
Not regularly	4 (25.0)	99 (53.8)	215 (75.4)	173 (93.0)
Once a year	5 (31.3)	47 (25.5)	53 (18.6)	11 (5.9)
Twice a year	7 (43.7)	38 (20.6)	17 (6.0)	2 (1.1)
Awareness				
No	14 (87.5)	180 (97.8)	277 (97.2)	136 (100)
Yes	2 (12.5)	4 (2.2)	8 (2.8)	0 (0.0)
Diabetes				
Type 1	4 (25.0)	58 (31.5)	25 (8.8)	2 (1.1)
Type 2	12 (75.0)	126 (68.5)	260 (91.2)	184 (98.9)
HbA1c				
HbA1c ≤ 7.0%	12 (75.0)	140 (76.1)	5 (1.8)	2 (1.1)
HbA1c > 7.0%	4 (25.0)	44 (23.9)	280 (98.2)	184 (98.9)

Patients who did not attend routine oral check-ups had higher QGBI scores. In contrast, awareness of the link between diabetes and gingival health was more common among individuals without signs of inflammation or bleeding (QGBI = 0), though this finding is based on a limited number of cases.

Regarding diabetes type, patients with type 2 generally showed higher levels of gingival bleeding compared to those with type 1. Similarly, a higher prevalence of individuals with poorly controlled HbA1c levels (≥7.0%) was observed among those with higher QGBI scores. This trend is further supported by the distribution of HbA1c levels across QGBI categories, as shown in Figure 2.

Spearman's correlation analysis revealed a strong positive association between HbA1c levels and QGBI scores (r_s = 0.868, 95% CI: 0.848–0.885).

Multivariate linear regression analysis showed a positive association between QGBI levels, patient age (r_c = 0.247, 95% CI: 0.180–0.314), smoking (r_c = 0.121, 95% CI: 0.057–0.184), and HbA1c levels (r_c = 3.362, 95% CI: 3.145–3.580) (Table 5). A negative association was observed with sex (r_c = −0.211, 95% CI: −0.275 to −0.147) and, to a limited extent, with regular oral care (r_c = −0.071, 95% CI: −0.145 to 0.003). No significant associations were found for hypertension (r_c = −0.015, 95% CI: −0.074 to 0.043) or awareness of the link between diabetes and gingival health (r_c = −0.080, 95% CI: −0.282 to 0.123).

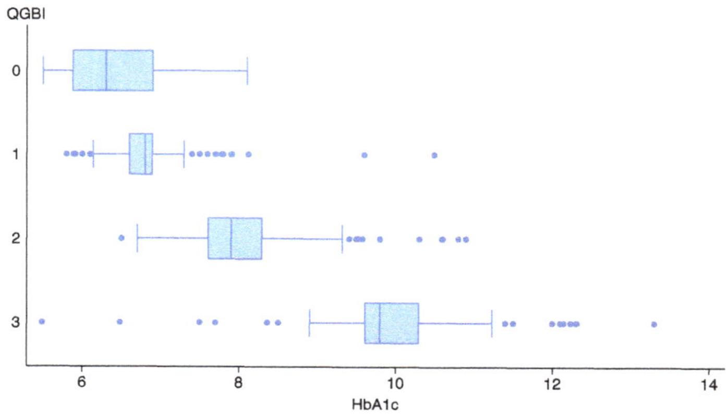

Figure 2. Box plot showing the relationship between HbA1c levels and QGBI scores, highlighting the trend of increasing glycemic levels with greater gingival bleeding severity.

Table 5. Results from linear regression and logistic models, respectively, between continuous QGBI scores and risk of moderate/severe gingival bleeding (QGBI ≥ 2) and patients' characteristics. Regression coefficient (r_c), odds ratio (OR), and 95% confidence interval (CI).

Characteristics	r_c	(95% CI)	OR	(95% CI)
HbA1c (1-unit increase)	3.362	(3.145; 3.58)	20.97	(11.10–39.62)
Age (1-year increase)	0.247	(0.18; 0.314)	1.05	(1.03–1.07)
Sex (females)	−0.211	(−0.275; −0.147)	0.13	(0.06–0.26)
Smokers	0.121	(0.057; 0.184)	4.23	(1.96–9.14)
Hypertension	−0.015	(−0.074; 0.043)	1.18	(0.57–2.44)
Regular oral care	−0.071	(−0.146; 0.003)	0.97	(0.43–2.19)
Awareness	−0.08	(−0.282; 0.123)	0.46	(0.05–4.36)

Logistic regression analysis for moderate to severe gingival bleeding (QGBI ≥ 2) showed a higher risk associated with increasing age (OR = 1.05, 95% CI: 1.03–1.07), smoking (OR = 4.23, 95% CI: 1.96–9.14), and elevated HbA1c levels (OR = 20.97, 95% CI: 11.10–39.62). In contrast, female patients had a significantly lower risk (OR = 0.13, 95% CI: 0.06–0.26) (Table 5). Routine dental check-ups were linked to a slightly reduced risk, while awareness of the link between diabetes and gingival health showed a stronger protective effect.

4. Discussion

Our study highlights a significant correlation between HbA1c levels and QGBI scores in hospitalized diabetic patients, suggesting that gingival health may serve as a simple and accessible indicator of glycemic control. This aligns with existing research on the bidirectional relationship between diabetes and periodontal disease, in which systemic inflammation, driven by hyperglycemia and the accumulation of advanced glycation end products (AGEs), worsens both conditions [13,23,24]. Oral health problems are recognized as potential complications of diabetes, with evidence suggesting they may adversely affect metabolic control [25,26].

While QGBI is a practical and patient-friendly tool for assessing gingival bleeding, it does not account for deeper periodontal conditions, such as clinical attachment loss and probing depth. Our study's lack of a plaque index limits a comprehensive assessment of gingival inflammation, as plaque accumulation plays a crucial role in gingival bleeding and periodontal disease progression [27,28]. Subsequent studies should incorporate plaque indices and inflammatory biomarkers to better understand the link between periodontal health and glycemic control.

Our findings show a significant and somewhat unexpected positive association between smoking and QGBI. Although smoking is traditionally associated with vasoconstriction and reduced clinical signs of gingival bleeding, recent evidence, including our results, suggests that smoking may not always suppress visible inflammation as previously believed. Instead, in certain populations, it may enhance inflammatory responses, contributing to elevated bleeding indices. This aligns with existing research showing that smoking impairs immune function, increases oxidative stress, and accelerates the destruction of periodontal tissues [29,30]. Moreover, population-based studies conducted in three South American cities reinforce the link between smoking and increased gingival inflammation across diverse groups, suggesting that the effect may vary depending on exposure level, duration, and individual susceptibility [30]. Among individuals with diabetes, smoking has an even greater impact, being strongly associated with poor metabolic control, which may further worsen periodontal inflammation and bleeding [30,31]. Because of these complex interactions, the following studies should broaden the focus beyond tobacco use to consider other lifestyle factors, such as dietary habits, physical activity, psychosocial stress, and examine their combined effects on periodontal health in diabetic populations. This approach could help identify important behavioral and metabolic factors involved in periodontal disease and support the development of more effective, coordinated prevention strategies across both dental and medical practice.

Hypertension, a common comorbidity in diabetes, is a known contributor to gingival inflammation. It is well established that hypertension induces systemic inflammation, which may worsen periodontal conditions [32]. Additionally, certain antihypertensive medications, particularly calcium channel blockers, are linked to gingival hyperplasia, which complicates oral hygiene and increases the risk of gingival bleeding [33,34]. Other classes of antihypertensive drugs may also reduce salivary flow, further elevating the risk of periodontal disease [35,36].

However, hypertension was not included as a confounding variable in our study. Future research should stratify patients based on hypertension status and medication use to better understand their impact on gingival health.

Age was also a significant factor influencing gingival health, with older patients showing higher QGBI scores. This aligns with findings that aging is linked to declining periodontal health due to cumulative plaque exposure, weakened immune response, and slower healing [37,38]. These findings emphasize the importance of targeted education and preventive strategies for older diabetic patients, especially in promoting oral hygiene and regular dental visits.

In addition to age, our study highlights the influence of modifiable and non-modifiable risk factors on periodontal health. Factors such as smoking, oral hygiene habits, sex, and diabetes type were all associated with gingival inflammation. Notably, males showed greater susceptibility, which is consistent with previous studies showing sex-based differences in periodontal disease progression due to hormonal, immune, and behavioral factors [39,40].

Furthermore, research suggests that individuals with type 1 diabetes tend to have better periodontal health outcomes compared to those with type 2, likely due to differences in metabolic control and treatment approaches [39].

What makes this study novel is the use of QGBI as a skilled self-assessment tool, where patients, after being shown how to recognize different levels of gingival bleeding, reported their symptoms. This approach demonstrates the potential of QGBI as a cost-effective and accessible method for the early identification of poor glycemic control, without requiring direct dental examination. Its correlation with HbA1c enables patients to recognize that an increase in gingival bleeding (QGBI) may indicate poor diabetes management and elevated HbA1c levels. This highlights its potential role in diabetes self-monitoring, empowering patients to obtain timely medical or dental intervention when necessary.

However, our study also found a general lack of awareness among diabetic patients regarding the link between periodontal health and glycemic control. Previous research shows that better oral health awareness is associated with better gingival health outcomes in diabetes patients [41,42]. This underscores the urgent need for integrated education programs within healthcare systems that emphasize the importance of oral health in diabetes management.

A main limitation of this study is the absence of detailed clinical data, like probing depth and attachment loss, which are critical for a comprehensive evaluation of periodontal health. Due to difficult hospital conditions and patients not agreeing to visit our university dental clinic for a periodontal check-up, we could not perform a more detailed clinical evaluation. Additionally, relying on self-reported QGBI may introduce potential bias, even though standardized instructions were given. While earlier research suggests that self-reported gingival bleeding can serve as a useful screening tool [22], future studies should combine it with clinical measures to enhance accuracy.

Future research should use longitudinal study designs to investigate further how glycemic control, periodontal health, and lifestyle factors, particularly dietary habits, interact and influence both diabetes management and gingival health [43]. It would also be valuable to perform subgroup analyses based on factors such as obesity, smoking, hypertension, and the use of antihypertensive medications to better understand their impact on gingival bleeding.

5. Conclusions

This study highlights the link between HbA1c levels and QGBI in hospitalized diabetes patients, reinforcing the importance of gingival health in diabetes management. A key finding was the lack of awareness of this connection, pointing to the need for better patient education. Additionally, the positive link between smoking habits and regular dental visits suggests that informed patients are more likely to prioritize oral health.

Integrating structured educational programs, routine dental examinations, and interdisciplinary collaboration between medical and dental professionals is essential for enhancing glycemic control and periodontal health. These preventive measures can increase patient awareness, encourage healthier behaviors, and reduce periodontal complications in individuals with diabetes.

Author Contributions: Conceptualization, A.M. (Aida Meto), A.S. and A.A. (Adem Alushi); methodology, A.K. and T.F.; software, T.F.; validation, A.M. (Agron Meto), A.A. (Adela Alushi) and A.A. (Adem Alushi); formal analysis, A.M. (Aida Meto), A.A. (Adela Alushi) and T.F.; investigation, A.S.; data curation, A.K. and T.F.; writing—original draft preparation, A.M. (Aida Meto), A.S. and T.F.; writing—review and editing, A.A. (Adela Alushi) and A.M. (Agron Meto); visualization, A.M. (Aida Meto) and A.K.; supervision, A.M. (Agron Meto); project administration, A.A. (Adem Alushi) All authors have read and agreed to the published version of the manuscript.

Funding: This research received no external funding.

Institutional Review Board Statement: The study was conducted following the Declaration of Helsinki and was approved by the Research Ethics Committee of Aldent University, Tirana, AL, USA, (Protocol no. 144/23) on 3 April 2023.

Informed Consent Statement: Written informed consent has been obtained from the patients to publish this paper.

Data Availability Statement: The data presented in this study are available on request from the corresponding authors.

Conflicts of Interest: The authors declare no conflicts of interest.

ferences

Lovic, D.; Piperidou, A.; Zografou, I.; Grassos, H.; Pittaras, A.; Manolis, A. The Growing Epidemic of Diabetes Mellitus. *Curr. Vasc. Pharmacol.* **2020**, *18*, 104–109. [CrossRef] [PubMed]

Magliano, D.J.; Boyko, E.J.; IDF Diabetes Atlas 10th Edition Scientific Committee. *IDF DIABETES ATLAS [Internet]*, 10th ed.; International Diabetes Federation: Brussels, Belgium, 2021. [PubMed]

American Diabetes Association Professional Practice Committee. 2. Classification and Diagnosis of Diabetes: Standards of Medical Care in Diabetes-2022. *Diabetes Care* **2022**, *45*, S17–S38. [CrossRef] [PubMed]

Skyler, J.S.; Bakris, G.L.; Bonifacio, E.; Darsow, T.; Eckel, R.H.; Groop, L.; Groop, P.-H.; Handelsman, Y.; Insel, R.A.; Mathieu, C.; et al. Differentiation of Diabetes by Pathophysiology, Natural History, and Prognosis. *Diabetes* **2017**, *66*, 241–255. [CrossRef] [PubMed]

Zaccardi, F.; Webb, D.R.; Yates, T.; Davies, M.J. Pathophysiology of type 1 and type 2 diabetes mellitus: A 90-year perspective. *Postgrad. Med. J.* **2016**, *92*, 63–69. [CrossRef]

Kusunoki, Y.; Konishi, K.; Tsunoda, T.; Koyama, H. Significance of Glycemic Variability in Diabetes Mellitus. *Intern. Med.* **2022**, *61*, 281–290. [CrossRef]

Faselis, C.; Katsimardou, A.; Imprialos, K.; Deligkaris, P.; Kallistratos, M.; Dimitriadis, K. Microvascular Complications of Type 2 Diabetes Mellitus. *Curr. Vasc. Pharmacol.* **2020**, *18*, 117–124. [CrossRef]

Moreno, A.; Lozano, M.; Salinas, P. Diabetic retinopathy. *Nutr. Hosp.* **2013**, *28*, 53–56. [CrossRef]

Zaino, B.; Goel, R.; Devaragudi, S.; Prakash, A.; Vaghamashi, Y.; Sethi, Y.; Patel, N.; Kaka, N. Diabetic neuropathy: Pathogenesis and evolving principles of management. *Dis. Mon.* **2023**, *69*, 101582. [CrossRef]

Viigimaa, M.; Sachinidis, A.; Toumpourleka, M.; Koutsampasopoulos, K.; Alliksoo, S.; Titma, T. Macrovascular Complications of Type 2 Diabetes Mellitus. *Curr. Vasc. Pharmacol.* **2020**, *18*, 110–116. [CrossRef]

Sun, H.; Saeedi, P.; Karuranga, S.; Pinkepanka, M.; Ogurtsovab, K.; Duncanc, B.B.; Steinc, C.; Basitd, A.; Chane, J.C.N.; Mbanya, J.C.; et al. IDF Diabetes Atlas: Global, regional and country-level diabetes prevalence estimates for 2021 and projections for 2045. *Diabetes Res. Clin. Pract.* **2022**, *183*, 109119. [CrossRef]

Russo, M.P.; Grande-Ratti, M.F.; Burgos, M.A.; Molaro, A.A.; Bonella, M.B. Prevalence of diabetes, epidemiological characteristics and vascular complications. *Arch. Cardiol. Mex.* **2023**, *93*, 30–36. [CrossRef] [PubMed]

Preshaw, P.M.; Bissett, S.M. Periodontitis and diabetes. *Br. Dent. J.* **2019**, *227*, 577–584. [CrossRef] [PubMed]

Zheng, M.; Wang, C.; Ali, A.; Shih, Y.A.; Xie, Q.; Guo, C. Prevalence of periodontitis in people clinically diagnosed with diabetes mellitus: A meta-analysis of epidemiologic studies. *Acta Diabetol.* **2021**, *58*, 1307–1327. [CrossRef] [PubMed]

Polak, D.; Shapira, L. An update on the evidence for pathogenic mechanisms that may link periodontitis and diabetes. *J. Clin. Periodontol.* **2018**, *45*, 150–166. [CrossRef]

Stöhr, J.; Barbaresko, J.; Neuenschwander, M.; Schlesinger, S. Bidirectional association between periodontal disease and diabetes mellitus: A systematic review and meta-analysis of cohort studies. *Sci. Rep.* **2021**, *11*, 13686. [CrossRef]

Garg, S.; Kapoor, K.K. The quantitative gingival bleeding index. *J. Indian. Dent. Assoc.* **1985**, *57*, 112–113. [PubMed]

Bessa Rebelo, M.A.; de Queiroz, A.C. Chapter 3: Gingival Indices: State of Art. In *Gingival Diseases*; Panagakos, F.S., Davies, R.M., Eds.; IntechOpen: London, UK, 2011. [CrossRef]

Rosenauer, T.; Wagenschwanz, C.; Kuhn, M.; Kensche, A.; Stiehl, S.; Hannig, C. The Bleeding on Brushing Index: A novel index in preventive dentistry. *Int. Dent. J.* **2017**, *67*, 299–307. [CrossRef]

Novaes, A.B., Jr.; de Lima, F.R.; Novaes, A.B. Compliance with supportive periodontal therapy and its relation to the bleeding index. *J. Periodontol.* **1996**, *67*, 976–980. [CrossRef]

Deng, K.; Pelekos, G.; Jin, L.; Tonetti, M.S. Diagnostic accuracy of self-reported measures of periodontal disease: A clinical validation study using the 2017 case definitions. *J. Clin. Periodontol.* **2021**, *48*, 1037–1050. [CrossRef]

22. Deng, K.; Pelekos, G.; Jin, L.; Tonetti, M.S. Gingival bleeding on brushing as a sentinel sign of gingival inflammation: A diagno accuracy trial for the discrimination of periodontal health and disease. *J. Clin. Periodontol.* **2021**, *48*, 1537–1548. [CrossRef]
23. Kinane, D.F.; Stathopoulou, P.G.; Papapanou, P.N. Periodontal diseases. *Nat. Rev. Dis. Primers* **2017**, *3*, 17038. [CrossRef] [PubM
24. Lalla, E.; Papapanou, P.N. Diabetes mellitus and periodontitis: A tale of two common interrelated diseases. *Nat. Rev. Endocri* **2011**, *7*, 738–748. [CrossRef] [PubMed]
25. National Institute for Health and Care Excellence (NICE). *Evidence Review D for Periodontal Treatment to Improve Diabetic Con in Adults with Type 1 or Type 2 Diabetes: Periodontal Treatment to Improve Diabetic Control in Adults with Type 1 or Type 2 Diabe Evidence Review D*; National Institute for Health and Care Excellence (NICE): London, UK, 2022. [PubMed]
26. Tricco, A.C.; Ivers, N.M.; Grimshaw, J.M.; Moher, D.; Turner, L.; Galipeau, J.; Halperin, I.; Vachon, B.; Ramsay, T.; Manns, B.; e Effectiveness of quality improvement strategies on the management of diabetes: A systematic review and meta-analysis. *La* **2012**, *379*, 2252–2261. [CrossRef] [PubMed]
27. Buhlin, K.; Gustafsson, A.; Andersson, K.; Håkansson, J.; Klinge, B. Validity and limitations of self-reported periodontal hea *Community Dent. Oral Epidemiol.* **2002**, *30*, 431–437. [CrossRef]
28. Renvert, S.; Persson, G.R. A systematic review on the use of residual probing depth, bleeding on probing and furcation sta following initial periodontal therapy to predict further attachment and tooth loss. *J. Clin. Periodontol.* **2002**, *29*, 82–89. [CrossR
29. Alkahtani, A.; Anderson, P.; Baysan, A. The impact of sociodemographic determinants and diabetes type-2 on oral hea outcomes: An analytical cross-sectional study. *Clin. Exp. Dent. Res.* **2024**, *10*, e846. [CrossRef]
30. Rösing, C.K.; Gomes, S.C.; Carvajal, P.; Gómez, M.; Costa, R.; Toledo, A.; Solanes, F.; Romanelli, H.; Gamonal, J.; Oppermann, Impact of smoking on gingival inflammation in representative samples of three South American cities. *Braz. Oral Res.* **2019**, e090. [CrossRef]
31. Borojevic, T. Smoking and periodontal disease. *Mater. Sociomed.* **2012**, *24*, 274–276. [CrossRef]
32. Natarajan, P.; Madanian, S.; Marshall, S. Investigating the link between oral health conditions and systemic diseases: A cr sectional analysis. *Sci. Rep.* **2025**, *15*, 10476. [CrossRef]
33. Zini, A.; Mazor, S.; Timm, H.; Barker, M.L.; Grender, J.M.; Gerlach, R.W.; Biesbrock, A.R. Effects of an oral hygiene regimen progression of gingivitis/early periodontitis: A randomized controlled trial. *Can. J. Dent. Hyg.* **2021**, *55*, 85–94. [PubMed]
34. Tonsekar, P.; Tonsekar, V. Calcium-Channel-Blocker-Influenced Gingival Enlargement: A Conundrum Demystified. *Oral* **202** 236–249. [CrossRef]
35. Ramírez Martínez-Acitores, L.; Hernández Ruiz de Azcárate, F.; Casañas, E.; Serrano, J.; Hernández, G.; López-Pintor, R Xerostomia and salivary flow in patients taking antihypertensive drugs. *Int. J. Environ. Res. Public Health* **2020**, *17*, 2478. [CrossR [PubMed]
36. Pająk-Łysek, E.; Polak, M.; Kopeć, G.; Podolec, M.; Desvarieux, M.; Pająk, A.; Zarzecka, J. Associations between pharmacothera for cardiovascular diseases and periodontitis. *Int. J. Environ. Res. Public Health* **2021**, *18*, 770. [CrossRef] [PubMed]
37. Zhu, L.; Tang, Z.; Hu, R.; Gu, M.; Yang, Y. Ageing and inflammation: What happens in periodontium? *Bioengineering* **2023**, 1274. [CrossRef] [PubMed]
38. Lipsky, M.S.; Singh, T.; Zakeri, G.; Hung, M. Oral health and older adults: A narrative review. *Dent. J.* **2024**, *12*, 30. [CrossRe
39. Costa, R.; Ríos-Carrasco, B.; Monteiro, L.; López-Jarana, P.; Carneiro, F.; Relvas, M. Association between type 1 diabetes melli and periodontal diseases. *J. Clin. Med.* **2023**, *12*, 1147. [CrossRef]
40. Liu, Y.; Yu, Y.; Nickel, J.C.; Iwasaki, L.R.; Duan, P.; Simmer-Beck, M.; Brown, L. Gender differences in the association periodontitis and type 2 diabetes. *Int. Dent. J.* **2018**, *68*, 433–440. [CrossRef]
41. Pranckeviciene, A.; Siudikiene, J.; Ostrauskas, R.; Machiulskiene, V. Severity of periodontal disease in adult patients with diab mellitus in relation to the type of diabetes. *Biomed. Pap. Med. Fac. Univ. Palacky Olomouc Czech Repub.* **2014**, *158*, 117– [CrossRef]
42. Kocher, T.; König, J.; Borgnakke, W.S.; Pink, C.; Meisel, P. Periodontal complications of hyperglycemia/diabetes melli Epidemiologic complexity and clinical challenge. *Periodontology 2000* **2018**, *78*, 59–97. [CrossRef]
43. Smith, H.; Thomas, D.T.; Vázquez-Morales, G.N.; Puckett, L.; Del Mar Rodriguez, M.; Stromberg, A.; Shaddox, L.M.; Santama M.P.; Pearce, K.; Andriankaja, O.M. Cross-sectional association among dietary habits, periodontitis, and uncontrolled diabetes Hispanics: The LLIPDS study. *Front. Oral Health* **2025**, *6*, 1468995. [CrossRef]

Journal of
Clinical Medicine

MDPI

icle

ssociations Between Lifestyle Factors, Oral Health Behaviors, ıd Glycemic Control in Type 2 Diabetic Patients

essa Bolchis [1,2], Iulia Alexa [1,3], Nicoleta A. Toderas [4], Ramona Dumitrescu [1,2], Ruxandra Sava-Rosianu [1,2,*], avia Balean [1,2], Vlad Tiberiu Alexa [1,2], Simona Popescu [5,6], Daniela Jumanca [1,2], Atena Galuscan [1,2], Iosif Ilia [7] Doina Chioran [8]

1 Translational and Experimental Clinical Research Centre in Oral Health, Department of Preventive, Community Dentistry and Oral Health, University of Medicine and Pharmacy "Victor Babes", 300040 Timisoara, Romania; vanessa.bolchis@umft.ro (V.B.); iulia.alexa@umft.ro (I.A.); dumitrescu.ramona@umft.ro (R.D.); balean.octavia@umft.ro (O.B.); vlad.alexa@umft.ro (V.T.A.); jumanca.daniela@umft.ro (D.J.); galuscan.atena@umft.ro (A.G.)

2 Clinic of Preventive, Community Dentistry and Oral Health, Department I, University of Medicine and 13 Pharmacy "Victor Babes", Eftimie Murgu Sq. no 2, 300041 Timisoara, Romania

3 Department of Dentistry, Faculty of Dental Medicine, "Vasile Goldis" Western University of Arad, 310045 Arad, Romania

4 Department of Psychology, Faculty of Sociology and Psychology, West University of Timisoara, 300223 Timisoara, Romania; nicoleta.toderas01@e-uvt.ro

5 Second Department of Internal Medicine, "Victor Babes" University of Medicine and Pharmacy, 300041 Timisoara, Romania; popescu.simona@umft.ro

6 Department of Diabetes, "Pius Brinzeu" Emergency Hospital, 300723 Timisoara, Romania

7 Faculty of Physical Education and Sport, "Aurel Vlaicu" University of Arad, 310130 Arad, Romania; iosif.ilia@uav.ro

8 Faculty of Dental Medicine, "Victor Babeș" University of Medicine and Pharmacy from Timisoara, 9 Revolutiei 1989 Ave., 300070 Timisoara, Romania; chioran.doina@umft.ro

* Correspondence: sava-rosianu.ruxandra@umft.ro

Abstract: Introduction: T2DM mellitus (T2DM) is a major global health issue associated with significant morbidity, mortality, and economic burden. While the role of lifestyle factors in glycemic control is well-established, the influence of oral health behaviors remains underexplored. **Objective:** This study aimed to investigate the interplay between lifestyle habits, oral health behaviors, and glycemic control in patients with T2DM. **Methodology:** A cross-sectional study was conducted on 132 patients (66 men and 66 women) with T2DM at the Pius Brînzeu Emergency Hospital in Timișoara, Romania. Data on smoking, physical activity, alcohol consumption, tooth brushing frequency, and dental visits were collected using structured questionnaires, and glycemic control was assessed through HbA1c measurements. Statistical analyses, including Pearson correlations and linear regression, were performed. **Results:** Among men, HbA1c levels were negatively associated with exercise frequency (ß = −0.26, $p < 0.05$) and education level (correlation coefficient −0.27, $p < 0.05$), and positively associated with dental visits and tooth brushing frequency (correlation coefficient 0.26, $p < 0.05$). In the combined analysis, education level positively correlated with both dental visits (correlation coefficient 0.24, $p < 0.01$) and alcohol consumption (correlation coefficient 0.22, $p < 0.05$). **Conclusions:** These findings underscore the importance of integrating oral health and lifestyle interventions into diabetes management to optimize patient outcomes.

Keywords: T2DM; oral health behaviors; lifestyle factors; glycemic control; HbA1c; prevention

 https://doi.org/10.3390/jcm14020450

1. Introduction

Type 2 diabetes mellitus (T2DM) is a chronic metabolic disorder characterized by persistent hyperglycemia due to relative or absolute insulin deficiency, affecting the metabolism of carbohydrates, proteins, and fats. In addition to its systemic complications, T2DM significantly impacts oral health, manifesting through conditions such as periodontal diseases, tooth loss, delayed wound healing, candidiasis, dry mouth, and burning mouth syndrome, which may serve as early indicators for undiagnosed diabetes or markers for glycemic control in diagnosed patients [1]. Acording to the WHO the expected values for normal fasting blood glucose concentration are between 70 mg/dL (3.9 mmol/L) and 100 mg/dL (5.6 mmol/L). The American Diabetes Association (ADA) defines normal fasting plasma glucose as below 100 mg/dL (5.6 mmol/L), with values between 100 and 125 mg/dL (5.6 to 6.9 mmol/L) indicating impaired fasting glucose (pre-diabetes). Diagnosis of T2DM is based on specific glucose thresholds, including fasting plasma glucose (FPG) levels of $\geq$126 mg/dL (7.0 mmol/L), 2-h plasma glucose (2-h PG) levels of $\geq$200 mg/dL (11.1 mmol/L) during a 75-g oral glucose tolerance test (OGTT), or an HbA1c level of $\geq$6.5% (48 mmol/mol). In individuals presenting with classic hyperglycemic symptoms or during a hyperglycemic crisis, a random plasma glucose level of $\geq$200 mg/dL (11.1 mmol/L) confirms the diagnosis. These thresholds are crucial for understanding glycemic control and provide essential context for analyzing diabetes-related data [2,3]. As a progressive condition, it negatively affects health-related quality of life, leads to severe comorbidities, and increases the risk of premature mortality. In addition to its health impact, this disease places a significant economic burden on individuals, healthcare systems, and society. However, research shows that it can be effectively prevented through lifestyle changes, underscoring the importance of early prevention efforts. Moreover, the positive effects of lifestyle interventions can last for several years. Despite more than two decades of evidence supporting the effectiveness of these approaches, healthcare systems still struggle to implement scalable, individual-level support for lifestyle changes in routine practice [4–7].

Optimal health behaviors include avoiding smoking, limiting alcohol intake and engaging in regular physical activity. These habits, along with balanced nutrition and managing mental stress, are linked to stronger immune function, particularly through enhanced natural killer cell activity, the body's first line of defense [8,9].

For individuals with diabetes, lifestyle factors play an even more critical role. Men with diabetes who adopt healthier behaviors and experience fewer microvascular complications are often those with higher educational levels. Among diabetic women, those with more education tend to perceive themselves as healthier, regardless of their actual medical status. However, diabetic patients with poor metabolic control and lower educational attainment frequently report more complications, mental health issues, sick leave, and reduced physical activity, highlighting the importance of both education and lifestyle in managing the condition. Additionally, social class and gender disparities further complicate outcomes, with lower-class diabetic women facing a higher mortality risk compared to both non-diabetic women and diabetic men from similar backgrounds [9,10].

In addition to its systemic effects, T2DM significantly impacts oral health, with a well-established bidirectional relationship between diabetes and periodontal disease. Poor glycemic control exacerbates periodontal inflammation through mechanisms such as oxidative stress, delayed wound healing, and heightened inflammatory responses. Conversely, untreated periodontitis amplifies systemic inflammation, complicating glycemic management and increasing the risk of diabetes-related complications. Decompensated diabetic patients often exhibit a diminished response to non-surgical periodontal therapy, such as scaling and root planing, due to delayed tissue healing and altered immune function. This underscores the critical role of achieving glycemic control to enhance periodontal treatment outcomes. Lifestyle choices, including proper oral hygiene, balanced nutrition, and regular physical activity, are essential for addressing the interconnected impacts of T2DM and periodontitis. Adopting healthier habits not only aids in controlling blood glucose levels but also mitigates systemic and oral health challenges associated with diabetes [11–14].

Adopting healthier habits, such as improving diet and increasing physical activity, is essential for controlling blood glucose levels and reducing the global prevalence of diabetes. A healthy lifestyle, as defined by the World Health Organization, involves daily habits and behaviors that reduce the risk of disease or premature death by addressing critical factors such as balanced nutrition and regular exercise. This multifaceted concept encompasses various aspects of life, including diet, physical activity, sleep, stress management, and substance use, all of which are influenced by social, economic, and environmental factors. By adopting these preventive measures, individuals can mitigate chronic diseases, enhance overall well-being, and improve long-term health outcomes. In the case of periodontitis, immune responses are key to the severity of inflammation, as bacteria trigger the release of inflammatory mediators like TNF-α and interleukin-1, which contribute to tissue and bone damage [15,16].

Poor blood sugar control in diabetes also induces oxidative stress, slowing tissue repair in the gums and making infections harder to heal, which worsens periodontal conditions. Additionally, complications like reduced blood flow further impede recovery in diabetic patients, increasing susceptibility to periodontal damage. These connections highlight the significant impact of lifestyle on both oral and systemic health [9,15,17,18].

Good oral hygiene habits include brushing teeth at least twice daily, visiting the dentist annually, using interdental devices like floss, and limiting snacking and cariogenic foods. These habits are associated with healthy food consumption, regular exercise, and vitamin use, particularly among adolescents. Physical activity supports better brushing habits; while smoking and alcohol consumption are linked to poorer oral health. Poor oral hygiene leads to plaque buildup and worsens periodontal health, while frequent brushing is linked to reduced sugar intake. Although diabetic patients tend to have poor oral health behaviors, the absence of a control group limits conclusions about the connection between oral health and type-2 diabetes. Interestingly, even non-diabetic periodontitis patients have been found to have elevated fasting blood glucose levels [19,20].

A complementary literature review analyzed 52 studies using Web of Science, with keyword co-occurrence analysis in VOSviewer identifying emerging links between lifestyle factors, oral health, and glycemic control.

This study aimed to investigate the interplay between T2DM, oral health behaviors, and lifestyle factors such as smoking, alcohol consumption, and physical activity. By exploring how these elements intersect with diabetes management, we sought to identify key areas for improving the quality of life and comprehensive care of diabetic individuals. The absence of similar studies in Romania underscores the importance of this research in addressing local knowledge gaps and providing a foundation for developing targeted public health strategies tailored to the Romanian context.

2. Background of the Study

The current research aimed to explore the relationships between T2DM, oral health behaviors, and lifestyle factors starting from a detailed analysis of existing literature. The process of screening the literature was initiated by using Web of Science, a globally recognized academic database that provides access to thousands of high-quality research articles across multiple disciplines, including medicine, public health, and life sciences. Through the Web of Science Core Collection, which includes highly cited journals, conference proceedings, and patent records a basic search was conducted focusing on three main keywords: T2DM, Oral Health Behaviors, and Lifestyle Factors.

After the initial screening of 52 relevant scientific articles that focused on the core themes of this research were selected. These articles were chosen based on their relevance, citation impact, and the quality of the journals in which they were published. Web of Science's advanced filtering options, including citation network analysis and the ability to track emerging trends in the field, helped ensure that the selected studies provided a comprehensive overview of the latest research.

To better understand the relationships between key concepts in the literature, VOSviewer (version 1.6.20), a powerful visualization software designed to map co-occurrences of keywords from these selected articles was utilized. VOSviewer allows for the identification and analysis of relationships between key terms, providing a clear perspective on emerging trends and significant areas of interest in T2DM research.

The co-occurrence analysis of keywords helped to identify the most critical themes within the selected literature. Through this mapping, strong connections between terms such as T2DM, obesity, physical activity, insulin resistance, oral health behaviors, and smoking were discovered. These connections highlight the complex interplay between lifestyle factors and the management of diabetes. This approach not only emphasized the individual importance of each factor but also showed how they interact to influence glycemic control and the prevention of diabetes-related complications.

Thus, by analyzing the co-occurrence and visualizing the relationships between these concepts, the importance of this subject in the context of public health and clinical management could be underscored. The findings provide important insights into how lifestyle, smoking, and oral health behaviors directly influence the management of T2DM.

The co-occurrence map generated from 52 Web of Science articles highlights key thematic connections in T2DM research (Figure 1). Central terms like T2DM and obesity emphasize their critical relationship, with strong links to insulin resistance and glycemic control, underscoring their importance in disease management. The map also reveals the significance of lifestyle factors, such as physical activity and diet, which play a crucial role in improving health outcomes. Peripheral but notable themes include oral health behaviors and inflammation, illustrating emerging research areas exploring how chronic conditions like periodontitis impact diabetes. This comprehensive visualization reflects the need for an integrative approach to diabetes care, incorporating both lifestyle and systemic health factors.

In the next phase, the co-occurrence map was refined by raising the threshold to include only keywords with a minimum of 3 occurrences, narrowing the analysis to 51 key terms (Figure 2). This adjustment helped to highlight the most central and frequently discussed themes in the literature. Core topics such as diabetes management, lifestyle interventions, and risk factors remained prominent, reflecting the ongoing research focus. The streamlined analysis also reinforced the importance of behavioral and physiological aspects of T2DM care, emphasizing how lifestyle changes and patient engagement play critical roles in disease management.

The final analysis focused on identifying trends in the evolution of research topics over time. Using a time-overlay visualization in VOSviewer, the color gradient in the map—from blue to yellow—reveals the shifts in research emphasis from 2012 to 2020 (Figure 3). Early research (highlighted in blue and green) predominantly focused on general risk factors for T2DM, such as obesity, insulin resistance, and cardiovascular disease. These foundational topics laid the groundwork for understanding the broader scope of diabetes-related complications and the role of lifestyle in disease progression.

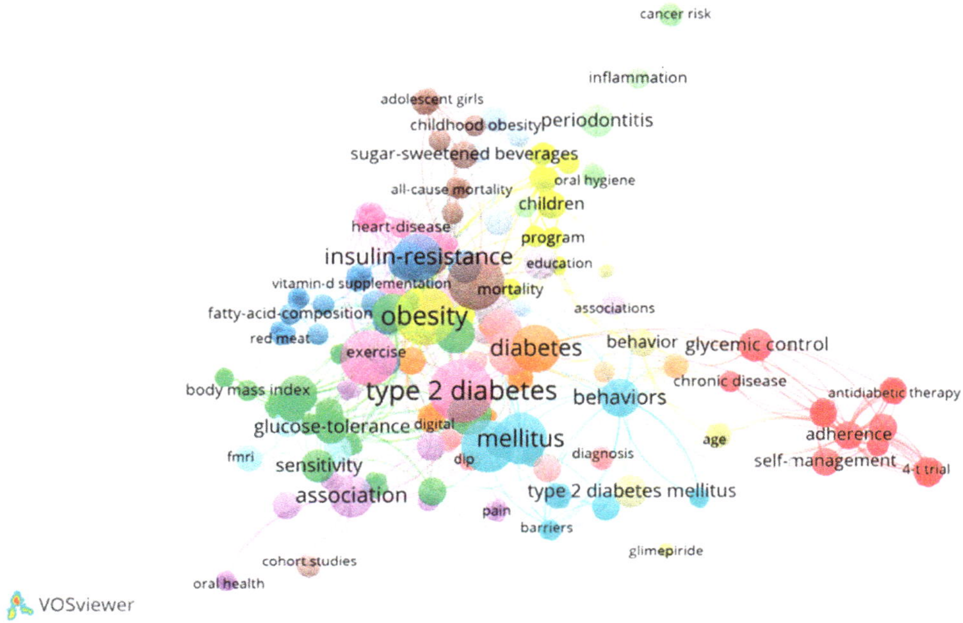

Figure 1. Clustered Network Visualization of Key Concepts in T2DM Research.

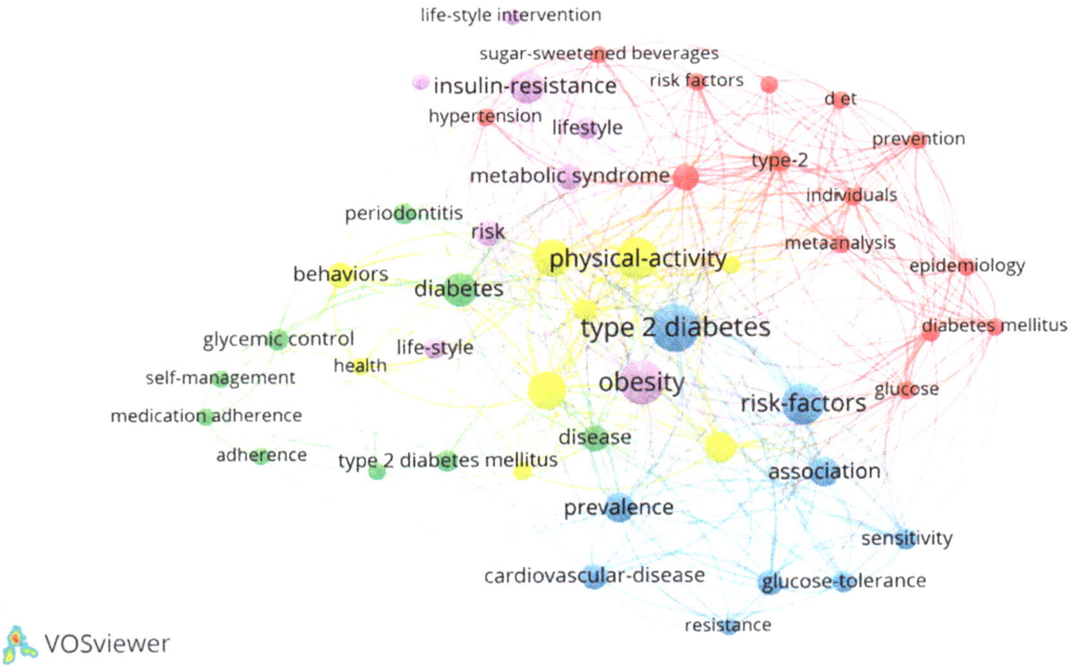

Figure 2. Refined Co-occurrence Map Highlighting Central Themes in T2DM Research.

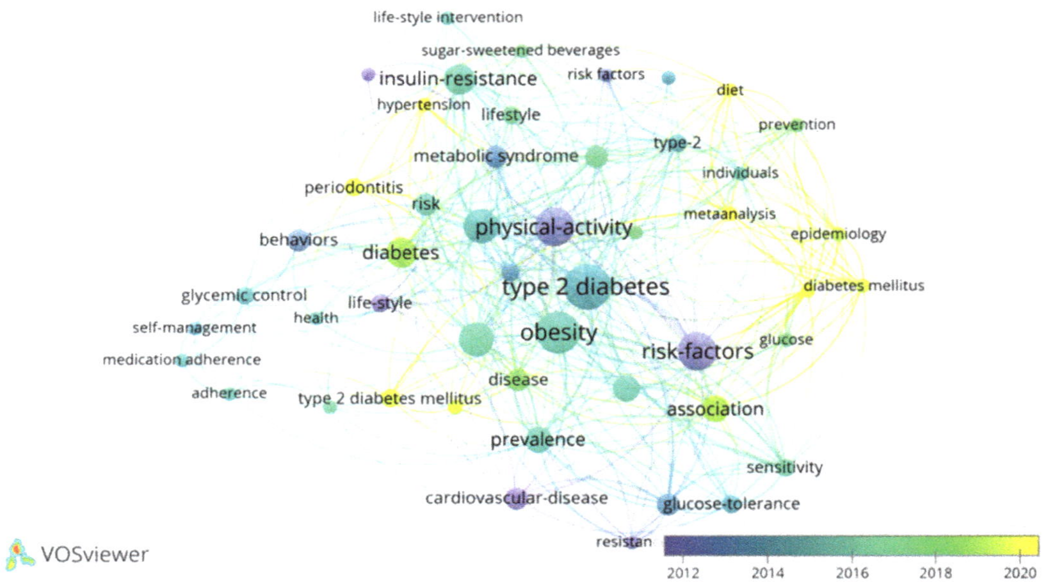

Figure 3. Temporal Evolution of Research Focus in T2DM.

As the years progressed, newer research (depicted in yellow) shifted towards more specific interventions and public health strategies, with increasing attention on epidemiology, meta-analyses, and preventive measures like diet and lifestyle interventions. This shift underscores a growing recognition of the importance of early prevention and tailored interventions in diabetes care. Additionally, keywords related to self-management, medication adherence, and periodontitis show the expanding focus on patient-centered care and the integration of oral health into diabetes management.

This temporal analysis not only highlights the dynamic nature of diabetes research but also demonstrates a forward-looking trend toward prevention and holistic care. By tracing these shifts in research focus, we gain a deeper understanding of how the field has evolved, paving the way for more comprehensive and effective approaches to managing T2DM.

3. Materials and Methods

3.1. Study Design

This cross-sectional, observational and correlational study was conducted at the Outpatient Diabetes Care Facility of the Pius Brînzeu County Emergency Hospital in Timișoara, Romania, between February and April 2024. A total of 132 patients with T2DM (66 women and 66 men) participated, reflecting a diverse demographic representative of diabetic patients in the region. All participants provided informed consent prior to their inclusion in the study, ensuring ethical compliance and voluntary participation. None of the participants were involved in the design or development of the research, maintaining the integrity and objectivity of the study process. The research was conducted in full alignment with the ethical principles outlined in the 2013 revision of the Declaration of Helsinki, which governs ethical standards for research involving human subjects. Furthermore, the study received formal approval from the Ethics Committee of the University of Medicine and Pharmacy Victor Babes, Timisoara, Romania, under protocol number 05/30.01.2024, affirming its adherence to rigorous ethical guidelines. For drafting the manuscript, GenAI tools have been used solely for English editing, given the fact that none of the authors are native English speakers.

This study was conducted in Romania, focusing on the western region, which reflects the country's notable regional and local disparities in human development. The research examines areas with varying levels of socioeconomic development, as indicated by education attainment, income levels, and access to healthcare services. The western region, characterized by a mix of industrial, agricultural, and service-based economic activities, includes urban centers like Timișoara that serve as regional economic hubs with relatively high education levels and well-developed healthcare infrastructure, particularly in Timiș County, which specializes in chronic care such as diabetes management. In contrast, rural areas in the region face challenges related to poverty, limited connectivity, and reduced access to healthcare and resources. Geographically, the combination of plains and mountainous terrains influences lifestyle behaviors, including agricultural practices and recreational activities, providing a nuanced context for studying the interplay between lifestyle, oral health behaviors, and glycemic control in diabetic patients [21,22].

The participants were drawn from the western region of Romania, where the prevalence of diabetes is estimated at 8.23%, as reported by the PREDATORR study. To ensure that the study captured a broad spectrum of experiences, a stratified random sampling method was employed, balancing representation based on age, gender, and residential environment (urban vs. rural). This approach minimized selection bias and enhanced the applicability of the findings to the wider population of diabetic patients.

3.2. *Inclusion/Exclusion Criteria*

The study included individuals aged 18 and older, all diagnosed with T2DM. Exclusion criteria encompassed patients with type 1 diabetes, those who did not provide informed consent, individuals with severe cognitive or psychiatric impairments that hindered their ability to consent, pregnant or breastfeeding women, and those who had undergone major surgery or experienced significant physical trauma within the previous six months.

3.3. *Data Collection*

The data collection process was conducted by a team of three healthcare professionals, including a diabetologist (S.P.) and two dentists (V.B. and R.D). Participants were provided with an information sheet detailing the study's objectives and procedures, addressing any questions they had. Participation was voluntary, and individuals who met the inclusion criteria and consented to participate signed a written consent form. Subsequently, they were asked to complete a self-administered questionnaire while waiting for their medical appointment. Completing the questionnaire required approximately 8 to 15 min. The questionnaire was developed following a thorough review of existing literature and prior studies [23,24]. It consisted of sections assessing lifestyle factors, oral hygiene behaviors, and demographic and clinical characteristics. The lifestyle factors section included questions on smoking habits, alcohol consumption, and the frequency of physical activity. Oral hygiene behaviors were evaluated by examining the frequency of toothbrushing, the use of fluoride toothpaste, and the utilization of auxiliary cleaning methods, such as dental floss or interdental brushes. The questionnaire used was developed based on the WHO adult questionnaire, ensuring its validity and relevance for assessing health behaviors and lifestyle in the target population [25]. Clinical data, such as glycated hemoglobin (HbA1c) levels, were extracted from participants' medical records to ensure accuracy and standardization. Demographic data collected included age, gender, place of residence (urban or rural), diabetes duration, and education level. This structured and comprehensive approach ensured the collection of high-quality data on the relationships between lifestyle factors, oral health behaviors, and glycemic control among individuals with T2DM, allowing for a nuanced analysis of these interrelated variables.

3.4. Variables and Study Outcomes

The primary dependent variable in this study was glycemic control, measured by glycated hemoglobin (HbA1c) levels obtained from participants' medical records. Secondary dependent variables included oral health behaviors, specifically the frequency of tooth brushing and dental visits. Independent variables encompassed lifestyle factors such as smoking status, alcohol consumption, and frequency of physical activity; demographic characteristics, including age, gender, place of residence (urban or rural), and educational level; as well as clinical characteristics, such as the duration of diabetes and the use of oral hygiene aids like dental floss or interdental brushes. This framework allowed for a comprehensive analysis of the relationships between lifestyle, oral health behaviors, and glycemic control among diabetic patients.

3.5. Statistical Analysis

The statistical analysis combined insights from a comprehensive literature review with the evaluation of empirical data. The primary objective of the statistical tests was to comprehensively analyze and elucidate the intricate relationships between various lifestyle factors, oral health behaviors, and HbA1c levels, while simultaneously investigating potential gender-specific differences within the study population. These analyses aimed to provide a deeper understanding of how these variables interact and influence one another, contributing to the overall health outcomes of individuals with diabetes.

Descriptive statistics summarized the demographic and behavioral characteristics of the 132 participants, while Pearson correlations assessed relationships between variables such as exercise frequency, education level, dental visits, and HbA1c levels. A split-file analysis by gender further highlighted specific trends, including significant negative correlations between HbA1c and exercise frequency or education among men, and a positive correlation between education and dental visits among women. Linear regression models identified predictors of HbA1c variability, with exercise frequency emerging as the strongest negative predictor. All analyses were conducted using SPSS version 23, with statistical significance set at $p < 0.05$.

4. Results

To further ensure representativeness, the sample reflected the regional demographic profile of diabetic patients, with approximately equal numbers of participants from urban (53%) and rural (47%) areas, mirroring the distribution reported in national health surveys. Additionally, age distribution ranged from 34 to 87 years, with the majority of patients in the 50–65 age group, a demographic most affected by T2DM. This stratification provided a nuanced understanding of the diverse challenges faced by diabetic individuals across different socioeconomic and geographical backgrounds, strengthening the external validity of the study's findings (Table 1).

The values of Skewness and Kurtosis for the variables of interest fall within the parametric range (−2, 2), indicating that the dataset follows a normal distribution and is parametric. The participants were equally distributed by gender, with 66 males and 66 females (N = 132). The majority of participants had completed either secondary education (10 classes) or high school (12 classes), accounting for 64.4% (N = 85) of the sample, followed by 20.5% (N = 27) who had a maximum of 8 years of education (gymnasium).

The mean age of the sample was 63.45 years (SD = 10.48), with the youngest participant aged 34 and the oldest aged 87. Regarding alcohol consumption, 50% of participants

(N = 66) reported occasional or monthly consumption, while 9.1% (N = 12) consumed alcohol daily, and 33.3% (N = 44) abstained entirely.

Table 1. Descriptive Statistics for Key Variables in the Study Sample (N = 132).

Variables	N (%)
Gender	
Male	66 (50.0)
Female	66 (50.0)
Age	
34–44	4 (2.7)
45–54	18 (16.2)
55–64	33 (29.8)
65–74	45 (40.5)
75–87	12 (10.8)
Missing age	20 (15.2)
Residence	
Rural area	51 (38.6)
Urban area	81 (61.4)

In terms of exercise frequency, defined as any type of physical activity performed for an extended duration, the majority of participants (49.2%, N = 65) reported being inactive. Among the remaining participants, 22.7% (N = 30) engaged in physical activity 1–2 times per week, 15.9% (N = 21) exercised 3–4 times per week, and 12% (N = 16) reported exercising 5 or more times per week.

Oral health was assessed through two variables: the frequency of dental visits and the frequency of tooth brushing. Most participants (47.7%, N = 63) reported not visiting the dentist in the past year, while 44.7% (N = 59) visited once or twice, and a minority of 7.6% (N = 10) visited three or more times annually. Regarding tooth brushing habits, 38.6% (N = 51) brushed their teeth twice daily, 31.1% (N = 41) brushed once daily, 16.7% (N = 22) brushed less than once daily, and 13.6% (N = 18) brushed more than twice daily (Table 2).

Table 2. Descriptive Statistics for Behavioral, Demographic, and Health Variables (N = 132).

Variables	Mean	Std. Deviation
Studies	1.88	0.55
HbA1C	7.95	1.51
Alcohol consumption	1.73	0.62
Dental visit	1.59	0.62
Exercise	2.87	1.24
Age	63.45	10.48
Tooth brushing	2.49	0.92
Gender	1.50	0.50

4.1. Gender-Specific Correlations

For gender specific correlation the Pearson correlation was used after splitting the groups between females and males. The results show that regarding males, there's a significative positive correlation between tooth brushing frequency and dental visits R (66) = 0.26, $p < 0.05$, with a small effect size of $r^2 = 0.06$, meaning the frequency of tooth brushing increases as males attend more dental check-ups. Regarding the value of HbA1, there are two variable that correlate negatively to this. First, there is a negative significative correlation between frequency of exercise and value of HbA1c, R (66) = −0.26, $p < 0.05$, with a small effect size of $r^2 = 0.06$, meaning that the value of HbA1c increases as the frequency exercise per week decreases. Secondly, there is a negative significative correlation between HbA1c and education level R (66) = −0.27, $p < 0.05$ with a small effect size of $r^2 = 0.06$, meaning that the HbA1c value increases as the education level o participants gets smaller (Table 3).

Table 3. Correlation Matrix of Lifestyle Factors, Oral Health Behaviors, and HbA1c Levels Among Participants (N = 66).

	Men			Women	Overall	
	Tooth Brushing Freq.	**Exercise**	**Studies**	**Dental Visits**	**Alcohol Consumption**	**Dental Visit**
Dental visit	0.26 *	0.02	0.15	-	0.10	-
Exercise	0.06	-	0.07	0.05	−0.10	0.04
Alcohol consumption	0.00	−0.04	0.24	0.08	-	0.10
Studies	0.15	0.07	-	0.25 *	0.22 *	0.24 **
HbA1C	−0.07	−0.26 *	−0.27 *	−0.09	−0.13	−0.16

p * < 0.05; p ** < 0.01.

For the female subgroup (N = 66), the analysis identified a single significant positive correlation. Specifically, the frequency of dental visits was positively correlated with the level of education achieved R (66) = 0.25, $p < 0.05$ with a small effect of $r^2 = 0.06$, meaning that women with higher education also have higher rate of dental visits in the last year.

Although no other statistically significant correlations were identified within this subgroup, this result underscores the potential influence of education on oral health behaviors. Women with higher educational attainment may have increased awareness of the importance of regular dental care, access to better resources, or a stronger inclination toward preventive health behaviors, contributing to this observed trend.

When analyzing at the correlation between the variables without taking into account the gender, we found the following results regarding studies: there is a positive significative correlation between level of studies and frequency of dental visits R (132) = 0.24, $p < 0.01$, with a small effect size of $r^2 = 0.05$, meaning that overall, when the level of studies increases so does the frequency of dental visits. Additionally, the last significative result we found was regarding level of studies and alcohol intake, we found a positive significative correlation of R (132) = 0.22, $p < 0.05$ with a small effect of $r^2 = 0.04$. These findings highlight the potential influence of education on health-related behaviors, such as oral hygiene and lifestyle habits. While the effect sizes are small, the consistent association between higher education levels and both dental visits and alcohol intake suggests the need for further research to explore the underlying mechanisms and potential socioeconomic or cultural factors influencing these behaviors.

To explore the nuances between variances and variables, a split-file analysis based on gender was conducted. A linear regression analysis was performed with HbA1c as the dependent variable and the following predictors: frequency of dental visits, exercise frequency, alcohol consumption, and education level, analyzed separately for men and women.

The relationships between these predictors and HbA1c levels are further illustrated in the linear regression model displayed in Table 3, which provides a visual representation of their relative contributions to the variability in glycemic control.

For the whole sample the results of the linear regression analysis shows that the level of studies, frequency of dental visits and exercise frequency significantly predict the variability of HbA1c $F(3, 120) = 3.23$, $p < 0.05$. These variables predict in proportion of 0.075% of the total variability of HbA1c, $R^2 = 0.07$. The strongest negative predictor was level of exercise with a $\beta = -0.17$, $p = 0.05$ explaining 2.89% of the total variability of HbA1c, $R^2 = 0.02$ (Table 4).

Table 4. Linear Regression Analysis Predicting HbA1c Levels Based on Education, Dental Visits, and Exercise Frequency.

	HbA1c		
	Beta	**Std Err.**	***p***
Overall			
Studies	−0.09	0.24	0.28
Dental visits	−0.15	0.22	0.08
Exercise	−0.17 *	0.12	0.05
Alcohol Consumption	−0.79	0.23	0.40
Tooth Washing	−0.05	0.15	0.56
Men			
Alcohol consumption	0.12	0.28	0.34
Studies	−0.24	0.32	0.07
Dental visits	−0.26 *	0.32	0.05
Tooth washing	0.07	0.21	0.56
Exercise	−0.21	0.18	0.09
Women			
Alchool consumption	−0.20	0.40	0.21
Dental visits	−0.12	0.33	0.35
Tooth Washing	−0.18	0.23	0.32
Exercise	−0.12	0.19	0.32

Note: * $p < 0.005$.

The results of the linear regression analysis for men showed us that there are some significant predictors of HbA1c, F (5, 50) = 2.49, $p < 0.05$, with the strongest negative significant predictor for men being dental visit frequency, $\beta = -0.26$, $p = 0.05$, explaining 5% of the total variability of HbA1c for men, $R^2 = 0.05$.

No significant results were observed for women in relation to any of the chosen predictors (dental visits, level of exercise, level of education, teeth brushing frequency, and alcohol consumption).

4.2. Correlations Between Age and Oral Health Status, Glycemic Control (HbA1c) and Lifestyle Factors

To further explore the nuances in the relationships between the variables, a Pearson correlation analysis was conducted based on age. The only significant correlations identified within this study sample were between age and level of education, as well as age and frequency of dental visits. The results showed a significative correlation R (105) = −0.33, $p < 0.01$, with a medium to large effect size $R^2 = 0.11$, between age distribution and the level of studies, meaning as the age increases, the level of studies decreases. Another significative correlation was found between age and frequency of dental visits, with a R (112) = −0.32, $p < 0.01$, with a medium to large effect size of $R^2 = 0.10$, meaning as the age of participants increased, the frequency of dental visits decreased. As indicated in Table 5, no other significant correlations were observed between age and the remaining variables.

Table 5. Correlations between age and socio-demographic and clinical parameters.

	Age	**HbA1c**	**Studies**	**Alchool Consumption**	**Exercise Freqeuncy**	**Dental Visit**	**Teeth Washing**
earson Correlation	1.00	0.03	−0.33	−0.12	−0.10	−0.33	0.17
Sig. (2-tailed)		0.78	0.00	0.22	0.30	0.00	0.06
N	112.00	111.00	106.00	102.00	112.00	112.00	112.00

5. Discussion

This study explored the intricate relationships between T2DM mellitus, lifestyle factors, and oral health behaviors, providing new insights into the determinants of glycemic control (HbA1c) and their variability among diabetic patients in Romania. Our findings underscore the critical role of lifestyle and education in managing T2DM mellitus, aligning with global research trends while addressing gaps specific to the Romanian population.

The primary goal of diabetes management is achieving optimal glycemic control, yet our study revealed that a substantial proportion of patients with T2DM had poor glycemic control, with a mean HbA1c of 7.95% (SD = ±1.52). This finding aligns with earlier studies that reported high rates of poor glycemic control, ranging from 65% to 81.9% [26,27], further emphasizing the persistent challenge in managing diabetes effectively. However, the proportion remains significantly higher compared to developed countries, such as the United States, where only 12.9% of patients have poor glycemic control [28]. This disparity likely reflects differences in healthcare infrastructure, patient education, and access to resources. For instance, in developed settings, uniform clinical guidelines, comprehensive health insurance, and robust primary care systems likely contribute to better glycemic outcomes. In contrast, our findings suggest that gaps in awareness, adherence to lifestyle modifications, and limited access to dental and medical care may hinder effective management in our study population. This is further supported by the observed negative correlation between HbA1c levels and education level, as well as exercise frequency, highlighting the pivotal role of socioeconomic and behavioral factors in glycemic control.

Previous research has highlighted the relationship between glycemic control and lifestyle factors [29,30].

Similarly, our study identified significant associations between glycemic control and key lifestyle components such as exercise and medical adherence. These findings underscore the critical importance of patient awareness and adherence to disease management and lifestyle modifications in achieving effective diabetes control.

Our study sheds light on the role of physical activity in glycemic control, contributing valuable data to the existing body of research. Previous studies have consistently linked physical inactivity to higher glucose levels and poor glycemic control [31–33].

Our findings confirm this association, demonstrating a significant negative correlation between exercise frequency and HbA1c levels, particularly among male participants (R (66) = −0.26, $p < 0.05$). This suggests that consistent physical activity is associated with better glycemic outcomes. However, a concerning 49.2% of our participants (N = 65) were categorized as physically inactive, with only 22.7% (N = 30) engaging in exercise 1–2 times weekly and 12% (N = 16) exercising five or more times weekly. Furthermore, adherence to both dietary and exercise regimens was limited, with just 30 participants adhering to recommended practices, highlighting a significant gap in lifestyle management. These results emphasize the urgent need for targeted interventions to promote regular exercise and dietary adherence among patients with T2DM. Barriers to physical activity, including lack of awareness, accessibility, or motivation, must be addressed through structured educational programs and individualized support systems. The observed associations reinforce the broader evidence advocating for lifestyle modifications as critical components of effective diabetes management. Interventions tailored to the unique challenges faced by this population could significantly enhance self-management capabilities, reduce HbA1c levels, and ultimately improve health outcomes.

The observed correlations between higher education levels and improved health behaviors, such as more frequent dental visits, reflect the importance of education in fostering awareness and access to preventive care. These results are consistent with existing literature, which highlights education as a significant determinant of health outcomes. This study reinforces the influence of sociodemographic factors on glycemic control, in line with previous findings that younger and less-educated individuals tend to exhibit higher HbA1c levels compared to their older, better-educated counterparts [34]. In our analysis, a significant negative correlation was observed between education level and HbA1c values, indicating that higher education is associated with better glycemic control. This disparity underscores the importance of educational interventions targeted at enhancing diabetes self-management, particularly among younger and less-educated populations, to mitigate the observed gaps in glycemic outcomes.

For men, the negative correlation between education and HbA1c levels emphasizes the broader impact of educational attainment on metabolic control, suggesting that educational interventions might be particularly beneficial for improving diabetes management among this subgroup. Physical activity emerged as a strong negative predictor of HbA1c levels, reinforcing the importance of exercise in diabetes care. This finding aligns with global evidence that regular physical activity improves insulin sensitivity and glycemic control. However, nearly half of the participants reported being inactive, highlighting a critical area for targeted public health interventions. Gender-specific strategies may be necessary, as exercise frequency was significantly associated with HbA1c in men but not in women. This difference suggests potential sociocultural or biological factors influencing health behaviors, which warrant further investigation.

The present study revealed significant gaps in oral hygiene behaviors and dental care among patients with diabetes, paralleling findings from another research. Specifically, 38.6% of our participants brushed their teeth twice daily, slightly below the 49.3% average reported in a systematic review of diabetes patients' oral hygiene practices [35]. Moreover, only 7.6% of participants in our study visited a dentist three or more times annually, with 47.7% not visiting a dentist at all in the past year. This aligns with broader findings showing just over half (54%) of diabetes patients worldwide visit a dentist annually [36], a rate substantially lower than the general population in high-income countries such as England (73%), the U.S. (64%), and Australia [35].

Regarding oral health behaviors, our diabetic group showed suboptimal practices compared to international standards but slightly better adherence to dental visits compared to other Romanian study [37]. For instance, while Sadeghi et al. [38] reported that 83% of participants attended regular dental checkups, our study found that 65.27% of diabetic participants did so, a significant improvement compared to previous local data but still indicative of barriers to consistent preventive care. Additionally, brushing frequency in our diabetic cohort was less frequent than ideal, with only a minority adhering to the recommended twice-daily brushing regimen.

Our findings further support the notion that barriers to regular dental care—such as lack of perceived need, limited awareness, and accessibility issues—are prevalent among diabetic patients. This is particularly concerning given the established bidirectional relationship between periodontal health and glycemic control, where poor oral health can exacerbate diabetes complications. The low adherence to flossing practices, with only a quarter of global diabetes patients flossing daily [35], mirrors our results, suggesting a critical need for improved education on the importance of interdental cleaning.

Interestingly, the frequency of dental visits also predicted HbA1c variability in men, highlighting the link between oral health and systemic health. Periodontal inflammation, which is exacerbated by poor glycemic control, can worsen diabetes outcomes, creating a bidirectional relationship. The present findings suggest that men who visit the dentist more frequently may experience better metabolic control, possibly due to reduced inflammation or heightened health awareness. This connection underscores the need for integrating oral health education and care into diabetes management programs.

For women, while no significant predictors of HbA1c were identified, the positive correlation between education and dental visits suggests a critical role for educational attainment in shaping preventive health behaviors. Women with higher education levels may have better access to dental care and a greater understanding of its importance in overall health. This finding aligns with existing research suggesting that women's health behaviors are influenced by socioeconomic and educational factors, further emphasizing the need for targeted educational programs.

Overall, this study highlights the multifaceted nature of diabetes care, emphasizing the interplay between lifestyle factors, education, and oral health. These findings suggest that effective management of T2DM mellitus requires a holistic approach that integrates lifestyle interventions, educational support, and oral health care. Given the limited focus on these factors in Romania, our results provide a strong foundation for developing tailored public health strategies and patient-centered care models. Future research should aim to explore the underlying mechanisms driving these relationships and evaluate the effectiveness of integrative interventions in improving outcomes for diabetic patients.

This study has several limitations that should be considered when interpreting the findings. First, the cross-sectional design limits the ability to infer causal relationships between lifestyle factors, oral health behaviors, and glycemic control, highlighting the need for longitudinal studies to confirm these associations. Second, reliance on self-reported data for variables such as exercise, alcohol consumption, and oral hygiene behaviors introduces potential reporting bias, as participants may have under- or overreported their habits. The study's focus on a single outpatient facility in western Romania may also restrict the generalizability of findings to other regions or populations with differing socioeconomic or healthcare contexts. Additionally, the relatively small sample size, though reflective of the local population, may have reduced the statistical power to detect smaller effects, especially in subgroup analyses. The p-value requirement for inclusion ($p < 0.05$) was emphasized; however, it should be noted that this predictor is at the upper threshold of significance with a p-value of $p = 0.05$. Consequently, the conclusion should be interpreted with caution.

Another notable limitation is the absence of clinical oral examination data, such as DMFT, plaque index, or gingival index, which could have provided deeper insights into participants' oral health and its relationship with lifestyle and glycemic control. While self-reported oral health behaviors were valuable, they lack the objectivity and detail clinical measures could offer. This omission may have limited the study's ability to explore specific mechanisms linking oral and systemic health. Future research should address these limitations by incorporating larger, more diverse samples, longitudinal designs, and both self-reported and objective measures of lifestyle and health behaviors for a more comprehensive understanding.

6. Conclusions

This study highlights the intricate relationships between lifestyle factors, oral health behaviors, and glycemic control in patients with T2DM mellitus (T2DM). The findings emphasize that both lifestyle and oral health practices play crucial roles in managing glycemic levels, with education emerging as a consistent determinant influencing both metabolic outcomes and preventive health behaviors.

These results underscore the necessity of integrative approaches in diabetes care, combining lifestyle modifications with oral health interventions to optimize metabolic control and improve overall health outcomes in the present sample. Future research should further explore the underlying mechanisms driving these associations and assess the efficacy of combined educational and behavioral interventions. Tailored strategies addressing socioeconomic disparities and fostering patient engagement are essential to achieving comprehensive care for individuals with T2DM.

Author Contributions: Conceptualization, S.P. and A.G.; methodology, R.D. and O B.; software, N.A.T., I.I. and V.T.A.; validation, V.B., R.D. and O.B.; formal analysis, R.S.-R. and D.C.; investigation, S.P., R.D. and V.B.; resources, D.J.; data curation, D.C., V.T.A. and I.A.; writing—original draft preparation, V.B., I.A. and R.D.; writing—review and editing, A.G. and R.S.-R.; visualization, R.D. and S.P.; supervision, A.G.; project administration, A.G.; funding acquisition, D.J. All authors have read and agreed to the published version of the manuscript.

Funding: We would like to acknowledge Victor Babes University Of Medicine and Pharmacy Timisoara for their support in covering the costs of publication for this research paper (Grant Number 4814/02.10.2023). This research is part of a project underway at the "Translational and Experimental Clinical Research Centre in Oral Health, Department of Preventive, Community Dentistry, and Oral Health, University of Medicine and Pharmacy "Victor Babes", Timisoara," which aims to study the risk factors in oral health and their relationship with the quality of life.

Institutional Review Board Statement: The study was conducted in accordance with the Declaration of Helsinki, and approved by the Ethics Committee of the University of Medicine and Pharmacy "Victor Babes", Timisoara, Romania (No. 05/30.01.2024).

Informed Consent Statement: Informed consent was obtained from all subjects involved in the study.

Data Availability Statement: The data presented in this study are available on request from the corresponding author.

Acknowledgments: We would like to acknowledge Victor Babes University of Medicine and Pharmacy Timisoara for their support in covering the costs of publication for this research paper. The authors are really grateful to the staff of the Faculty of Dental Medicine, University of Medicine and Pharmacy "Victor Babes", Timisoara, Romania and The Outpatient Diabetes Care Facility of the Pius Brinzeu County Emergency Hospital Timisoara, Romania. The authors used ChatGPT, an AI language model developed by OpenAI, to exclusively improve the manuscript's language and readability. All the scientific content, the interpretations and conclusions are the original work of the authors.

Conflicts of Interest: The authors declare no conflicts of interest.

ferences

Oluwatoyin, A.E.; Arinola, E.; Olufemi, O.E.; Jokotade, A. Self-Reported Oral Health and Oral Health-Related Quality of Life among Patients with Diabetes Mellitus in a Tertiary Health Facility. *BMC Oral. Health* **2024**, *24*, 181. [CrossRef] [PubMed]

American Diabetes Association Professional Practice Committee; ElSayed, N.A.; McCoy, R.G.; Aleppo, G.; Balapattabi, K.; Beverly, E.A.; Briggs Early, K.; Bruemmer, D.; Ebekozien, O.; Echouffo-Tcheugui, J.B.; et al. 2. Diagnosis and Classification of Diabetes: Standards of Care in Diabetes—2025. *Diabetes Care* **2025**, *48*, S27–S49. [CrossRef] [PubMed]

American Diabetes Association Professional Practice Committee; ElSayed, N.A.; Aleppo, G.; Bannuru, R.R.; Bruemmer, D.; Collins, B.S.; Ekhlaspour, L.; Hilliard, M.E.; Johnson, E.L.; Khunti, K.; et al. 1. Improving Care and Promoting Health in Populations: Standards of Care in Diabetes—2024. *Diabetes Care* **2024**, *47*, S11–S19. [CrossRef] [PubMed]

Available online: https://diabetesatlas.org/ (accessed on 24 October 2024).

Jalkanen, K.; Aarnio, E.; Lavikainen, P.; Jauhonen, H.-M.; Enlund, H.; Martikainen, J. Impact of Type 2 Diabetes Treated with Non-Insulin Medication and Number of Diabetes-Coexisting Diseases on EQ-5D-5 L Index Scores in the Finnish Population. *Health Qual. Life Outcomes* **2019**, *17*, 117. [CrossRef] [PubMed]

Huang, Y.; Cai, X.; Mai, W.; Li, M.; Hu, Y. Association between Prediabetes and Risk of Cardiovascular Disease and All Cause Mortality: Systematic Review and Meta-Analysis. *BMJ* **2016**, *355*, i5953. [CrossRef] [PubMed]

Williams, R.; Karuranga, S.; Malanda, B.; Saeedi, P.; Basit, A.; Besançon, S.; Bommer, C.; Esteghamati, A.; Ogurtsova, K.; Zhang, P.; et al. Global and Regional Estimates and Projections of Diabetes-Related Health Expenditure: Results from the International Diabetes Federation Diabetes Atlas, 9th Edition. *Diabetes Res. Clin. Pract.* **2020**, *162*, 108072. [CrossRef]

Payne, B.J.; Locker, D. Relationship Between Dental and General Health Behaviors in a Canadian Population. *J. Public Health Dent.* **1996**, *56*, 198–204. [CrossRef] [PubMed]

9. Movva, L.R.; Ho, D.K.L.; Corbet, E.F.; Leung, W.K. Type-2 Diabetes Mellitus, Metabolic Control, Serum Inflammatory Fact Lifestyle, and Periodontal Status. *J. Dent. Sci.* **2014**, *9*, 1–9. [CrossRef]
10. Liu, G.; Li, Y.; Pan, A.; Hu, Y.; Chen, S.; Qian, F.; Rimm, E.B.; Manson, J.E.; Stampfer, M.J.; Giatsidis, G.; et al. Adherence t Healthy Lifestyle in Association With Microvascular Complications Among Adults With Type 2 Diabetes. *JAMA Netw. Open* 2(*6*, e2252239. [CrossRef] [PubMed]
11. Stoica, S.A.; Valentini, G.; Dolci, M.; D'Agostino, S. Diabetes and Non-Surgical Periodontal Therapy: What Can We Hope F *Hygiene* **2022**, *2*, 85–93. [CrossRef]
12. Stewart, J.E.; Wager, K.A.; Friedlander, A.H.; Zadeh, H.H. The Effect of Periodontal Treatment on Glycemic Control in Patie with Type 2 Diabetes Mellitus. *J. Clin. Periodontol.* **2001**, *28*, 306–310. [CrossRef] [PubMed]
13. Hopealaakso, T.K.; Thomas, J.T.; Pätilä, T.; Penttala, M.; Sakellari, D.; Grigoriadis, A.; Gupta, S.; Sorsa, T.; Räisänen, Periodontitis, Metabolic Syndrome and Diabetes: Identifying Patients at Risk for Three Common Diseases Using the aMM Rapid Test at the Dentist's Office. *Diagnostics* **2024**, *14*, 2878. [CrossRef]
14. Păunică, I.; Giurgiu, M.; Dumitriu, A.S.; Păunică, S.; Pantea Stoian, A.M.; Martu, M.-A.; Serafinceanu, C. The Bidirectio Relationship between Periodontal Disease and Diabetes Mellitus—A Review. *Diagnostics* **2023**, *13*, 681. [CrossRef] [PubMed
15. Berniyanti, T.; Wening, G.R.S.; Palupi, R.; Setyowati, D.; Putri, C.R. Low Levels of Tumor Necrosis Factor-α Will Prev Periodontitis Exacerbation in Type 2 Diabetes Mellitus. *Eur. J. Dent.* **2022**, *16*, 443–448. [CrossRef]
16. Brivio, F.; Viganò, A.; Paterna, A.; Palena, N.; Greco, A. Narrative Review and Analysis of the Use of "Lifestyle" in Hea Psychology. *Int. J. Environ. Res. Public Health* **2023**, *20*, 4427. [CrossRef]
17. Schellenberg, E.S.; Dryden, D.M.; Vandermeer, B.; Ha, C.; Korownyk, C. Lifestyle Interventions for Patients With and at Risk Type 2 Diabetes: A Systematic Review and Meta-Analysis. *Ann. Intern. Med.* **2013**, *159*, 543. [CrossRef]
18. American Diabetes Association. Diagnosis and Classification of Diabetes Mellitus. *Diabetes Care* **2009**, *32*, S62–S67. [CrossR [PubMed]
19. Commisso, L.; Monami, M.; Mannucci, E. Periodontal Disease and Oral Hygiene Habits in a Type 2 Diabetic Populati Periodontal Disease in Diabetics. *Int. J. Dent. Hyg.* **2011**, *9*, 68–73. [CrossRef] [PubMed]
20. Skamagas, M.; Breen, T.; LeRoith, D. Update on Diabetes Mellitus: Prevention, Treatment, and Association with Oral Disea *Oral Dis.* **2008**, *14*, 105–114. [CrossRef] [PubMed]
21. Available online: https://insse.ro/cms/sites/default/files/field/publicatii/anuarul_statistic_al_romaniei_carte-ed.2022. (accessed on 6 January 2025).
22. Sandu, D. *Actualizarea Indicelui Dezvoltării Umane Locale: De Ce, Cum Și Cu Ce Rezultate (Updating Local Human Development In Why, How and with What Results)*; Research Gate: Berlin, Germany, 2021. [CrossRef]
23. Kamath, D.G.; Nayak, S.U.; Pai, K.K.; Shenoy, R. Knowledge and Awareness of Oral Health among Diabetic Patients- Cross-Sectional Study from Mangalore City. *Int J Diabetes Dev Ctries* **2015**, *35*, 71–75. [CrossRef]
24. Poudel, P.; Griffiths, R.; Wong, V.W.; Arora, A.; George, A. Knowledge and Practices of Diabetes Care Providers in Oral Hea Care and Their Potential Role in Oral Health Promotion: A Scoping Review. *Diabetes Res. Clin. Pract.* **2017**, *130*, 266– [CrossRef] [PubMed]
25. Sayili, U.; Sak, K.; Aydin, S.N.; Kara, B.; Turgut, D.; Bisgin, O. Development, Validity and Reliability of the Healthy Lifest Behavior Scale. *Discov. Public Health* **2024**, *21*, 62. [CrossRef]
26. Teklay, G.; Hussien, J.; Tesfaye, D. Non-Adherence and Associated Factors among Type 2 Diabetic Patients at Jimma Univers Specialized Hospital, Southwest Ethiopia. *J. Med. Sci.* **2013**, *13*, 578–584. [CrossRef]
27. Hailu, E.; Mariam, W.H.; Belachew, T.; Birhanu, Z. Self-Care Practice and Glycaemic Control amongst Adults with Diabetes at Jimma University Specialized Hospital in South-West Ethiopia: A Cross-Sectional Study. *Afr. J. Prim. Health Care Fam. Med.* 2(*4*, a311. [CrossRef]
28. Ali, M.K.; McKeever Bullard, K.; Imperatore, G.; Barker, L.; Gregg, E.W.; Centers for Disease Control and Prevention (CD Characteristics Associated with Poor Glycemic Control among Adults with Self-Reported Diagnosed Diabetes–National Hea and Nutrition Examination Survey, United States, 2007–2010. *MMWR Morb. Mortal Wkly. Rep.* **2012**, *61*, 32–37.
29. Che, M.; Zhou, Q.; Lin, W.; Yang, Y.; Sun, M.; Liu, X.; Liu, H.; Zhang, C. Healthy Lifestyle Score and Glycemic Control in Typ Diabetes Mellitus Patients: A City-Wide Survey in China. *Healthcare* **2023**, *11*, 2037. [CrossRef]
30. Ünver, N. Relationship between the Poor Glycemic Control and Risk Factors, Life Style and Complications. *Biomed. Res.* **2017**, 1581–1586.
31. Sanal, T.; Nair, N.; Adhikari, P. Factors Associated with Poor Control of Type 2 Diabetes Mellitus: A Systematic Review a Meta-Analysis. *J. Diabetol.* **2011**, *2*, 4. [CrossRef]
32. Khattab, M.; Khader, Y.S.; Al-Khawaldeh, A.; Ajlouni, K. Factors Associated with Poor Glycemic Control among Patients w Type 2 Diabetes. *J. Diabetes Its Complicat.* **2010**, *24*, 84–89. [CrossRef] [PubMed]
33. Wang, J.; Li, J.; Wen, C.; Liu, Y.; Ma, H. Predictors of Poor Glycemic Control among Type 2 Diabetes Mellitus Patients Treated w Antidiabetic Medications: A Cross-Sectional Study in China. *Medicine* **2021**, *100*, e27677. [CrossRef]

Badedi, M.; Solan, Y.; Darraj, H.; Sabai, A.; Mahfouz, M.; Alamodi, S.; Alsabaani, A. Factors Associated with Long-Term Control of Type 2 Diabetes Mellitus. *J. Diabetes Res.* **2016**, *2016*, 2109542. [CrossRef] [PubMed]
Poudel, P.; Griffiths, R.; Wong, V.W.; Arora, A.; Flack, J.R.; Khoo, C.L.; George, A. Oral Health Knowledge, Attitudes and Care Practices of People with Diabetes: A Systematic Review. *BMC Public Health* **2018**, *18*, 577. [CrossRef]
Mohd Khairuddin, A.N.; Bogale, B.; Kang, J.; Gallagher, J.E. Impact of Dental Visiting Patterns on Oral Health: A Systematic Review of Longitudinal Studies. *BDJ Open* **2024**, *10*, 18. [CrossRef] [PubMed]
Badea (Paun), A.G.; Bocanet, V.I.; Badea, I.C.; Chifor, R.; Duma, L.T.; Borzan, C.M. Relationship between Behavior and Periodontal Health Self-Perception in Diabetic and Non-Diabetic Patients from Transylvania, Romania—A Self-Report Study, Including the Desire to Use a Mobile App for Oral Care Improvements. *Medicina* **2023**, *59*, 1419. [CrossRef] [PubMed]
Sadeghi, R.; Taleghani, F.; Farhadi, S. Oral Health Related Quality of Life in Diabetic Patients. *J Dent. Res. Dent. Clin. Dent. Prospect.* **2014**, *8*, 230–234. [CrossRef]

Journal of
Clinical Medicine

Article

Comparison of the Effects of Oral Hygiene Instruction Method on Oral Hygiene and Self-Perception in Older Adults: A Randomized Controlled Trial

Inês Caetano Santos [1,2,3,*], Catarina Colaço [1], Giancarlo De la Torre Canales [1,4,5], Luís Proença [1], Mário Polido [1], José João Mendes [1], Helena Canhão [2,3,6] and Ana Cristina Manso [1]

1 Egas Moniz Center for Interdisciplinary Research (CiiEM), Egas Moniz School of Health & Science, 2829-511 Almada, Portugal; ccolaco@egasmoniz.edu.pt (C.C.); gcanales@egasmoniz.edu.pt (G.D.l.T.C.); lproenca@egasmoniz.edu.pt (L.P.); mpolido@egasmoniz.edu.pt (M.P.); jmendes@egasmoniz.edu.pt (J.J.M.); cmanso@egasmoniz.edu.pt (A.C.M.)
2 NOVA Medical School, Faculdade de Ciências Médicas, Universidade Nova de Lisboa, 1169-056 Lisbon, Portugal; helena.canhao@nms.unl.pt
3 Comprehensive Health Research Center (CHRC), Universidade Nova de Lisboa, 1169-056 Lisbon, Portugal
4 Division of Oral Diagnostics and Rehabilitation, Department of Dental Medicine, Karolinska Institutet, SE-14104 Huddinge, Sweden
5 Department of Dentistry, Ingá University Center, Uningá, Paraná 87035-510, Brazil
6 LA REAL, ULS São José, 1900-028 Lisbon, Portugal
* Correspondence: isantos@egasmoniz.edu.pt

Abstract: Background: Age-related conditions, such as being misinformed, having limited oral health literacy, and the loss of manual dexterity, autonomy, or visual acuity, may act as barriers to oral health. The aim of this study was to evaluate the effectiveness of two different oral hygiene instruction methods on oral hygiene and the self-perception of oral health in older adults. **Methods:** This randomized controlled trial included participants aged 65 and older who completed a questionnaire on socio-economic factors, self-perceived oral health, and oral hygiene behaviours. Oral hygiene status was assessed using the Oral Hygiene Index—Simplified (OHI-S). Participants were randomly allocated into two different groups, according to the method of oral hygiene instruction: a "General Approach" (GA) ($n = 28$) and a "Personalized Technique" (PT) ($n = 26$). After two months, a follow-up session was conducted. Data were analysed using descriptive and inferential methodologies. **Results:** The GA and PT methods were effective in promoting oral hygiene behaviours, with a significant increase in the use of interdental devices, but no significant differences were found between the two methods. Self-perceived oral health did not change significantly, neither after the instruction nor between methods. Significant improvements were achieved with both methods for the OHI-S, with significant differences between the two methods for the Calculus Index, where the PT achieved better results. **Conclusions:** Oral hygiene education leads to improvements in the adoption of oral hygiene behaviours and clinical indicators. Furthermore, a personalized approach promoted better results in clinical indicators.

Keywords: oral health; oral hygiene; older; health motivation; self-assessment

1. Introduction

The demographic transition to an ageing society has become a global challenge, with the number of older people expected to increase to 1.5 billion, 16.0% of the total population, by 2050 [1,2]. Despite this rapid worldwide growth, too-limited attention has been given to how older people live, what and how they can contribute to society, and what services and support they may need. Regarding the ageing population, the world remains inadequately prepared to meet the challenges and opportunities of global demographic change [3].

In terms of oral health, there is an increased susceptibility to oral diseases in this age group, such as dental caries and periodontal disease, which can lead to tooth loss, affecting aesthetics, phonetics, and chewing function. Poor oral health also affects overall health, well-being, and quality of life, and oral diseases have been associated with some chronic diseases, such as diabetes and cardiovascular and respiratory diseases [4–7]. In addition, while there are structural factors that promote oral health inequalities, leading to financial constraints on treatment and limited access to oral health care, there are also individual factors, often age-related, that can act as barriers to good oral health, such as misinformation or limited oral health literacy and the loss of manual dexterity, autonomy, or visual acuity, which can lead to some neglect of oral hygiene in terms of toothbrushing and interdental cleaning and oral care concerns [7–10]. This highlights the importance of improving oral health care for vulnerable older adults.

The maintenance of oral health, which is directly related to proper oral hygiene, is highly dependent on two factors: the patient's motivation/cooperation and the patient's ability to perform oral hygiene effectively. Given that bacterial plaque can be effectively removed by proper oral hygiene, there is a need to enhance oral hygiene behaviours and to invest in education and motivation with appropriate oral health interventions that consider the specific needs of this ageing group [11,12]. Oral health education promotes the improvement of general knowledge, which may lead to the adoption of favourable oral health behaviours, which in turn could contribute to a reduction in the prevalence of oral diseases [13].

The results of oral health education can be measured by objective clinical measures of oral health, but self-perceived oral health is a subjective measure that has been shown to be associated with clinical indicators and psychosocial factors and should, therefore, be considered a complementary indicator [14–16]. In addition, subjective measures of oral health involve multiple factors, not only personal experiences but also the environment and social context. In older adults, some studies reported that their self-perception of health is negative, while others report a good self-perception, even with poor oral health [14–19]. It is, therefore, important to assess whether oral health self-perception is modified by education techniques [20]. Notwithstanding this, there is still no consensus on which factor has the greatest impact on improving oral hygiene behaviours, as several studies have tested different theory-based behavioural models, but all of them point to the importance of education and subjective indicators of oral health in patients' compliance with oral hygiene behaviours [21–23].

Although some studies have been conducted on the importance of oral health instruction methods, the literature suggests that the results are still insufficient and that there is a need to implement effective oral health programs that ensure the involvement of the older population to fully assess their impact on oral health [13,24]. In addition, self-perceived oral health has not been included in the assessment of post-intervention changes in previous studies. Furthermore, behavioural studies in older populations are important for introducing or modifying oral health policies to address oral health barriers in this age group [21,22,25]. Thus, the aim of this study was to evaluate the effectiveness of two different oral hygiene instruction methods on oral hygiene and self-perception of oral health in older adults.

2. Materials and Methods

This two-armed randomized controlled trial (RCT) was conducted at a university dental hospital (Egas Moniz Dental Clinic, Almada, Portugal) from 30 January 2023 to 29 May 2023. This study was approved by the Ethics Committee of the Egas Moniz School of Health & Science, Portugal (No. 1131 of 26 January 2023), registered at ClinicalTrials.gov (NCT06444490) and conducted according to the tenets of the Declaration of Helsinki. All participants were thoroughly informed about the aims of this study and provided written consent to participate in the clinical trial. The reporting of data followed the CONSORT checklist [26].

2.1. Participants

A total of 60 participants were recruited as a convenience sample at Egas Moniz Dental Clinic. Inclusion criteria were being over 65 years of age, not being totally edentulous, not being institutionalized, and being able to understand and sign an informed consent form. Participants also had to be able to speak and understand Portuguese, be literate, and be able to comply with the study protocol, i.e., not have disabilities such as blindness, deafness, or dementia.

2.2. Study Protocol, Randomization, and Blinding

In this study, participants completed a questionnaire focusing on socio-economic data, oral hygiene behaviours, and self-perceived oral health (Part A) at baseline. Clinical parameters of participants' oral hygiene were then obtained by intraoral examination (Part B). At this stage, oral hygiene instruction was provided ("General Approach (GA)" or "Personalized Technique (PT)"), depending on the instruction method assigned. Two months later, a follow-up session was conducted. The study flow diagram is shown in Figure 1.

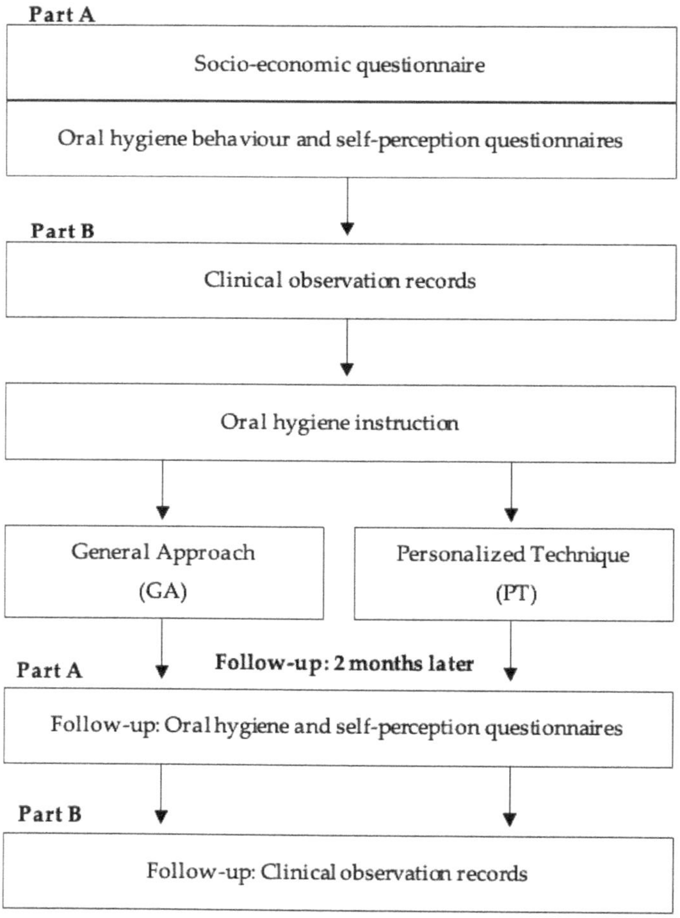

Figure 1. Study flow diagram.

For the oral hygiene instruction, participants were randomly allocated into two groups, with 30 participants (n = 30) in each group, and exposed to different methods of professional education. A computer-generated random number list with allocation concealment was used to assign participants to 1 of the 2 groups (1:1 proportion). This allocation was kept in a sealed envelope, which was not opened until the instruction session. The randomization was performed by an external investigator, not involved in the intervention or assessment. In addition, the researcher responsible for outcome assessment was blinded to intervention allocation.

2.3. Intervention

For oral hygiene instruction, we defined two groups: The first group, identified as the "General Approach" (GA) group, focused more broadly on the different topics of oral diseases and oral hygiene care. Instruction for the second group, identified as the "Personalized Technique" (PT), was based on the specific needs of each participant and was considered the "Tell-Show-Do" method [27]. All oral hygiene instructions were performed by the same dentist in both groups, using a checklist to ensure that the same procedures and topics were covered.

Instruction for the first group, GA, consisted of a 15 min single session in which the dentist attempted to impart knowledge about oral hygiene in general, highlighting some of the most common conditions in this age group, namely the difficulty in achieving correct brushing and interdental cleaning, demonstrating the correct technique on a typodont (model), and alerting them to the importance of oral health to systemic health. Periodontal disease, dental caries and denture care were also covered in general terms. Participants were then given a written explanatory guide to reinforce good oral hygiene habits and an explanation of these diseases. Oral hygiene tools were also provided to encourage the expected improvement in oral health. Finally, there was a question-and-answer session to clarify any doubts the participant might have.

As for the method applied to the second group, the PT is more patient-centred. This approach began with a self-examination using an extraoral mirror by the participant to allow the professional to understand each participant's perception of their oral health and their concerns, and the use of a plaque-disclosing solution to allow the participant to be more sensitive to the areas where brushing and interdental cleaning were not as effective. After understanding the participant's oral hygiene behaviour, the aim was to alert them to the most inappropriate aspects of their oral hygiene and to explain and define the best solutions to adopt to improve it, adapting the oral hygiene tools to their clinical conditions. At this stage, conditions such as dental caries, major gingival recessions, areas of greater inflammation, areas where dental plaque accumulation or even tartar was more visible (both in the mouth and on the denture), xerostomia symptoms, and further denture care were highlighted. The typodont (model) was then used to demonstrate the correct toothbrushing and interdental cleaning techniques, allowing participants to practice brushing and cleaning interdental spaces until they were proficient. In the case of periodontal disease and dental caries, an explanation of these diseases and the benefits of good oral hygiene in preventing their rapid progression was given. The session ended in the same way as the first method, with the participant receiving an explanatory guide and more appropriate tools to promote the expected improvement in oral health. In addition, a personalized plan was created for the participant to take home to improve their oral hygiene techniques. The same question-and-answer session was used to clarify any doubts. This PT method consisted of a single session of approximately 20 min.

2.4. Outcomes

Participants' outcomes were assessed at two time points (baseline and 2 months) over the 2-month study period. Both subjective and objective outcomes were conducted at each evaluation period by a researcher not involved in any other study procedures. For the subjective assessment, a structured questionnaire about socio-economic data, oral hygiene behaviours, and self-perceived oral health was used, while oral hygiene clinical indicators were the objective assessments. The primary outcomes of this study were oral hygiene behaviours and self-perceived oral health. The secondary outcomes were clinical oral hygiene indices (DI-S, CI-S, and OHI-S).

2.4.1. Part A—Socio-Economic Data, Oral Hygiene Behaviours, and Self-Perceived Oral Health

A self-reported structured questionnaire collected information on socio-economic data, including age (years), sex (female/male), whether participants lived alone or not, education level, categorized as primary school or less (≤4 years), or more than primary school (>4 years), and monthly income (<800 EUR/≥800 EUR).

The oral hygiene behaviours questionnaire included brushing frequency (<2x/day/≥2x/day) and use of interdental devices ("Do you use an interdental brush or dental floss?", with yes/no responses). For denture users, the questions surveyed about denture hygiene and care were "Do you clean your denture every day?"; "Do you usually sleep with your dentures on?", with dichotomous (yes/no) responses.

Self-perceived oral health was assessed through the following questions: "How would you describe your oral health?", "How would you describe the condition of your teeth?", and "How would you describe the condition of your gums?". The answers to the questions were classified as poor ("neither satisfied nor unsatisfied", "unsatisfied", and "very unsatisfied") or good ("very satisfied" and "satisfied") [14]. For xerostomia assessment, the survey question was "Do you feel your mouth dry: yes/no?".

2.4.2. Part B—Oral Hygiene Clinical Indicators

Clinical recordings were collected by a single, blinded, and experienced general dentist who had previously been subjected to a calibration procedure on ten patients not included in the study. Measurement reliability and reproducibility were assessed by the intra-class correlation coefficient (ICC), and the intra-examiner agreement was 0.96. The room used for the observations had both natural and artificial lighting. The equipment used included an intraoral mirror, a CPI probe, gloves, a mask, and compresses [28]. Data on the Oral Hygiene Index—Simplified (OHI-S), which is the sum of the arithmetic mean of the Debris Index—Simplified (DI-S) and the Calculus Index—Simplified (CI-S), could be obtained from the clinical records. We then applied the terms "good", "fair", and "poor" to correspond to selected levels of debris and calculus as follows: 0.0 to 0.6 is considered good, 0.7 to 1.8 is deemed fair, and 1.9 to 3.0 is considered poor, with the OHI-S value being the sum of the two: 0.0 to 1.2 (good), 1.3 to 3.0 (fair), and 3.1 to 6.0 (poor) [29].

2.5. Data Analysis

Statistical analyses were performed using IBM SPSS Statistics v.29 software and included descriptive and inferential methodologies. For descriptive analysis, categorical data were presented as frequency and percentage distributions and numerical data as mean and standard deviation (SD). Inferential methodologies included the application of statistical tests, depending on the characteristics of the variables and the type of comparison (Chi-squared test/Fisher's exact test, McNemar test, Student's *t*-tests for independent and paired samples). Effect sizes were identified by calculating Cohen's d and Cramer's V values. A significance level of 5% ($p \leq 0.05$) was established in all inferential analyses.

3. Results

A total of 60 participants were assessed for eligibility. Of these, six participants were lost to follow-up. For the GA, 28 participants completed the follow-up, and for the PT, 26 participants completed this assessment (Figure 2).

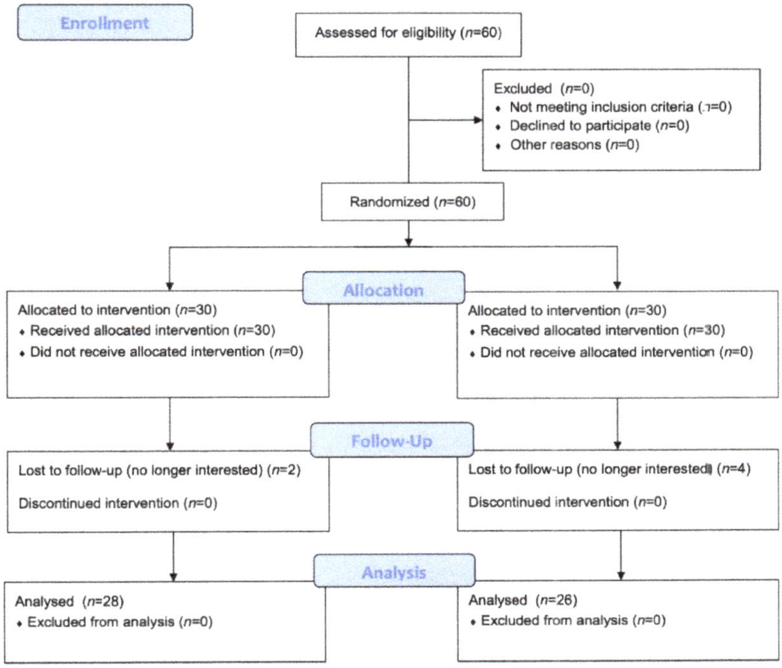

Figure 2. RCT study CONSORT diagram.

3.1. Socio-Economic Characteristics of the Study Participants

Participant characteristics regarding the socio-economic variables are shown in Table 1. Inter-group comparisons showed that the GA group was older (t(df = 53) = 2.021, p = 0.048) and had a lower level of education (χ2(df = 3) = 8.620, p = 0.003) compared to the PT group. No significant differences were found in other socio-economic variables.

Table 1. Socio-economic characteristics and denture use of study participants.

		Total (n = 54)	GA (n = 28)	PT (n = 26)	t Value *	χ2 Value *	Effect Size *	p-Value *
ge (years), mean (± SD)		73.2 (±6.6)	74.9 (±6.6)	71.4 (±6.2)	2.021	-	6.44 [a]	0.048
Sex, n (%)	Female Male	23 (42.6) 31 (57.4)	12 (42.9) 16 (57.1)	11 (42.3) 15 (57.7)	-	0.002	0.006 [b]	0.967
Living alone, n (%)	No Yes	37 (68.5) 17 (31.5)	19 (67.9) 9 (32.1)	18 (69.2) 8 (30.8)	-	0.012	0.015 [b]	0.914
ducation level, n (%)	≤4 years >4 years	19 (35.2) 35 (64.8)	15 (53.6) 13 (46.4)	4 (15.4) 22 (84.6)	-	8.620	0.40 [b]	0.003
Ionthly income (EUR), n (%)	<800 ≥800 NA	7 (13.0) 38 (70.3) 9 (16.7)	6 (21.4) 17 (60.7) 5 (17.9)	1 (3.8) 21 (80.2) 4 (15.4)	-	-	-	-
enture use, n (%)	Yes No	51 (94.4) 3 (5.6)	26 (92.9) 2 (7.1)	25 (96.2) 1 (3.8)	-	0.279	0.07 [b]	0.597

* GA vs. PT (Chi-squared (χ2) test), except for age (Student's t-test for independent samples). Effect size: [a] Cohen's d; [b] Cramer's V. Abbreviations: GA—General Approach; n—number of participants; NA—not answered; PT—Personalized Technique; SD—standard deviation.

3.2. Oral Hygiene Behaviours

Regarding intra-group comparisons and considering oral hygiene behaviours, only the use of an interdental device showed statistically significant improvements between baseline and follow-up in the two instruction method groups (GA: $\chi2(df = 3) = 5.143$, $p = 0.016$; PT: $\chi2(df = 3) = 4.167$, $p = 0.031$). Considering inter-group comparisons, no statistically significant differences were found between the two methods of instruction (Table 2).

Table 2. Changes in oral hygiene behaviours (baseline vs. follow-up) according to instruction method and comparison of oral hygiene behaviours between the two instruction methods.

		GA (*n* = 28)		PT (*n* = 26)			
		Baseline	**Follow-Up**	**Baseline**	**Follow-Up**	**χ2 Value ****	***p*-Value ****
Brushing frequency, *n* (%)	<2x/day ≥2x/day	24 (85.7) 4 (14.3)	1 (3.6) 27 (96.4)	4 (15.4) 22 (84.6)	1 (3.8) 25 (96.2)	0.090	1.000
	χ2 value *	0.800		1.333			
	p-value *	0.375		0.250			
Interdental device, *n* (%)	No Yes	13 (46.4) 15 (53.6)	6 (21.4) 22 (78.6)	10 (38.5) 16 (61.5)	4 (15.4) 22 (84.6)	0.027	0.869
	χ2 value *	5.143		4.167			
	p-value *	0.016		0.031			
Daily denture hygiene, *n* (%)	No Yes	6 (23.1) 20 (76.9)	1 (3.8) 25 (96.2)	0 (0.0) 25 (100.0)	0 (0.0) 25 (100.0)	-	-
	χ2 value *	2.286		-			
	p-value *	0.125		-			
Sleeping with denture, *n* (%)	No Yes	23 (88.5) 3 (11.5)	25 (96.2) 1 (3.8)	20 (80.0) 5 (20.0)	25 (100.0) 0 (0.0)	0.690	0.465
	χ2 value *	0.250		-			
	p-value *	0.625		-			

* Follow-up vs. baseline (McNemar test). ** GA vs. PT (Chi-squared (χ2) test/Fisher's exact test). Abbreviations: GA—General Approach; *n*—number of participants; PT—Personalized Technique.

3.3. Self-Perception of Oral Health

Regarding self-perception of oral health, no significant differences were found for both instruction methods between baseline and follow-up assessments in intra-group comparisons, nor were any found between the two instruction methods (Table 3).

Table 3. Changes in self-perception (baseline vs. follow-up) according to instruction method and comparison of self-perception between the two instruction methods.

		GA(*n* = 28)		PT (*n* = 26)			
		Baseline	**Follow-Up**	**Baseline**	**Follow-Up**	**χ2 Value ****	***p*-Value ***
Oral health perception, *n* (%)	Good Poor	24 (85.7) 4 (14.3)	23 (82.1) 5 (17.9)	23 (88.5) 3 (11.5)	22 (84.6) 4 (15.4)	0.003	1.000
	χ2 value *	0.000		0.000			
	p-value *	1.000		1.000			
Teeth perception, *n* (%)	Good Poor	24 (85.7) 4 (14.3)	24 (85.7) 4 (14.3)	24 (92.3) 2 (7.7)	25 (96.2) 1 (3.8)	0.436	0.604
	χ2 value *	0.000		0.000			
	p-value *	1.000		1.000			

Table 3. *Cont.*

		GA(n = 28)		PT (n = 26)			
		Baseline	Follow-Up	Baseline	Follow-Up	χ2 Value **	*p*-Value **
Gum perception, *n* (%)	Good Poor	24 (85.7) 4 (14.3)	26 (92.9) 2 (7.1)	24 (92.3) 2 (7.7)	25 (96.2) 1 (3.8)	0.147	1.000
	χ2 value *	0.167		0.000			
	p-value *	0.625		1.000			
Xerostomia, *n* (%)	No Yes	16 (57.1) 12 (42.9)	13 (46.4) 15 (53.6)	10 (38.5) 16 (61.5)	9 (34.6) 17 (65.4)	0.436	0.604
	χ2 value *	0.800		0.000			
	p-value *	0.375		1.000			

* Follow-up vs. baseline (McNemar test). ** GA vs. PT (Chi-squared (χ2) test/Fisher's exact test). Abbreviations: GA—General Approach; *n*—number of participants; PT—Personalized Technique.

3.4. Oral Clinical Indicators

Considering intra-group comparisons, the DI-S (GA: t(df = 27) = 8.131, $p < 0.001$; PT: t(df = 25) = 5.447, $p < 0.001$), CI-S (GA: t(df = 27) = 2.299, $p = 0.029$; PT: t(df = 25) = 4.750, $p < 0.001$), and OHI-S (GA: t(df = 27) = 7.485, $p < 0.001$; PT: t(df = 25) = 5.691, $p < 0.001$) ($p < 0.001$) baseline scores decreased at follow-up for both instruction methods (Table 4).

Table 4. Changes in clinical indicators (baseline vs. follow-up) according to instruction method and comparison between the two instruction methods (GA vs. PT).

	Instruction Method	Baseline (b)	Score	Follow-Up (f)	Score	Diff. (f–b)	*t* Value *	Effect Size *	*p*-Value *	*t* Value **	Effect Size **	*p*-Value **
DI-S, Mean (±SD)	GA	0.95 (±0.47)	Fair	0.38 (±0.37)	Good	−0.56 (±0.37)	8.131	0.37	<0.001	−0.526	0.42	0.601
	PT	0.95 (±0.47)	Fair	0.45 (±0.34)	Good	−0.50 (±0.47)	5.447	0.47	<0.001			
CI-S, Mean (±SD)	GA	0.35 (±0.41)	Good	0.23 (±0.30)	Good	−0.12 (±0.27)	2.299	0.27	0.029	2.804	0.35	0.007
	PT	0.55 (±0.41)	Good	0.16 (±0.21)	Good	−0.39 (±0.41)	4.750	0.41	<0.001			
OHI-S, Mean (±SD)	GA	1.30 (±0.71)	Fair	0.61 (±0.59)	Good	−0.68 (±0.48)	7.485	0.48	<0.001	1.162	0.65	0.250
	PT	1.50 (±0.83)	Fair	0.61 (±0.45)	Good	−0.89 (±0.80)	5.691	0.79	<0.001			

* Follow-up vs. baseline (Student's *t*-test for paired samples). ** Difference (f–b): GA vs. PT (Student's *t*-test for independent samples). Effect size: Cohen's d. Abbreviations: b—baseline; CI-S—Calculus Index—Simplified; Diff. (f–b)—difference between follow-up and baseline score values; DI-S—Debris Index–Simplified; f—follow-up; GA—General Approach; OHI-S—Oral Hygiene Index—Simplified; PT—Personalized Technique; SD—standard deviation.

Regarding inter-group comparisons, we found no statistically significant differences between the two methods for DI-S and OHI-S scores. However, a statistically significant difference was observed for the CI-S (t(df = 53) = 2.804, $p = 0.007$), with a higher reduction in the PT method (Table 4).

4. Discussion

To the best of our knowledge, this is the first study conducted in Portugal to assess the effectiveness of two instruction methods on subjective and objective indicators of oral hygiene among older adults. Our findings showed that both instruction methods applied in this study increased the use of interdental cleaning devices, although there were no differences between the methods. However, the PT method obtained significantly better results for the CI-S improvements, even though both methods improved all clinical indicators.

Despite the scientific consensus that brushing is the most effective method of removing plaque, empirical evidence suggests that brushing alone may only remove up to 60% of total plaque during each cleaning session [30]. Additionally, several reports suggest that brushing is more effective at cleaning the facial surfaces of teeth and less effective on the interdental surfaces. This finding is significant because interdental areas are at the highest risk for plaque accumulation on both anterior and posterior teeth [30,31]. Therefore, interdental cleaning devices play a crucial role in the prevention of oral diseases and conditions, such as gingivitis, coronal and interproximal caries, and tooth loss [12,32]. In our study, dental floss and interdental brushes were evaluated collectively, which may have contributed to higher baseline adherence levels than those reported in most studies [33–35], as patient compliance with daily flossing is typically low, largely due to a lack of motivation or difficulties in using dental floss, especially among older adults who may experience decreased dexterity and motor skills [30]. However, the use of interdental brushes is considered to be the most effective for interdental cleaning due to greater ease of use, better ergonomic handlers, and patient acceptance [30]. Therefore, demystifying the existence of easier-to-use interdental cleaning devices appears to be sufficient for patient compliance, which may explain the success of both methods without favouring one over the other.

Despite some variation in reported daily denture care practices in the literature [33,36,37], they tend to be generally high and favourable, aligning with this study's findings and potentially explaining the lack of significant differences between groups. The widespread practice of denture care can be attributed to its accessibility, simplicity, and affordability [33,36]. Moreover, proper denture cleaning is crucial for maintaining good oral health, as it helps prevent unpleasant odours, maintains aesthetic appearance, and prevents the accumulation of dental plaque and calculus, which can lead to oral mucosal lesions that affect overall health, particularly in older adults [38]. It is also recommended to remove dentures when sleeping to prevent stomatitis caused by microorganisms, particularly *Candida albicans*, or by trauma [36,37]. Therefore, education about denture care practices remains essential in daily clinical practice.

Regarding self-perceived oral health, contrary to our results, some studies suggest that knowledge of oral hygiene practices and oral health literacy can impact how patients perceive their oral health [14]. However, it is interesting to note that the perception of gum health in this study showed a tendency to achieve better results after both instruction methods, which could be attributed to better oral hygiene, often associated with a reduction in gingival inflammation [12,22], increasing the perception of gum health.

When examining clinical oral indicators, the PT method obtained significant and the most favourable results for the CI-S. This finding could be because a more individualized approach allowed participants to visibly recognize the accumulation of calculus, which was more apparent than debris, potentially influencing their attitudes towards visiting the dentist for a check-up or professional tooth cleaning. However, it is important to note that participants in the GA group were significantly older and had lower levels of education. These factors might have affected the effectiveness of this instructional method, since older age is often associated with reduced autonomy and dexterity, and lower education levels are linked with reduced oral health literacy, which can be a barrier to maintaining proper oral hygiene practices [9,10,39,40]. Moreover, we observed significant improvements in all oral hygiene clinical indices for both instruction methods at follow-ups, indicating the success and effectiveness of both interventions. Regular interdental cleaning is known to reduce dental plaque, calculus, and gingivitis [30]. Thus, significant improvements in clinical indicators are likely to result from the substantial adherence to interdental cleaning devices found in this study.

As a final note, this study's results indicate that oral hygiene instruction can improve the oral hygiene of older adults, regardless of the method used. This underscores the importance of motivating older adults during dental visits and through educational programs. However, the PT method showed slightly better outcomes, suggesting that personalized and detailed attention enhances results. Nevertheless, the improvements in the GA group demonstrate that benefits can also be achieved through training, lectures, workshops, or even teledentistry. Our results aim to contribute to future national public oral health strategies by demonstrating the importance of expanding oral health motivational and educational interventions to ensure improvements in oral health for older adults. Furthermore, in countries with still-low public sector coverage of dental services and with unequal geographical distributions of oral health care, such as Portugal, preventive dentistry focused on education could help reduce dental treatment costs and inequalities in the burden of oral diseases.

Limitations

This study is not free from limitations. In the present study, the small sample size and the fact that it was a convenience sample limit the generalizability of our findings and our ability to detect minor effects. However, this did not prevent our study from obtaining statistically significant differences in some parameters within and between groups. In addition, we performed an a posteriori power analysis to confirm the adequacy of the sample size. Using the CI-S as a clinical outcome, considering the differences between groups after follow-up, a Cohen's d effect of 0.78 was determined. According to this value, to establish an alpha error of 5% and a power of 80%, a total sample size of 52 participants ($n = 26$ per group) was required. The follow-up period of this study may also be too short to show more robust results. However, we consider it important that this evaluation in this specific population be shorter, so that we do not lose contact with the study participants. Future research on this topic should involve a larger population and a longer period of time. Therefore, this study could be a basis for planning such trials, as there are no studies in the Portuguese elderly population involving oral health education. Another limitation is that the participants in the GA group were significantly older and had lower levels of education than those in the PT group, which may have influenced the more positive results in the latter group. In addition, we did not have a control group without intervention. There may also have been some sample bias due to the fact that this population attends a university clinic, which is often motivated by dental students, and this may have influenced the results. Finally, this study did not consider participants' oral health literacy before and after the intervention and did not include a cognitive–behavioural approach in the intervention evaluation. Further studies could include these aspects when assessing the attitudes and perceptions of older adults.

5. Conclusions

The study results suggest that both the GA and PT instruction methods effectively promote improvements in using interdental cleaning devices and oral hygiene score levels in older adults, with a personalized approach potentially maximizing the clinical outcomes. However, self-perceived oral health did not change significantly either after the instruction method or between methods.

As the global older population continues to grow and life expectancy increases, it is becoming increasingly important to invest in preventative oral and systemic health measures in these patients. A more personalized approach through regular dental visits would be ideal, but a generalized approach could also be considered to improve oral hygiene in this population, providing education and literacy to enable the patient to adopt appropriate behaviours and, thus, prevent potential oral diseases. This generalized approach could be further evaluated in more detail, and, if proven successful and cost-effective in a wider range of studies, it could be useful for national oral health strategies aiming to include older adults with less accessibility to oral health care services.

Author Contributions: Conceptualization, I.C.S., C.C. and H.C.; methodology, I.C.S.; software, I.C.S.; validation, I.C.S., G.D.l.T.C., M.P., H.C., A.C.M. and J.J.M.; formal analysis, I.C.S. and L.P.; investigation, I.C.S. and C.C.; resources, I.C.S.; data curation, I.C.S.; writing—original draft preparation, I.C.S., C.C. and G.D.l.T.C.; writing—review and editing, I.C.S., G.D.l.T.C. and A.C.M.; visualization, I.C.S.; supervision, H.C., M.P., A.C.M. and J.J.M.; project administration, I.C.S. All authors have read and agreed to the published version of the manuscript.

Funding: This research was financed by national funds through the FCT—Foundation for Science and Technology, I.P., under project 10.54499/UIDB/04585/2020.

Institutional Review Board Statement: The study was conducted in accordance with the Declaration of Helsinki and was approved by the Institutional Review Board (or Ethics Committee) of Egas Moniz (ID no. 1131 on 26 January 2023).

Informed Consent Statement: Informed consent was obtained from all subjects involved in the study.

Data Availability Statement: The entirety of the data examined throughout this study can be found in this document. The datasets analysed in the current study are available from the corresponding author upon reasonable request.

Acknowledgments: The authors wish to thank the Egas Moniz—Cooperativa de Ensino Superior, CRL, for scientific and logistical support. We also thank Isabel Varela for her invaluable help during the fieldwork.

Conflicts of Interest: The authors declare no conflicts of interest.

References

1. United Nations: World Population Ageing 2020. Available online: https://www.un.org/development/desa/pd/sites/www.un.org.development.desa.pd/files/undesa_pd-2020_world_population_ageing_highlights.pdf (accessed on 28 May 2024).
2. Poudel, P.; Paudel, G.; Acharya, R.; George, A.; Borgnakke, W.S.; Rawal, L.B. Oral health and healthy ageing: A scoping revi *BMC Geriatr.* **2024**, *24*, 33. [CrossRef]
3. World Health Organization. Progress Report on the United Nations Decade of Healthy Ageing, 2021–2023. Available onli https://iris.who.int/bitstream/handle/10665/374192/9789240079694-eng.pdf?sequence=1 (accessed on 28 May 2024).
4. World Health Organization. Global Oral Health Status Report: Towards Universal Health Coverage for Oral Health by 20 Available online: https://www.who.int/publications/i/item/9789240061484 (accessed on 28 May 2024).
5. Valdivia, A.D.C.M.; Sánchez, M.A.V.; Cortés, D.E.A.; Cortés, E.G. Oral Health: Fundamentals, Importance, and Perspecti In *Human Teeth—From Function to Esthetics*, 1st ed.; Ardelean, L.C., Rusu, L.C., Eds.; IntechOpen: London, UK, 2023; pp. 1- [CrossRef]
6. Gil-Montoya, J.; Ferreira de Mello, A.L.; Barrios, R.; Gonzalez-Moles, M.A.; Bravo, M. Oral health in the elderly patient and impact on general well-being: A nonsystematic review. *Clin. Interv. Aging* **2015**, *10*, 461–467. [CrossRef] [PubMed]
7. Lamster, I.B.; Asadourian, L.; Del Carmen, T.; Friedman, P.K. The aging mouth: Differentiating normal aging from dise *Periodontology 2000* **2016**, *72*, 96–107. [CrossRef] [PubMed]
8. Tuuliainen, E.; Nihtilä, A.; Komulainen, K.; Nykänen, I.; Hartikainen, S.; Tiihonen, M.; Suominen, A.L. The association of fra with oral cleaning habits and oral hygiene among elderly home care clients. *Scand. J. Caring Sci.* **2020**, *34*, 938–947. [CrossRe
9. Chan, A.K.Y.; Tamrakar, M.; Jiang, C.M.; Lo, E.C.M.; Leung, K.C.M.; Chu, C.H. Common Medical and Dental Problems of Ol Adults: A Narrative Review. *Geriatrics* **2021**, *6*, 76. [CrossRef]
10. Schensul, J.J.; Salvi, A.; Ha, T.; Grady, J.; Li, J.; Reisine, S. Evaluating Cognitive/Emotional and Behavioral Mediators of O Health Outcomes in Vulnerable Older Adults. *J. Appl. Gerontol.* **2022**, *41*, 187–197. [CrossRef]
11. Lee, K.H.; Choi, Y.Y.; Jung, E.S. Effectiveness of an oral health education programme for older adults using a workbo *Gerodontology* **2020**, *37*, 374–382. [CrossRef]
12. Murakami, S.; Mealey, B.L.; Mariotti, A.; Chapple, I.L.C. Dental plaque–induced gingival conditions. *J. Periodontol.* **2018**, S17–S27. [CrossRef]
13. Ghaffari, M.; Rakhshanderou, S.; Ramezankhani, A.; Noroozi, M.; Armoon, B. Oral Health Education and Promotion Programm Meta-Analysis of 17-Year Intervention. *Int. J. Dent. Hyg.* **2018**, *16*, 59–67. [CrossRef]
14. Fagundes, M.L.B.; do Amaral Júnior, O.L.; Menegazzo, G.R.; do Nascimento Tôrres, L.H. Factors associated with self-percei oral health in different age groups. *Community Dent. Oral Epidemiol.* **2022**, *50*, 476–483. [CrossRef]
15. Shim, H.; Koo, J.; Ahn, J. Association between Rheumatoid Arthritis and Poor Self-Perceived Oral Health in Korean Adu *Healthcare* **2022**, *10*, 427. [CrossRef]
16. Vettore, M.V.; Ahmad, S.F.H.; Machuca, C.; Fontanini, H. Socio-economic status, social support, social network, dental status, a oral health reported outcomes in adolescents. *Eur. J. Oral Sci.* **2019**, *127*, 139–146. [CrossRef]
17. McNally, M.E.; Matthews, D.C.; Clovis, J.B.; Brillant, M.; Filiaggi, M.J. The oral health of ageing baby boomers: A comparison adults aged 45– 64 and those 65 years and older. *Gerodontology* **2014**, *31*, 123–135. [CrossRef]
18. Andrade, F.B.D.; Teixeira, D.S.C.; Frazão, P.; Duarte, Y.A.O.; Lebrão, M.L.; Antunes, J.L.F. Oral health profile among commun dwelling elderly and its association with self-rated oral health. *Rev. Bras. Epidemiol.* **2018**, *21*, e180012. [CrossRef] [PubMed]
19. Silva, J.V.D.; Oliveira, A.G.R.D.C. Individual and contextual factors associated to the self-perception of oral health in Brazil adults. *Rev. Saude Publica* **2018**, *52*, 29. [CrossRef]

Adunola, F.; Garcia, I.; Iafolla, T.; Boroumand, S.; Silveira, M.L.; Adesanya, M.; Dye, B.A. Self-perceived oral health, normative need, and dental services utilization among dentate adults in the United States: National Health and Nutrition Examination Survey (NHANES) 2011-2014. *J. Public Health Dent.* **2019**, *79*, 79–90. [CrossRef] [PubMed]

Fishbein, M. A Reasoned Action Approach to Health Promotion. *Med. Decis. Mak.* **2008**, *28*, 834–844. [CrossRef] [PubMed]

Schensul, J.; Reisine, S.; Salvi, A.; Ha, T.; Grady, J.; Li, J. Evaluating mechanisms of change in an oral hygiene improvement trial with older adults. *BMC Oral Health* **2021**, *21*, 362. [CrossRef]

Watt, R.G.; Daly, B.; Allison, P.; Macpherson, L.M.D.; Venturelli, R.; Listl, S.; Weyant, R.J.; Mathur, M.R.; Guarnizo-Herreño, C.C.; Celeste, R.K.; et al. Ending the neglect of global oral health: Time for radical action. *Lancet* **2019**, *394*, 261–272. [CrossRef]

Carvalho, C.; Manso, A.C.; Escoval, A.; Salvado, F.; Nunes, C. Self-perception of oral health in older adults from an urban population in Lisbon, Portugal. *Rev. Saude Publica* **2016**, *50*, 53. [CrossRef]

Kakudate, N.; Morita, M.; Sugai, M.; Kawanami, M. Systematic cognitive behavioral approach for oral hygiene instruction: A short-term study. *Patient Educ. Couns.* **2009**, *74*, 191–196. [CrossRef]

Schulz, K.F.; Altman, D.G.; Moher, D.; CONSORT Group. CONSORT 2010 Statement: Updated guidelines for reporting parallel group randomised trials. *BMJ* **2010**, *340*, c332. [CrossRef]

Razak, P.A.; Richard, K.M.J.; Thankachan, R.P.; Hafiz, K.A.A.; Kumar, K.N.; Sameer, K.M. Geriatric oral health: A review article. *J. Int. Oral Health* **2014**, *6*, 110–116.

World Health Organization. Oral Health Surveys: Basic Methods (5th ed). Available online: https://iris.who.int/bitstream/handle/10665/97035/9789241548649_eng.pdf?sequence=1 (accessed on 28 May 2024).

Greene, J.G.; Vermillion, J.R. The Simplified Oral Hygiene Index. *J. Am. Dent. Assoc.* **1964**, *68*, 7–13. [CrossRef] [PubMed]

Ng, E.; Lim, L.P. An Overview of Different Interdental Cleaning Aids and Their Effectiveness. *Dent. J.* **2019**, *7*, 56. [CrossRef]

Agrawal, A.; Sawhney, A.; Panda, S.; Gupta, N.; Amol Khale, P.; Rathod, V.; Singh Makkad, R. Comparison of the Efficacy of Different Oral Hygiene Aids in Maintaining Periodontal Health in Patients With Gingivitis. *Cureus* **2023**, *15*, e44391. [CrossRef] [PubMed]

Elhddad, A.I.; Elnaili, S.A.; Beaayou, H.S.; Bushwigeer, S.S. Denture Hygiene Knowledge, Attitudes and Practices Toward Patient Education in Denture Care among Dental Clinicians in Benghazi City, Libya. *Libyan J. Dent.* **2023**, *7*, 31–37. [CrossRef]

Konstantopoulou, K.; Kossioni, A.E. Association between Oral Hygiene Information Sources and Daily Dental and Denture Care Practices in Urban Community-Dwelling Older Adults. *J. Clin. Med.* **2023**, *12*, 2881. [CrossRef]

Melo, P.; Marques, S.; Silva, O.M. Portuguese self-reported oral-hygiene habits and oral status. *Int. Dent. J.* **2017**, *67*, 139–147. [CrossRef]

Botelho, J.; Machado, V.; Proença, L.; Alves, R.; Cavacas, M.A.; Amaro, L.; Mendes, J.J. Study of Periodontal Health in Almada-Seixal (SoPHiAS): A cross-sectional study in the Lisbon Metropolitan Area. *Sci. Rep.* **2019**, *9*, 15538. [CrossRef]

Algabri, R.; Alqutaibi, A.Y.; Altayyar, S.; Mohammed, A.; Khoshafa, G.; Alryashi, E.; Al-Shaher, S.; Hassan, B.; Hassan, G.; Dammag, M.; et al. Behaviors, hygiene habits, and sources of care among removable complete and partial dentures wearers: A multicenter cross-sectional study. *Clin. Exp. Dent. Res.* **2024**, *10*, e867. [CrossRef]

Cankaya, Z.T.; Yurdakos, A.; Kalabay, P.G. The association between denture care and oral hygiene habits, oral hygiene knowledge and periodontal status of geriatric patients wearing removable partial dentures. *Eur. Oral Res.* **2020**, *54*, 9–15. [CrossRef]

Atri, M.; Lamba, G.S. Assessment of Oral Health Status and Treatment Needs in Geriatric Day Care Centers in New Delhi. *Ann. Int. Med. Dent. Res.* **2023**, *9*, 59–80. [CrossRef]

Dibello, V.; Zupo, R.; Sardone, R.; Lozupone, M.; Castellana, F.; Dibello, A.; Daniele, A.; De Pergola, G.; Bortone, I.; Lampignano, L.; et al. Oral frailty and its determinants in older age: A systematic review. *Lancet Healthy Longev.* **2021**, *2*, e507–e520. [CrossRef]

Veladas, F.M.V.; De la Torre Canales, G.; de Souza Nobre, B.B.; Escoval, A.; Pedro, A.R.; de Almeida, A.M.; Assunção, V.A.; Manso, A.C. Do sociodemographic factors influence the levels of health and oral literacy? A cross-sectional study. *BMC Public Health* **2023**, *23*, 2543. [CrossRef]

Journal of
Clinical Medicine

MDPI

Article

Oral Health-Related Quality of Life in a Paediatric Population i[n] the Dominican Republic

David Ribas-Perez [1,*], Carlos Muñoz-Viveros [2], Angel Luis Formoso-Veloso [1], Francisco Jesus Carrillo-Sanchez [1], Luis El Khoury-Moreno [1], Julio Torrejon-Martinez [1] and Antonio Castaño-Seiquer [1]

1 Department of Stomatology, University of Seville, 41004 Seville, Spain; pacocarrillo11@gmail.com (F.J.C.-S.); lelkhoury@us.es (L.E.K.-M.); jtorrejon1@us.es (J.T.-M.); acastano@us.es (A.C.-S.)
2 Kerr Corporation, Orange, CA 91766, USA; cmunozviveros@yahoo.com
* Correspondence: dribas@us.es

Abstract: Introduction: During the summer of 2019 and within the framework of a social dentistry program carried out in the low-income town of San Francisco de Macorís (Dominican Republic), a descriptive study was carried out on oral health-related quality of life (OHRQoL), aiming to find out the oral health status of a population of children in the aforementioned Dominican city. **Objective:** The aim of this study was to describe the oral health status of a child population and its relationship with the quality of life perceived by these children in the aforementioned population of San Francisco de Macorís in order to develop an specific oral health program taking into account not only the existing oral health status but also the perceptions and feelings of the child population in this regard. **Method:** A descriptive cross-sectional study was carried out on a representative sample of children who were examined on their oral health status, following WHO guidelines, by professionals from the University of Seville (Spain) together with professionals from private practice (USA) and students from the Universidad Católica Nordestana (UCNE, Dominican Republic). Likewise, the children's parents voluntarily completed the Oral Quality of Life questionnaire COHIP-19 in its culturally adapted Spanish version. **Results:** For this purpose, 94 children with a mean age of 10.34 (SD 3.38) were observed in our study following WHO recommendations for oral health studies and evaluating OHQoL using the specific questionnaire validated in Spanish COHIP-19 in its short format (SF). The results show a state of oral health with a significant prevalence of caries (80.9%) and a DMFT of 1.70 (SD 1.90). The OHQoL perceived by these children shows that pain, bad breath or feeling sad because of the condition of their teeth were the factors with the worst evaluation score. **Conclusions:** The conclusion that mainly emerges from this study is that caries continues to be the main problem to be solved (more than other variables studied, such as malocclusion or fluorosis), and this ailment also causes pain, dysfunction, and bad breath and is therefore perceived as a problem to be solved in the children of this Dominican city.

Keywords: oral health-related quality of life (OHRQoL); Child Oral Health Impact Profile-19 Short Form (COHIP-19SF); Dominican Republic

1. Introduction

Oral health is an indivisible part of the general health of any child. As we know, depending on the age of the child, they can be in a stage of primary, mixed, or permanent dentition. According to the Global Burden of Disease Study, in 2017, more than 530 million children worldwide had dental caries in their primary teeth. Traditionally, dental treatment of primary dentition has not been given sufficient attention, even though it can cause a large number of infections with their significant associated repercussions. There is also a clear relationship between caries in the primary dentition and its appearance in the permanent dentition [1,2].

Caries can have a significant impact on children, families, and societies. The disease begins in the primary teeth, may continue in the permanent teeth, and has an inescapable impact on overall health and oral quality of life throughout life. Caries may be related to other common childhood diseases, mainly due to risk factors in common with other non-communicable diseases, e.g., high sugar intake, and with diseases related to other health disorders such as obesity [3,4].

Dental problems may make chewing and sleeping difficult and restrict children's life activity. Severe dental caries is associated with growth deficiencies, and in addition, caries can become an economic burden on the family and society; treatment of caries for extensive dental repair is particularly costly and unaffordable for many families [5].

All this can be obviously related to an inadequate oral quality of life, since the functions performed within the oral cavity can be altered and, in many cases, severely hindered or even prevented by oral disorders such as caries, which are easily preventable. On the other hand, the self-esteem of children suffering from oral diseases can be affected by this alteration of oral functions [6,7].

When establishing a situational analysis prior to the implementation of specific oral health programs, it is necessary to carry out epidemiological surveys to evaluate the human and economic resources necessary to carry out the program, thus better linking the program to the real and perceived needs of the population [8].

Traditionally, cross-sectional oral health studies have been carried out with a description of the health–disease status of the community, with data showing caries, periodontal diseases, and/or malocclusions to be the dominant conditions [9]. Recent studies have shown that other sociocultural factors, such as self-esteem and self-perception in community health, should also be considered for the structuring, design, and implementation of this type of oral health program. This is where the inclusion of oral quality of life surveys comes in for the prior and much-needed situational analysis.

A variety of questionnaires have been developed to measure oral quality of life for adults [10–12]. However, because children and adolescents have different quality of life issues compared to adults [13], several instruments have been developed in recent decades to measure oral quality of life in paediatric populations, despite the difficulties associated with the development and validation of such instruments [14].

These include the Oral Health Outcome Scale for 5-year-olds, the Paediatric Oral Health-Related Quality of Life Measure [15,16], and the Child Oral Impacts on Daily Performance Index [17]. However, the most frequently used self-completed quality of life scales for children are the Children's Perceptions Questionnaire (CPQ) and the Children's Oral Health Impact Profile (COHIP) [18,19].

The COHIP (Community Oral Health Improvement Plan), which was originally developed to assess "oral–facial well-being" across a range of ages (8–15 years) and ethnicities [19–22], is also a comprehensive and well-validated questionnaire for determining children's OHRQoL. It contains 34 questions and 5 subscales (oral health, functional well-being, socio-emotional well-being, school environment, and self-image). The COHIP questions cover areas in the area of oral and maxillofacial health, as well as the inclusion of positive aspects of oral quality of life such as self-confidence and looking attractive).

The COHIP Short Form (COHIP-SF) 19 is an abbreviated version of the scale, developed in 2012, which contains 19 items and 4 subscales (self-image, oral health, functional well-being and socio-emotional well-being). In this abbreviated form, the psychometric properties of the original version are well maintained, and it can be administered more quickly, which facilitates the assessment of oral quality of life in clinical studies. For the interpretation of this questionnaire, we have, on the one hand, to analyze the final score of the questionnaire. On the other hand, we must also analyze the average score of each dimension and the score of each question individually [19–24].

In certain areas of the world that are more socioeconomically maligned, poorer oral health has been shown, and we assume that this results in poorer quality of life. Studies such as the one we have carried out in children to demonstrate this relationship between poor oral health and a low quality of oral life, which in principle would be a presupposition, are lacking.

The objective of the present study was to describe the oral health status of a population of children in the Dominican Republic (in terms of caries, fluorosis, and malocclusions) and its relationship with the oral quality of life perceived by these children using the COHIP 19 SF, with the final objective of carrying out an oral health program focused on the population studied.

2. Materials and Methods

2.1. Study Type and Settings

A cross-sectional study was carried out in the city of San Francisco de Macorís (Dominican Republic), Urbanización Vista del Valle, the subjects of which were 94 children between 4 and 16 years of age. These children attended the Dental Outreach Program co-organized by professionals from private practice (USA), the University of Seville, and the Universidad Católica Nordestana (UCNE, Dominican Republic) and were selected during the summer of 2019. All the children whose parents agreed to participate in the study and who did not present any type of severe systemic pathology that could alter the study were considered.

For the start of the measurements, written informed consent was requested from the parents or legal guardians, considering the international provisions of the Declaration of Helsinki (modification of Edinburgh 2000).

2.2. Data Collection

Data collection was carried out in two stages: first, clinical examinations were performed in portable dental units to obtain diagnoses of oral health status, applying the methodology recommended by the WHO in its book *Oral Health Surveys Basic Methods*, fourth edition [25]. Following these indications, caries, fluorosis (Dean's index) and malocclusion indices were obtained.

In a second phase, the children's parents completed the COHIP-19SF questionnaire that assessed levels of perception of Quality of Life related to oral health. Specifically, this questionnaire assesses four dimensions (functional well-being, socio-emotional well-being, oral health and self-image).

This questionnaire was previously evaluated for face validity by two examiners in a pilot test to assess its comprehension and to compare the different scores obtained with the theory. It contains 19 questions with a single response option on a 5-point Likert scale (ranging from never to always) and includes information on associated sociodemographic factors (age, sex, birth place).

2.3. Study Variables and Statistical Analysis

To conduct the statistical analysis for the oral health status and levels of perception of oral health-related quality of life, the means, standard deviation, frequency distribution, and percentages were calculated.

Relationships between variables were evaluated using the Chi-square test to test for statistical significance, assuming a statistically significant association when the p value was less than 0.05. All estimator values were adjusted from the sample design. The statistical program SPSS version 27 for Windows was used for the analysis.

3. Results

Of the 94 children seen in the operation, the mean age was 10.34 (SD 3.38). To facilitate the analysis, we grouped the children into small (under 6 years), medium (between 6 and 12 years), and large (over 12 years, up to 16 years). Of these three groups, the most frequent was the medium group with more than 50% of the children seen (57.4%) (Table 1).

Table 1. Distribution of the sample by age group.

	Frequency (n)	Percentage (%)
Small < 6 years	15	16.0
Medium	54	57.4
Large > 12 years	25	26.6
Total	94	100.0

A similar number of boys and girls (55.3% of children) were seen, almost all of whom were from San Francisco de Macoris (74.5%) and to a lesser extent from adjacent neighbourhoods.

Regarding dental anomalies, fluorosis was very rare (only clearly perceptible in 5.4% of the children) and it can be affirmed that more than half of the children had orthodontic needs (55.4% with slight or moderate malocclusions), as seen in Table 2.

Table 2. Distribution of the sample by sex, origin, fluorosis, and malocclusion.

		Frequency (n)	Percentage (%)
Gender	Boys	52	55.3
	Girls	42	44.7
	Total	94	100.0
City	San Francisco de Macoris	70	74.5
	Santiago	16	17.0
	La Vega	8	8.5
	Total	94	100.0
Fluorosis (Dean index)	No fluorosis	82	87.2
	1 Dean	7	7.4
	2 Dean	4	4.3
	3 Dean	1	1.1
	Total	94	100.0
Malocclusion	None	42	44.7
	Light	48	51.0
	Mild or severe	4	4.3
	Total	94	100.0

The prevalence of caries found was significant (80.9%) with a mean DMFT of 1.70 (SD 1.90) and a dft of 1.86 (SD 2.04) for the total sample, although it is true that this index needs to be analyzed by age (Table 3).

Table 3. dft and DMFT in the sample.

	Mean	Dev.
dft (temporary)	1.86	2.040
DMFT (permanent)	1.70	1.905

When analysing each of the questions in the COHIP SF-19 questionnaire, we see the distribution in percentage of each answer to each question, as well as the mean and SD. In each of the 19 questions that make up the COHIP19 SF questionnaire, there are five possible answers that can be given, using a Likert scale from 0 to 4 where 0 corresponds to never and 4 to always (in terms of the frequency of occurrence with respect to the question asked). For each question, a mean was found with its corresponding standard deviation, as shown in Table 4.

Table 4. COHIP 19SF responses distribution; mean and SD.

Question	0 Never	1 Hardly Ever	2 Sometimes	3 Frequently	4 Always	Mean	SD
P1. Had pain in your teeth/toothache	44 (46.8%)	29 (30.8%)	16 (17%)	4 (4.3%)	1 (1.1%)	0.82	0.939
P2. Had crooked teeth or spaces between your teeth	52 (55.3%)	21 (22.3%)	15 (16%)	6 (6.4%)	0	0.73	0.952
P3. Had discoloured teeth or spots on your teeth	33 (35.1%)	31 (33%)	18 (19.1%)	7 (7.4%)	5 (5.4%)	1.15	1.145
P4. Had bad breath	29 (30.9%)	32 (34%)	20 (21.3%)	9 (9.6%)	4 (4.3%)	1.22	1.118
P5. Had bleeding gums	44 (46.8%)	22 (23.4%)	20 (21.3%)	6 (6.4%)	2 (2.1%)	0.94	1.066
P6. Been unhappy or sad	47 (50%)	20 (21.3%)	19 (20.2%)	3 (3.2%)	5 (5.3%)	0.93	1.148
P7. Missed school for any reason	31 (33%)	46 (48.9%)	13 (13.8%)	4 (4.3%)	0	0.89	0.796
P8. Been confident	32 (34.1%)	40 (42.5%)	19 (20.2%)	2 (2.1%)	1 (1.1%)	0.94	0.853
P9. Had difficulty eating foods you would like to eat	55 (58.5%)	19 (20.2%)	13 (13.8%)	7 (7.5%)	0	0.7	0.971
P10. Felt worried or anxious	37 (39.4%)	34 (36.2%)	17 (18.1%)	4 (4.3%)	2 (2%)	0.94	0.971
P11. Not wanted to speak/read out loud in class	60 (63.8%)	16 (17%)	17 (18.1%)	1 (1.1%)	0	0.56	0.824
P12. Avoided smiling or laughing with other children	64 (68.1%)	14 (14.9%)	14 (14.9%)	1 (1.1%)	1 (1%)	0.52	0.864
P13. Had trouble sleeping	64 (68.1%)	14 (15.9%)	15 (16%)	0	0	0.5	0.8
P14. Been teased, bullied, or called names by other children	66 (70.2%)	13 (13.8%)	11 (11.7%)	3 (3.2%)	1 (1.1%)	0.51	0.901
P15. Felt that you were attractive (good-looking)	26 (27.7%)	50 (53.1%)	17 (18.1%)	1 (1.1%)	0	0.93	0.707
P16. Felt that you look different	21 (22.3%)	47 (50.1%)	24 (25.5%)	2 (2.1%)	0	1.07	0.751
P17. Had difficulty saying certain words	29 (30.9%)	39 (41.5%)	20 (21.3%)	6 (6.4%)	0	1.03	0.885
P18. Had difficulty keeping your teeth clean	20 (21.3%)	45 (47.9%)	24 (25.5%)	5 (5.3%)	0	1.15	0.816
P19. Been worried about what other people think about your...	31 (33%)	32 (34%)	26 (27.7%)	5 (5.3%)	0	1.05	0.908
Social–emotional well-being subscale (p6–7, p10–12, p14, p16, p19)						0.92	1.086
Functional well-being subscale (p9, p13, p17–18)						0.84	0.88
Oral health subscale (p1–p5)						0.97	1.044
Self-image subscale (p8 y p15)						0.93	0.78

For the analysis of this table and taking into account the results obtained from the measure of centralization that can provide us with the most information (mean with its SD), we see that there is a generalized tendency for the answers to be never or almost never, in many cases comprising almost 80% of the answers to this question (this is true for questions p1 (77.6%), p2 (77.6%), p7 (81.9%), p9 (78.7%), p11 (80.8%), p12 (83%), p13 (84%), and p14 (84%).

More focused responses with more frequent values of 1 and 2 were given for the questions between p16 and p19, with values ranging from 75.6% for p16 to 61.7% for p19.

Negative values with answers of 3 and 4 were almost not seen in the sample, the most striking being for question p6 with a value of 5.3% for the answer of always.

The overall mean COHIP-19 SF for all the patients was 14.01, with an SD of 16.73. This gives us a mean COHIP-19 value with an acceptable self-perception of their oral health, as can be seen in Figure 1. In this same graph, it can be seen that the median is even lower than that (12.10), meaning that more than 50% of the respondents show very good values of self-perception of their oral health.

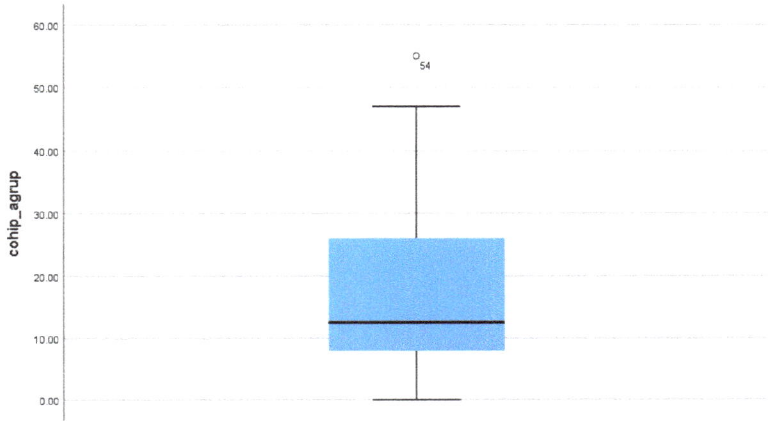

Figure 1. Final COHIP-19 cluster plot for the sample.

Within the areas of study that can be encompassed according to the COHIP 19 questions are oral health (from question p1 to p5), functional well-being (p6, p7 p9, p10 p11, p12 p14 and p19), socio-emotional well-being (p13, p16, p17 and p18) and self-image (p8 and p15). If we analyze the mean of each of these subareas, we can see that the mean of oral health is 0.97 (SD 1.044), that of functional well-being is 0.84 (SD 0.88), that of socio-emotional well-being 0.92 (SD 1.086), and that of self-image 0.93 (SD 0.78).

When we relate each of the answers to each question with the different sociodemographic variables and pathologies studied, we can assess whether the relationship between them is statistically significant or not (it will be when the p value is <0.05 (Table 5). For example, with respect to age, there is statistical significance in questions p4, p5, p6, p11, and p18. Regarding sex, the p value was less than 0.05 in questions p1, p4, p7, and p8. The population of origin was not a variable that caused statistically significant differences to appear with respect to the questions of the COHIP-19 questionnaire.

With regard to caries and its relationship with the questions, there are statistically significant differences in questions p1 to p8, p10, and p15. In this case, moreover, the higher the number of caries, the worse the overall COHIP-19 scores, as can be seen graphically in Figure 2a.

With regard to malocclusion, there are only differences in question p9. It can also be seen that the existing difference in terms of caries is not seen in terms of malocclusion, with the means being similar in the children's responses regarding their oral quality of life regardless of whether or not they have malocclusion (Figure 2b).

Table 5. Correlation between variables. * Statistical significance for d value at $p < 0.05$.

QUESTION	Age	Gender	City	Caries	Malocclusio
P1. Had pain in your teeth/toothache	0.263	0.026 *	0.144	0.012 *	0.115
P2. Had crooked teeth or spaces between your teeth	0.173	0.072	0.175	0.038 *	0.086
P3. Had discoloured teeth or spots on your teeth	0.158	0.101	0.186	0.000 *	0.489
P4. Had bad breath	0.030 *	0.034 *	0.593	0.001 *	0.160
P5. Had bleeding gums	0.001 *	0.080	0.328	0.042 *	0.454
P6. Been unhappy or sad	0.001 *	0.942	0.054	0.021 *	0.452
P7. Missed school for any reason	0.098	0.043 *	0.544	0.000 *	0.117
P8. Been confident	0.322	0.009 *	0.367	0.000 *	0.752
P9. Had difficulty eating foods you would like to eat	0.60	0.310	0.209	0.103	0.037 *
P10. Felt worried or anxious	0.155	0.661	0.450	0.046 *	0.106
P11. Not wanted to speak/read out loud in class	0.012 *	0.656	0.209	0.415	0.429
P12. Avoided smiling or laughing with other children	0.293	0.304	0.156	0.176	0.175
P13. Had trouble sleeping	0.330	0.463	0.322	0.179	0.330
P14. Been teased, bullied, or called names by other children	0.178	0.727	0.336	0.311	0.844
P15. Felt that you were attractive (good-looking)	0.246	0.382	0.137	0.026 *	0.567
P16. Felt that you look different	0.198	0.406	0.401	0.171	0.977
P17. Had difficulty saying certain words	0.298	0.824	0.911	0.152	0.986
P18. Had difficulty keeping your teeth clean	0.027 *	0.464	0.280	0.051	0.426
P19. Been worried about what other people think about your...	0.937	0.594	0.082	0.109	0.748
Socio-emotional well-being					
Functional well-being					
Oral health					
Self-image					

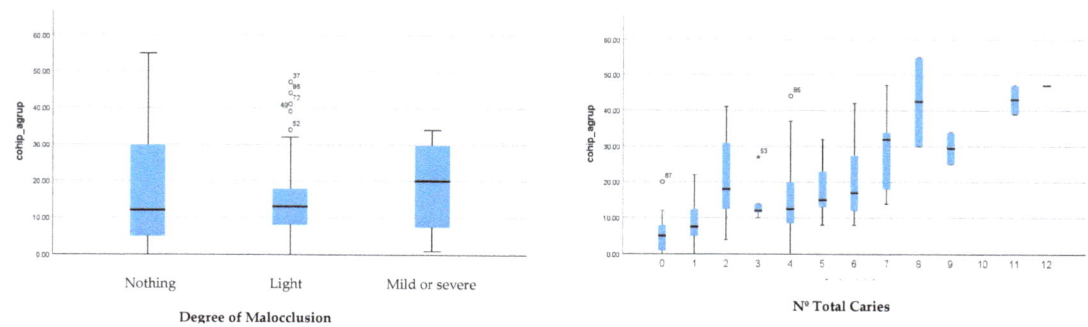

(a) (b)

Figure 2. Relationship between degree of malocclusion and (**a**) number of total caries and (**b**) final COHIP score14.

4. Discussion

One limitation of the study we have just presented is that it is a descriptive study in which the participants involved were those who attended the social project, so there was no sample selection. However, it does serve as a starting point for the future planning of oral health programs in the community.

4.1. Oral Quality of Life and Oral Pathology

In our study, the prevalence of caries was 80.9%. Taking (as a reference) the age of 12 years for comparison between the different studies, the prevalence is somewhat lower, with a percentage of 68.6%. In neighbouring countries, the prevalence values are very different, with data ranging from 35% in the study of Antigua and Barbuda to similar data in studies such as one in Haiti in 2005 [26]. If we compare them with data from the European Union, the prevalence values are far from those in countries such as Sweden, with 5.4%, or Spain, with 11.6% [25–27] (Table 6).

Table 6. Caries prevalence and DMFT in countries of the area at 12 years.

Country, Year	Caries Prevalence 12 Years	DMFT 12 Years
Bahamas 2000	54.5%	1.56
Antigua y Barbuda 2006	35.9%	0.90
Cuba 2000	54.5%	1.56
Dominican Republic 2008	--	8.66
Haiti 2005	71.9%	4.37
Jamaica 1995	41.0%	1.08
Puerto Rico 2011	69.0%	2.5
San Fco Macoris 2019	**68.6%**	**1.70**
Sweden 2020	5.4%	0.42
Spain 2020	11.6%	0.58

Access to healthcare should also be considered. Studies carried out in Sweden, the USA, Canada, and Australia [28–31] show that it is possible to achieve a significant reduction in the prevalence of dental caries when preventive strategies and improved accessibility to healthcare are taken into account.

As in our study, there are different studies that present similar results in terms of the correlation between the state of oral health and the socio-economic level of the individuals and in the demand for dental treatment. Although dentists are the main agents responsible for oral health, it is argued that there is also a duty of society to promote oral health education strategies, especially when there is an impact on quality of life and general health [32–34].

In this context, we believe that oral health education initiatives for young children implemented in general paediatrics and in the school setting should be valued. On the other hand, we also consider the education of the general population on the impact of oral disease on the quality of life when aesthetic and functional characteristics are compromised to be of great relevance.

Once again, we argue that prevention of childhood caries is essential, not only as a clinical problem for oral health professionals but also as a necessity in terms of oral health policy. Like other types of healthcare, considering the needs of children and families in oral healthcare will produce greater satisfaction and better compliance with medical recommendations [35–38].

As has been advocated in medical education and other health professionals' education, in the practice of dentistry, attitudes may be trained and developed according to patient-centred clinical models, which advocate consideration of the patient and family's needs, respect for their preferences and lifestyles, and participation in decision making for appropriate treatment plans. Patient-centred clinical methods and the attitudes consonant with them on the part of healthcare professionals result in an approach suitable to the child and his or her family as well as sound reasoning about aspects of quality of life [39–47].

The availability and accessibility of oral healthcare therefore depends not only on parental information and knowledge but also on the ability and financial resources of the family. In another study conducted in Italy and published in 2013 [48], it is stated that dental treatments are mainly provided by private health professionals; therefore, oral healthcare is mainly financed by direct payments from families or to a lesser extent through public schemes or private health insurance.

It is concluded that this fact endangers the most disadvantaged socio-economic populations because they do not manage to take care of their health; consequently, it leads to decreased resistance to oral and other diseases. Additionally, in Canada, there are discrepancies in access to oral healthcare because it is not included in the Canadian National Health Service, so the lower socio-economic classes have worse caries rates [49–51]. Thus, oral and dental health may be integrated into overall health promotion programs for families, using principles similar to the common risk factor approach [52–55].

Family-centred interventions aimed at health promotion suggest a suitable approach that can be incorporated into general health plans, always taking into consideration the specific characteristics of groups and communities [54,55]. Some studies argue that the family is the primary source of information on health, with mothers playing a fundamental role in modelling behaviours and attitudes related to healthy habits. In addition, the attitudes and values acquired in the early ages will influence the following stages and active responsibility for individual health [56].

Although health information in the family environment is developing, research also shows that some subjects never receive it. For this reason, the school has an important role in the creation of healthy environments and in the discussion of health-related topics [54,55].

As with caries, other oral pathologies also pose challenges regarding early interventions in prevention and health promotion. We also advocate for the need to resort to preventive strategies for malocclusion, since we recognize that some of the behaviours that are the basis of this type of pathology can be avoided and modified through the use of methodologies to provide information to parents and educators.

4.2. Oral Health Quality of Life: Early Intervention

Currently, there are no published studies regarding the Dominican Republic on oral health data in school children and no research on oral health-related quality of life. For this reason, it is difficult to compare the global results of the present study due to the lack of studies in the same geographic area. However, we know of different studies that assess oral health-related quality of life using scales such as the one used (COHIP-19 or ECOHIS) in early childhood in other countries—such as the USA, Turkey, Brazil, and China—either using non-probability samples or studying specific groups such as families of different socio-economic levels [57–63].

The results of our study confirm the hypothesis that alterations in oral health such as caries or alterations in occlusion affect the quality of life of preschool children and their families. Caries is the parameter that has the greatest impact on quality of life. As in other studies, malocclusions do not have such a great impact because there is no statistically significant association between COHIP 19 values and malocclusion [62–67].

This result shows that in the evaluation of oral health-related quality of life made by parents, they tend to consider caries first as a perceived health indicator. This fact is probably due to the consequences of caries perceived by parents as more severe and prolonged, causing them to neglect other oral health conditions that are as equally clinically complex [65].

The study by Martins-Júnior et al. conducted in Brazil with a population-based sample of preschool children corroborates the relationship between caries and oral health-related quality of life [59]. Analogous to what we found in our study, in this publication parents value caries in young children as a primary indicator of oral health-related quality of life. As in other age groups, oral health problems in children have an impact on quality of life because pain, discomfort, and functional limitation affect physical, psychological, and social capacity, which translates into difficulties in nutrition, language pronunciation, and socialization, as well as low self-esteem and irritability, among other issues [32,66].

The results in our work show an increase in the prevalence of caries with increasing age of the children, as it is related to the COHIP score. Thus, in older children, due to the permanence of the teeth for a longer period, they are subject to more aggressive pathologies and to developing more oral pathological symptoms. The age of the child influences the COHIP score, which agrees with the findings described in a Brazilian study [32].

The conclusion that older children have an increased likelihood of experiencing a negative impact on quality of life seems to be rooted in the fact that older children have more advanced-stage caries and have a greater and better ability to communicate with parents about the effect of oral health conditions on their quality of life.

This finding reinforces once again the need to consider early childhood oral health education as a priority. Caries lesions were associated with a negative impact on the quality of life of the students and their families, and traumatic dental lesions are also associated with worse quality of life [32].

Accordingly, the literature confirms that in children in whom a negative impact of oral health status on quality of life is found, the most frequently reported complaints are related to caries and to their developmental stage: pain, difficulty eating some foods and hot or cold drinks, sleep problems, irritability, and self-image problems when smiling [59,65–67].

Some authors argue that the mean COHIP score reflects an association between the presence of caries at different stages of development and impact on quality of life, with 40% to 69% of parents/caregivers reporting an impact on the child's quality of life according to the demand (or lack thereof) for treatment [66].

These data show that the demand for dental treatment may depend on the perception of the child's oral health conditions and eventual consequences [59]. In our study, perceptions of oral health were considered poorer than those of general health, which we can say is due to a concern on the part of parents who have been evaluated by oral health professionals because they are not as knowledgeable about the state of oral health because it is more specific. In addition, many of the children in our study had never been seen by a dentist, a fact that we verified empirically but which was also reported to us by those responsible for the school establishments.

For this reason, we believe that the commentary provided by us on the oral health of each child within his or her family will be very useful. Possibly, in this case, the socio-economic resources of the family will be reflected in the overall health of the child. The impact of oral disease on quality of life was perceived by parents to be negative; this occurred when the child presented caries or the need for treatment.

5. Conclusions

Although it must be taken into account that the data of this study correspond to a descriptive study without control of sample selection (since it was carried out on patients attending a social program), we can conclude that Dominican children have a prevalence of caries that is above the average of the surrounding countries and a perceived quality of oral health that does not correspond to this state of oral health.

These data show the need to carry out oral health programs focused on the treatment of caries (due to the damage it causes) rather than malocclusions, which do not have such a high impact on the quality of life of these disadvantaged populations.

Author Contributions: Conceptualization, D.R.-P. and C.M.-V.; methodology, A.C.-S.; software, D.R.-P.; validation, D.R.-P., A.L.F.-V. and J.T.-M.; investigation, D.R.-P. and L.E.K.-M.; resources, C.M.-V.; data curation, A.L.F.-V. and F.J.C.-S.; writing—original draft preparation, D.R.-P.; writing—review and editing, D.R.-P.; visualization, A.C.-S.; supervision, A.C.-S.; project administration, C.M.-V.; funding acquisition, C.M.-V. All authors have read and agreed to the published version of the manuscript.

Funding: The study was partially funded by The Envista Smiles Foundation, a non-profit organization.

Institutional Review Board Statement: The study was conducted in accordance with the Declaration of Helsinki and approved by the Fundacion Odontologia Social Ethics Committee (protocol code 002/19 approved 15 July 2019).

Informed Consent Statement: Informed consent was obtained from all parents or legal guardians of the subjects involved in the study.

Data Availability Statement: Data will be available from the corresponding authors if required.

Acknowledgments: Luis Esmurdoc, Vice-Rector for International Affairs, UCNE.

Conflicts of Interest: Author Carlos Muñoz-Viveros is a full time employee and Director of Clinical Affairs for Kerr Corporation, a division of Envista Holding Crop, the other authors declare no conflicts of interest.

References

1. Peres, M.A.; Macpherson, L.M.D.; Weyant, R.J.; Daly, B.; Venturelli, R.; Mathur, M.R.; Listl, S.; Celeste, R.K.; Guarnizo-Herre C.C.; Kearns, C.; et al. Oral diseases: A global public health challenge. *Lancet* **2019**, *394*, 249–260; Erratum in *Lancet* **2019**, *394*, 1([CrossRef] [PubMed]
2. Petersen, P.E.; Bourgeois, D.; Ogawa, H.; Estupinan-Day, S.; Ndiaye, C. The global burden of oral diseases and risks to oral hea *Bull. World Health Organ.* **2005**, *83*, 661–669. [PubMed] [PubMed Central]
3. Jin, L.J.; Lamster, I.B.; Greenspan, J.S.; Pitts, N.B.; Scully, C.; Warnakulasuriya, S. Global burden of oral diseases: Emerg concepts, management and interplay with systemic health. *Oral Dis.* **2016**, *22*, 609–619. [CrossRef] [PubMed]
4. Caplan, D.J.; Weintraub, J.A. The oral health burden in the United States: A summary of recent epidemiologic studies. *J. D Educ.* **1993**, *57*, 853–862. [CrossRef] [PubMed]
5. Bawaskar, H.S.; Bawaskar, P.H. Oral diseases: A global public health challenge. *Lancet* **2020**, *395*, 185–186. [CrossRef] [PubM
6. Chaffee, B.W.; Rodrigues, P.H.; Kramer, P.F.; Vítolo, M.R.; Feldens, C.A. Oral health-related quality-of-life scores differ socioeconomic status and caries experience. *Community Dent. Oral Epidemiol.* **2017**, *45*, 216–224. [CrossRef] [PubMed] [PubM Central]
7. Thomson, W.M.; Broder, H.L. Oral-Health-Related Quality of Life in Children and Adolescents. *Pediatr. Clin. N. Am.* **2018**, 1073–1084. [CrossRef] [PubMed]
8. Splieth, C.H.; Christiansen, J.; Foster Page, L.A. Caries Epidemiology and Community Dentistry: Chances for Future Impro ments in Caries Risk Groups. Outcomes of the ORCA Saturday Afternoon Symposium, Greifswald, 2014. Part 1. *Caries Res.* **2(** *50*, 9–16. [CrossRef] [PubMed]
9. Llodra Calvo, J.C.; Bourgeois, D. Estudio Prospectivo Delphi la Salud Bucodental en España 2020. In *Tendencias y Objetivos deSa Oral*; Revista del Consejo de Dentistas: Madrid, Spain, 2009.
10. Broder, H.L.; Wilson-Genderson, M.; Sischo, L. Reliability and validity testing for the Child Oral Health Impact Profile-Redu (COHIP-SF 19). *J. Public Health Dent.* **2012**, *72*, 302–312, Erratum in *J. Public Health Dent.* **2013**, *73*, 86. [CrossRef] [PubM [PubMed Central]
11. Gilchrist, F.; Rodd, H.; Deery, C.; Marshman, Z. Assessment of the quality of measures of child oral health-related quality of *BMC Oral Health* **2014**, *14*, 40. [CrossRef] [PubMed] [PubMed Central]
12. Tinanoff, N.; Reisine, S. Update on Early Childhood Caries since the Surgeon General's Report. *Acad. Pediatr.* **2009**, *9*, 396– [CrossRef]
13. Foster Page, L.; Thomson, W.M.; Baker, S.; Bekes, K. Chapter 10: Oral Health-Related Quality of Life and Coronal Caries. *Mon Oral Sci.* **2023**, *31*, 205–220. [CrossRef] [PubMed]
14. Minamidate, T.; Haruyama, N.; Takahashi, I. The development, validation, and psychometric properties of the Japanese vers of the Child Oral Health Impact Profile-Short Form 19 (COHIP-SF 19) for school-age children. *Health Qual. Life Outcomes* **2020**, 224. [CrossRef] [PubMed] [PubMed Central]
15. Birkeland, J.M.; Broch, L.; Jorkjend, L. Caries experience as predictor for caries incidence. *Community Dent. Oral Epidemiol.* **199** 66. [CrossRef]
16. Tesch, F.C.; Oliveira, B.H.; Leão, A. Mensuração do impacto dos problemas bucais sobre a qualidade de vida de crianças: Aspec conceptuais e metodológicos. *Cad. Saúde Pública* **2007**, *23*, 2555–2564. [CrossRef]
17. Contaldo, M.; Della Vella, F.; Raimondo, E.; Minervini, G.; Buljubasic, M.; Ogodescu, A.; Sinescu, C.; Serpico, R. Early Childhc Oral Health Impact Scale (ECOHIS): Literature review and Italian validation. *Int. J. Dent. Hyg.* **2020**, *18*, 396–402. [CrossR [PubMed]
18. De Stefani, A.; Bruno, G.; Irlandese, G.; Barone, M.; Costa, G.; Gracco, A. Oral health-related quality of life in children using child perception questionnaire CPQ11-14: A review. *Eur. Arch. Paediatr. Dent.* **2019**, *20*, 425–430. [CrossRef] [PubMed]
19. Broder, H.L.; Wilson-Genderson, M. Reliability and convergent and discriminant validity of the Child Oral Health Impact Pro (COHIP Child's version). *Community Dent. Oral Epidemiol.* **2007**, *35* (Suppl. S1), 20–31. [CrossRef] [PubMed]
20. Skandrani, A.; El Osta, N.; Pichot, H.; Eschevins, C.; Pereira, B.; Tubert-Jeannin, S. Validation of the French version of COHIP-SF among 12-years children in New Caledonia. *BMC Oral Health* **2022**, *22*, 358. [CrossRef] [PubMed] [PubMed Central]

Li, C.; Xia, B.; Wang, Y.; Guan, X.; Yuan, J.; Ge, L. Translation and psychometric properties of the Chinese (Mandarin) version of the Child Oral Health Impact Profile-Short Form 19 (COHIP-SF 19) for school-age children. *Health Qual. Life Outcomes* **2014**, *12*, 169. [CrossRef] [PubMed] [PubMed Central]
Arheiam, A.A.; Baker, S.R.; Ballo, L.; Elareibi, I.; Fakron, S.; Harris, R.V. The development and psychometric properties of the Arabic version of the child oral health impact profile-short form (COHIP-SF 19). *Health Qual. Life Outcomes* **2017**, *15*, 218. [CrossRef] [PubMed] [PubMed Central]
El Osta, N.; Pichot, H.; Soulier-Peigue, D.; Hennequin, M.; Tubert-Jeannin, S. Validation of the child oral health impact profile (COHIP) french questionnaire among 12 years-old children in New Caledonia. *Health Qual. Life Outcomes* **2015**, *13*, 176. [CrossRef] [PubMed] [PubMed Central]
BaniHani, A.; Deery, C.; Toumba, J.; Munyombwe, T.; Duggal, M. The impact of dental caries and its treatment by conventional or biological approaches on the oral health-related quality of life of children and carers. *Int. J. Paediatr Dent.* **2018**, *28*, 266–276. [CrossRef] [PubMed]
WHO. *Oral Health Surveys: Basic Methods*, 5th ed.; World Health Organization: Geneva, Switzerland, 2013.
Alburquerque, Y.; Teresa, M.; Méndez, M.L.A. Impacto de Las Enfermedades Orales en la Calidad de Vida Relacionada a Salud Oral en América Latina y El Caribe: Una Revisión Sistemática. Licentiate Thesis, Universidad Científica del Sur, Lima, Peru, 2021.
de Santos Rita, D.R.; María, I. Analisis de Salud Oral y su Impacto en la Calidad de Vida de la Población Preescolar del Municipio de Cascais, Portugal, en 2012. Ph.D. Thesis, Universidad de Sevilla, Seville, España, 2016.
Nunn, M.; Dietrich, T.; Singh, H.K.; Henshaw, M.M.; Kressin, N.R. Prevalence of Early Childhood Caries Among Very Young Urban Boston Children Compared with US Children. *J. Public Health Dent.* **2009**, *69*, 156–170. [CrossRef] [PubMed]
Wennhall, I. *The Rosengård Study: Outcome of an Oral Health Programme for Preschool Children in a Low Socio-Economic Multicultural Area in the City of Malmö, Sweden*; Department of Paediatric Dentistry, Faculty of Odontology, Malmo University: Holmbergs, Malmo, 2008.
Locker, D.; Matear, D. *Oral Disorders, Systemic Health, Well-Being and Quality of Life: A Summary of Recent Research Evidence*; University of Toronto: Toronto, ON, Canada, 2000.
Hallet, K.B.; O'Rourke, P.K. Pattern and severity of early childhood caries. *Community Dent. Oral Epidemiol.* **2006**, *34*, 25–35. [CrossRef]
Ramos-Jorge, J.; Pordeus, I.A.; Ramos-Jorge, M.L.; Marques, L.S.; Paiva, S.M. Impact of untreat dental caries on quality of life of preschool children: Different stages and activity. *Community Dent. Oral Epidemiol.* **2014**, *42*, 311–322. [CrossRef]
Bissar, A.; Schiller, P.; Wolff, A.; Niekusch, U.; Schulte, A.G. Factors contribute to severe early childhood caries in south-west Germany. *Clin. Oral Investig.* **2014**, *18*, 1411–1418. [CrossRef]
Agarwal, D.; Sunitha, S.; Reedy, C.V.K.; Machale, P. Early childhood caries prevalence, severity and pattern in 3–6 year old preschool children of Mysore City, Karnataka. *Pesqui. Bras. Odontopediatria Clínica Integr.* **2012**, *12*, 561–565. [CrossRef]
Abdel-Tawab, N.; Rotter, D. The relevance of client-centered communication to family planning settings in developing countries: Lessons from the Egyptian experience. *Soc. Sci. Med.* **2002**, *54*, 1357–1368. [CrossRef]
Cvengros, J.A.; Christensen, A.J.; Hillis, S.L.; Rosenthal, G.E. Patient and physician attitudes in the health care context: Attitudinal ssymmetry predicts patient satisfaction and adherence. *Ann. Behav. Med.* **2007**, *33*, 262–268. [CrossRef]
Krupat, E.; Rosenkranz, S.L.; Yeager, C.M.; Barnard, K.; Putman, S.M.; Inui, T.S. The practice orientation of physicians and patients: The effect of doctor-patient congruence on satisfaction. *Patient Educ. Couns.* **2000**, *39*, 49–59. [CrossRef]
Mast, M.S.; Kindlimann, A.; Langewitz, W. Recipients' perspective in breaking bad news: How you put it really makes a difference. *Patient Educ. Couns.* **2005**, *58*, 244–251. [CrossRef] [PubMed]
Laine, C.; Davidoff, F. Patient-centered medicine: A professional evolution. *J. Am. Med. Assoc.* **1996**, *275*, 152–156. [CrossRef]
Stewart, M. Towards a global definition of patient-centred care. *Br. Med. J.* **2001**, *322*, 444–445. [CrossRef] [PubMed]
Olsson, L.; Hansson, E.; Ekman, I.; Karlsson, J. A cost-effectiveness study of patient-centred integrated care pathway. *J. Adv. Nurs.* **2009**, *65*, 1626–1635. [CrossRef]
Stewart, M. Effective physician-patient communication and health outcomes. *Can. Med. Assoc. J.* **1995**, *152*, 1423–1443.
Zolnierek, K.B.H.; Di Matteo, M.R. Physician communication and patient adherence to treatment: A meta-analysis. *Med. Care* **2009**, *47*, 826–834. [CrossRef] [PubMed]
Street, R.L.; Krupat, E.; Bell, R.A.; Kravitz, R.; Haidet, P. Beliefs about control in the physician-patient relationship: Effect on communication in medical encounters. *J. Gen. Intern. Med.* **2003**, *18*, 609–616. [CrossRef] [PubMed]
Grilo, A.M.; Santos, M.C.; Rita, J.S.; Gomes, I.S. Assessment of nursing students and nurses' orientation towards patient-centeredness. *Nurse Educ. Today* **2014**, *34*, 35–39. [CrossRef] [PubMed]
Duggan, P.S.; Geller, G.; Cooper, L.A.; Beach, M.C. The moral nature of patient-centeredness: Is it "just the right thing to do"? *Patient Educ. Couns.* **2006**, *62*, 271–276. [CrossRef]
Mead, N.; Bower, P. Patient-centredness: A conceptual framework and review of the empirical literature. *Soc. Sci. Med.* **2000**, *51*, 1087–1110. [CrossRef]
Congiu, G.; Campus, G.; Sale, S.; Spano, G.; Cagetti, M.G.; Lugliè, P.F. Early childhood caries and associated determinants: A cross-sectional study on Italian preschool children. *J. Public Health Dent.* **2014**, *74*, 147–152. [CrossRef]
Leake, J.; Jozzy, S.; Uswak, G. Several dental caries, impacts and determinants among children 2–6 years of age in Inuvik Region, Northwest Territories, Canada. *J. Can. Dent. Assoc.* **2008**, *74*, 519.

50. Schroth, R.J.; Harrison, R.L.; Moffatt, M.E. Oral health of indigenous children and the influence of early childhood caries childhood health and well-being. *Pediatr. Clin. N. Am.* **2009**, *56*, 1481–1499. [CrossRef]
51. Rowan-Legg, A. Oral health care for children—A call for action. *Paediatr. Child Health* **2013**, *18*, 37–43. [CrossRef]
52. Oliveira, W.F.; Forte, F.D.S. Construindo o significado da saúde bucal a partir de experiência com mães. *Pesqui. Bras. Odontope tria Clínica Integr.* **2011**, *11*, 183–191. [CrossRef]
53. Wyne, A.H.; Al-Ghannam, N.A.; Al-Shammery, A.R.; Khan, N.B. Caries prevalence, severity and pattern in preschool child *Saudi Med. J.* **2002**, *23*, 580–584. [CrossRef]
54. Antonarakis, G.S. Integrating dental health into a family-oriented health promotion approach in Guatemala. *Health Promot. Pr* **2011**, *12*, 79–85. [CrossRef]
55. Smyth Chamosa, E.S.; González Novoa, M.C.; Taracido, S. Educación para la salud en Odontología Comunitaria. In *Odontolc Preventiva y Comunitaria: La Odontología Social. Un Deber, una Necesidad, un Reto*, 1st ed.; Castaño Seiquer, A., Ribas Pérez, D., E Fundación Odontología Social: Sevilla, Spain, 2012; pp. 725–737.
56. Blake, H.; Dawett, B.; Leighton, P.; Rose-Brady, L. School-based educational intervention to improve children's oral health-rela knowledge. *Health Promot. Pract.* **2015**, *16*, 571–582. [CrossRef]
57. Divaris, K.; Lee, J.Y.; Baker, A.D.; Vann, W.F., Jr. Caregivers' oral health literacy and their young children's oral health-real quality of life. *Acta Odontol. Scand.* **2012**, *70*, 390–397. [CrossRef]
58. Scarpelli, A.C.; Oliveira, B.H.; Tesch, F.C.; Leão, A.T.; Pordeus, I.A.; Paiva, S.M. Psychometric properties of the Brazilian vers of the Early Childhood Oral Health Impact Scale (B-ECOHIS). *BMC Oral Health* **2011**, *11*, 19. [CrossRef]
59. Martins-Júnior, P.A.; Vieira-Andrade, R.G.; Corrêa-Faria, P.; OliveiraFerreira, F.; Marques, L.S.; Ramos-Jorge, M.L. Impact of ea childhood caries on the oral health-related quality of life of preschool children and their parents. *Caries Res.* **2013**, *47*, 211– [CrossRef] [PubMed]
60. Lee, G.H.; McGrath, C.; Yiu, C.K.; King, N.M. Translation and validation of a Chinese language version of the Early Childhc Oral Health Impact Scale (ECOHIS). *Int. J. Paediatr. Dent.* **2009**, *19*, 399–405. [CrossRef] [PubMed]
61. Abanto, J.; Carvalho, T.S.; Mendes, F.M.; Wanderley, M.T.; Bönecker, M.; Raggio, D.P. Impact of oral diseases and disorders oral health-related quality of life of preschool children. *Community Dent. Oral Epidemiol.* **2011**, *39*, 105–114. [CrossRef] [PubM
62. Pani, S.C.; Badea, L.; Mirza, S.; Elbaage, N. Differences in perceptions of early childhood oral health-related quality of life betw fathers and mothers in Saudi Arabia. *Int. J. Paediatr. Dent.* **2011**, *22*, 244–249. [CrossRef] [PubMed]
63. Leal, S.C.; Bronkhorst, E.M.; Fan, M.; Frencken, J.E. Untreated cavitated dentine lesions: Impact on children's quality of *Caries Res.* **2012**, *46*, 102–106. [CrossRef] [PubMed]
64. Aldrigui, J.M.; Abanto, J.; Carvalho, T.S.; Mendes, F.M.; Wanderley, M.T.; Bönecker, M.; Raggio, D.P. Impact of traumatic der injuries and malocclusions on quality of life of young children. *Health Qual. Life Outcomes* **2011**, *9*, 78. [CrossRef] [PubMed]
65. Welbury, R.R.; Whitworth, J.M. Traumatic injuries to the teeth. In *Paediatric Dentistry*, 3rd ed.; Welbury, R.R., Duggal, M.S., Ho M.T., Eds.; Oxford University Press: Oxford, UK, 2008; pp. 257–294.
66. Montero, J.; Rosel, E.; Barrios, R.; López-Valverde, A.; Albaladejo, A.; Bravo, M. Oral health-related quality of life in 6- 12-year-old schoolchildren in Spain. *Int. J. Paediatr. Dent.* **2016**, *26*, 220–230. [CrossRef] [PubMed]
67. Ribas-Pérez, D.; Sevillano Garcés, D.; Rodriguez Menacho, D.; Hernandez-Franch, P.V.; Barbero Navarro, I.; Castaño Séiquer Cross-Sectional Study on Oral Health-Related Quality of Life Using OHIP-14 in Migrants Children in Melilla (Spain). *Child* **2023**, *10*, 1168. [CrossRef]

Journal of
Clinical Medicine

MDPI

icle

ıctors Influencing the Choice of Conservative and Surgical rocedures in Dental Patients from Poland: A Single-Center etrospective Analysis

cper Łaganowski [1], Martyna Ortarzewska [1], Kornela Cieślik [2], Jakub Jankowski [1]
l Kacper Nijakowski [1,*]

1 Department of Conservative Dentistry and Endodontics, Poznan University of Medical Sciences, 70 Bukowska Street, 60-812 Poznan, Poland; k.laganowski@ump.edu.pl (K.Ł.); mortarzewska@ump.edu.pl (M.O.); jjankowski41@wp.pl (J.J.)
2 University Center of Dentistry and Specialized Medicine, 70 Bukowska Street, 60-812 Poznan, Poland; k.cieslik@ucs.poznan.pl
* Correspondence: kacpernijakowski@ump.edu.pl

Abstract: Background/Objectives: Oral health behaviors can be shaped by various factors, both global (such as the COVID-19 pandemic) and individual (e.g., gender, age). This retrospective study aims to assess the factors influencing the choice between conservative and surgical dental procedures among patients based on the example of the university specialized center in Poznan. **Methods**: We explored the patient dataset from the University Center of Dentistry and Specialized Medicine (Poznan, Poland), covering the period from 1 January 2017 to 31 December 2023. A total of 182,654 medical records were analyzed, focusing on procedures such as restorations, endodontic interventions, and extractions. Multivariate logistic regression and multidimensional correspondence analyses were employed to assess the impact of demographic factors (age and gender) and tooth-specific characteristics on clinical decisions. **Results**: Females, particularly younger, were more likely to choose restorative procedures, while males, especially those over 50, predominantly underwent surgical procedures. Endodontic treatments were most common in males aged 18–30, primarily for maxillary anterior teeth and premolars. Molar extractions, especially in the mandible, were the most frequent surgical procedure. Maxillary teeth, particularly canines and premolars, were more likely to be treated conservatively. **Conclusions**: Economic factors, limited treatment access, and variations in patient preference influenced the observed patterns. Despite a national trend toward increased conservative treatments, disparities persisted based on age, gender, and tooth type. These findings emphasize the need for targeted prevention strategies and equitable access to advanced dental care.

Keywords: gender; tooth restoration; root canal treatment; dental surgery; age; decision making

1. Introduction

The general health status and health behaviors of individuals are shaped by various factors, both external and individual. While some of these factors, such as age or gender, are unmodifiable, others, like income, education, and lifestyle choices, can be influenced or modified. Individual characteristics, including gender, age, income, and education, play a significant role in determining health behaviors and decisions related to oral health and dental care. Research highlights the impact of these factors on oral health. Poor oral hygiene and less engagement in health maintenance are often linked to male gender, low income, rural residential area, and lower educational attainment [1–7].

Gender, in particular, stands out as a strong determinant. Males generally exhibit poorer oral health, less consistent hygiene practices, and fewer or less regular dental check-ups and treatment compared to females. These findings underscore the need for gender-specific strategies to enhance oral health and address gender disparities. Beyond hygiene habits, gender also influences emotional well-being and perceptions of oral health. Studies associate poorer self-assessment of oral health and higher dental anxiety levels with males, who also tend to have a greater prevalence of general diseases [5,6,8–10].

Dental fear remains a significant barrier to seeking care. Encouragingly, recent trends indicate a reduction in dental anxiety among schoolchildren and young adults benefiting from public dental health programs that emphasize prevention and psychological support. Despite these advancements, dental fear persists at concerning levels, necessitating further refinement of psychological approaches to patient care [11]. Additional determinants of health behaviors include living conditions, sociocultural factors, and access to healthcare services. These factors significantly affect patients' overall health and their willingness to engage in oral health practices [1,2,12]. The interplay of these external and individual influences highlights the complex nature of medical decision making and the importance of addressing diverse factors to improve health outcomes.

According to the latest report on the oral health of Poles, conducted between 2016 and 2020 in the Greater Poland region, the incidence of tooth decay (dmft/DMFT > 0) showed a concerning increase with age, rising from 21.0% in children aged 3 to 89.0% by the age of 18. Dental calculus was present in one out of four 12-year-olds and nearly half of 18-year-olds. Among adults aged 35–44, the prevalence of dental caries reached a staggering 98.7%, with a dental caries index of 16.5%. Additionally, only 31.5% of individuals in this age group had a healthy periodontium. In older adults aged 65–74, 18.8% were edentulous, and the DMFT index (decayed, missing, and filled teeth) was alarmingly high (24.9). The percentage of individuals with a healthy periodontium was nearly 25%, though edentulism or residual dentition limited precise analysis. The authors of this study highlight some improvements compared to earlier reports on the Polish population, including reductions in the percentage of edentulous individuals, decreased caries intensity, increased retention of natural teeth, reduced treatment needs, and improved periodontal health among adults [1]. However, despite these positive trends, the results remain troubling. The demographic and socioeconomic disparities highlight the need for targeted interventions to bridge gaps in oral healthcare access and outcomes.

Previous studies have shown the influence of global factors on the spectrum of dental procedures performed and thus indicated the need to take a closer look at individual factors depending on patients and their preferences [13,14]. This retrospective analysis aims to explore the impact of factors such as gender and age on the choice of specific dental procedures within restorative dentistry, endodontics, and surgery. Additionally, the study examines the relationship between particular dental services and the treatment of individual tooth groups or the extent of dental procedures required.

2. Materials and Methods

2.1. Study Design, Setting, and Sample

This retrospective analysis focused on patient records from the University Center of Dentistry and Specialized Medicine (Poznan, Poland). The University of Medical Sciences in Poznan is the leading academic center in central Poland. The analyzed period was between 1 January 2017 and 31 December 2023.

The patient dataset was provided from outpatient departments that maintained operations during the first wave of the COVID-19 pandemic in 2020, specifically the Clinic of Conservative Dentistry and Periodontology, the Clinic of Oral Surgery, and the Central Dental Clinic. All patients from these three clinics, both children and adults, were included. The number of patients was determined by year, divided by gender and age (Table 1).

Table 1. The number of patients from selected outpatient departments in the University Center of Dentistry and Specialized Medicine (Poznan, Poland) from 1 January 2017 to 31 December 2023.

	0–18		19–30		31–50		>51	
	F	**M**	**F**	**M**	**F**	**M**	**F**	**M**
2017	792	667	4800	3773	4716	3932	5354	3741
2018	715	629	4584	3499	4367	3711	4982	3488
2019	661	630	4468	3503	4305	3929	5044	3963
2020	568	461	3064	2175	3255	2935	3133	2216
2021	772	614	4193	2937	4293	3577	3809	3141
2022	980	723	4631	3023	5124	4321	4579	3551
2023	1138	1024	4563	3111	5764	4610	4861	3750

Legend: F, females; M, males.

2.2. Data Collection

The medical database of patients was based on the software KS-SOMED v.2024.03.0.07 (Kamsoft, Katowice, Poland). The system generated data on all visits from the examined period, taking into account demographic data (gender, age on the day of the visit) and visit data (date, clinic, performed procedure based on ICD-9, location in oral cavity). Selected procedures in restorative dentistry (i.e., temporary fillings, refunded, or commercial restorations), endodontics (i.e., intervention procedures, root canal fillings), and dental surgery (i.e., extractions) were analyzed in detail.

2.3. Data Analysis

The radar plot was used to present the percentages of procedures performed in the specific tooth number. Next, the distributions of these specific procedures were demonstrated depending on the gender and age group of patients, as well as the extent of them. The proportions between the two groups were compared with the Z test for independent proportions.

Also, the odds ratios were calculated for the surgical procedures vs. the conservative procedures (restorative and endodontic procedures) using univariate logistic regression modeling. To explore the relationship between personal factors and the spectrum of dental procedures, the multidimensional correspondence analysis was performed using the two-dimensional visualization based on the scree plot. The smaller the angle between the evaluated points, the stronger the dependence (with the vertex of the angle placed at the origin of the coordinate system).

The significance level was set at alfa = 0.05. All analyses were conducted using Statistica v.13.3 (Statsoft, Cracow, Poland) and PQStat v.1.8.6.122 (PQStat Software, Poznan, Poland).

3. Results

The number of patients categorized by gender and age for the years 2017–2023 is presented in Table 1. It is evident that in every period, females outnumbered males across all age groups. The lowest number of patients was recorded in 2020, likely due to the COVID-19 pandemic, while a significant increase in patient numbers was observed in 2022–2023, following Russia's invasion of Ukraine.

This study's analysis focused on the most common procedures performed on permanent teeth: conservative treatments (restorations and root canal fillings) and surgical procedures (extractions). A total of 182,654 patients' medical records from the University Center of Dentistry and Specialized Medicine (Poznan, Poland) were analyzed. The radar chart (Figure 1) illustrates the percentage distribution of these three treatment procedure groups depending on tooth numbers. The vast majority of procedures involved tooth restorations, except for wisdom teeth, which were most frequently extracted. Endodontic procedures were notably less common. The size of the chart fields highlights a tendency for more frequent conservative procedures in maxillary teeth compared to mandibular teeth.

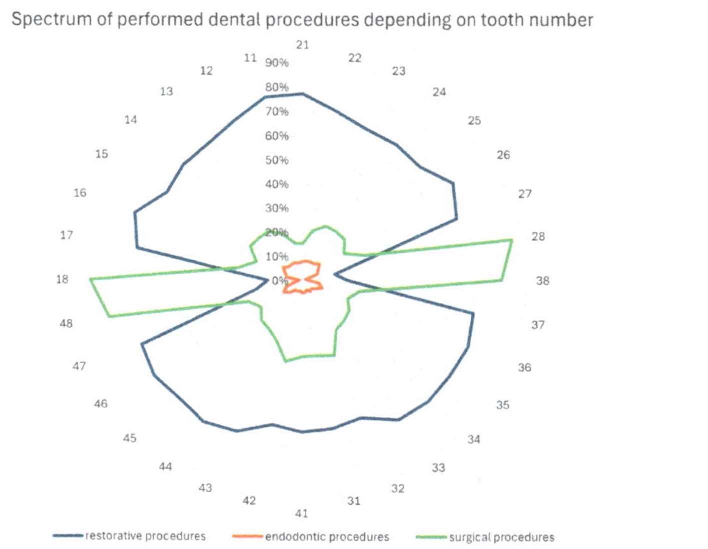

Figure 1. Radar plot for the percentage spectrum of performed dental procedures depending on the tooth number (as outer numbers according to the FDI numbering system).

The comparative analysis of gender's influence on the spectrum of dental procedures performed on individual teeth is shown in Table 2. Overall, females were more likely than males to opt for tooth restorations, regardless of tooth type. Interestingly, only males more frequently chose conservative treatment for wisdom teeth. Conversely, surgical procedures were generally more common among males, except in the case of wisdom teeth. Additionally, males were more prone to experiencing tooth pain that culminated in endodontic intervention, particularly in the anterior teeth and premolars of the maxilla.

On the other hand, a similar comparison considering the age of patients is provided in Table 3. As age increased, the percentage of teeth treated conservatively decreased, while the percentage of teeth removed increased. This trend was consistent across all teeth, except for wisdom teeth, which showed the opposite pattern compared to other teeth. Regarding endodontic treatment, interventional procedures were most commonly performed in the 18–30 age group. However, the percentage of teeth ultimately treated endodontically was slightly higher in the 18–30 and 31–50 age groups. Again, these procedures were predominantly performed on anterior teeth and maxillary premolars.

Table 2. Percentage distribution of performed dental procedures depending on the tooth number and gender.

Tooth	n		Filled Permanent Teeth			Temporary Filling			Endodontic Intervention Procedure			Root Canal Filling			Tooth Extraction		
	F	M	F	M	p-Value	F	M	p-Value	F	M	p-Value	F	M	p-Value	F	M	p-Value
11	3052	3064	73.1	67.9	<0.001 *	6.3	7.2	0.176	2.5	3.1	0.179	4.0	4.9	0.100	14.2	17.0	0.003 *
12	2462	2316	68.2	61.1	<0.001 *	6.5	7.3	0.301	2.9	3.6	0.199	4.3	4.9	0.357	18.1	23.2	<0.001 *
13	2221	2215	65.3	58.8	<0.001 *	5.8	6.3	0.525	2.8	4.4	0.005 *	3.7	4.5	0.205	22.3	26.0	0.004 *
14	3193	2904	62.1	56.5	<0.001 *	7.7	8.6	0.216	4.2	4.3	0.896	3.8	3.2	0.230	22.1	27.4	<0.001 *
15	3322	2731	56.6	53.2	0.009 *	10.9	9.9	0.221	5.4	4.9	0.415	4.1	4.1	0.948	23.0	27.9	<0.001 *
16	5505	4498	61.7	59.4	0.021 *	12.3	11.8	0.464	4.7	5.2	0.270	2.7	2.1	0.061	18.7	21.5	<0.001 *
17	3456	2914	59.6	55.2	<0.001 *	10.5	9.3	0.121	4.8	4.4	0.485	1.6	1.7	0.831	23.5	29.4	<0.001 *
18	2837	1953	10.3	14.4	<0.001 *	1.7	2.0	0.514	0.6	1.8	<0.001 *	0.1	0.1	0.642	87.3	81.6	<0.001 *
21	3031	3077	71.3	68.2	0.009 *	7.0	7.9	0.197	3.1	2.7	0.392	4.5	5.0	0.391	14.2	16.2	0.032 *
22	2495	2402	65.9	60.6	<0.001 *	8.0	7.8	0.836	4.0	3.9	0.915	3.8	4.5	0.247	18.4	23.3	<0.001 *
23	2244	2330	63.9	56.7	<0.001 *	7.0	7.8	0.329	3.7	4.5	0.198	3.7	4.3	0.338	21.7	26.7	<0.001 *
24	2900	2794	62.4	55.5	<0.001 *	8.4	8.8	0.491	4.8	4.9	0.909	3.0	3.5	0.322	21.3	27.3	<0.001 *
25	3100	2743	57.7	53.0	<0.001 *	11.3	10.6	0.417	4.8	5.1	0.640	4.2	5.1	0.116	22.0	26.2	<0.001 *
26	5135	4337	61.5	58.2	0.001 *	12.9	12.0	0.197	4.8	5.2	0.399	2.2	2.8	0.071	18.5	21.9	<0.001 *
27	3477	2918	59.2	54.3	<0.001 *	10.2	9.3	0.244	4.4	4.7	0.607	1.9	1.7	0.615	24.3	30.0	<0.001 *
28	2866	2009	8.9	14.3	<0.001 *	1.7	2.6	0.038 *	1.1	1.1	0.889	0.0	0.1	0.329	88.3	81.8	<0.001 *
31	1208	1070	61.1	57.9	0.131	3.3	3.6	0.782	2.4	2.5	0.985	2.9	2.6	0.758	30.3	33.4	0.123
32	1208	1102	60.9	55.5	0.010 *	3.1	4.5	0.098	1.8	2.7	0.186	1.9	2.4	0.493	32.3	34.8	0.220
33	1636	1432	67.9	62.1	<0.001 *	4.0	5.5	0.061	2.5	3.1	0.369	2.3	3.5	0.060	23.3	25.8	0.118
34	2368	1924	69.8	63.1	<0.001 *	5.3	3.9	0.037 *	2.7	3.1	0.492	2.3	1.7	0.202	19.9	28.2	<0.001 *
35	2923	2399	67.0	60.6	<0.001 *	7.0	6.8	0.817	3.3	4.4	0.044 *	2.4	2.8	0.407	20.3	25.4	<0.001 *
36	5871	4993	60.3	55.8	<0.001 *	13.8	13.2	0.377	5.7	5.8	0.856	2.7	2.8	0.796	17.6	22.4	<0.001 *
37	4415	3785	61.0	56.1	<0.001 *	11.6	10.4	0.090	5.1	5.4	0.577	1.4	1.7	0.312	20.9	26.4	<0.001 *
38	3902	2773	13.6	17.5	<0.001 *	2.9	2.8	0.867	1.7	2.4	0.054	0.0	0.2	0.018 *	81.8	77.1	<0.001 *
41	1187	1085	60.5	58.3	0.306	3.6	3.9	0.791	2.1	2.8	0.345	2.4	3.3	0.244	31.3	31.7	0.873
42	1140	1080	59.5	55.6	0.069	3.9	3.6	0.795	2.0	1.8	0.850	2.2	3.1	0.234	32.4	35.8	0.100
43	1429	1431	66.1	61.2	0.007 *	4.3	4.5	0.865	2.1	2.4	0.678	2.3	3.1	0.228	25.1	28.7	0.033 *
44	2297	1908	69.4	62.9	<0.001 *	5.0	4.1	0.189	2.7	3.2	0.387	2.1	1.6	0.282	20.8	28.1	<0.001 *
45	2992	2516	66.5	59.2	<0.001 *	7.3	5.6	0.013 *	4.1	4.5	0.507	2.8	3.0	0.718	19.3	27.7	<0.001 *
46	5996	5282	59.0	55.4	<0.001 *	14.1	13.8	0.666	5.5	6.4	0.048 *	3.0	2.8	0.565	18.4	21.6	<0.001 *
47	4187	3884	61.4	55.6	<0.001 *	11.8	10.1	0.016 *	4.7	5.5	0.113	1.6	2.5	0.005 *	20.5	26.3	<0.001 *
48	3876	2854	14.4	17.7	<0.001 *	2.3	4.2	<0.001 *	1.6	2.6	0.005 *	0.1	0.1	0.696	81.6	75.4	<0.001 *
	97,931	84,723	56.0	53.5	<0.001 *	8.4	8.3	0.446	3.8	4.2	<0.001 *	2.4	2.8	<0.001 *	29.4	31.2	<0.001 *

Legend: F, females; M, males; *, significant differences in Z test for independent proportions.

Table 3. Percentage distribution of performed dental procedures depending on the tooth number and age.

Tooth	*n*				Filled Permanent Teeth				Temporary Filling				Intervention Procedure				Root Canal Filling				Tooth Extraction			
	<18	18–30	31–50	>51	<18	18–30	31–50	>51	<18	18–30	31–50	>51	<18	18–30	31–50	>51	<18	18–30	31–50	>51	<18	18–30	31–50	>51
11	1167	915	1497	2537	77.8	72.6	71.8	65.6	9.3	11.4	6.1	4.3	3.4	5.9	2.9	1.3	7.9	4.9	4.1	2.9	1.6	5.2	15.2	26.0
12	510	758	1347	2163	79.6	68.9	64.1	60.2	8.8	11.2	7.6	4.4	3.5	5.5	3.8	2.0	5.3	6.1	4.8	3.7	2.7	8.3	19.7	29.6
13	139	384	1199	2714	87.1	67.7	65.7	58.4	2.9	10.2	5.3	6.0	2.2	6.8	4.0	3.1	2.9	5.2	3.8	4.1	5.0	10.2	21.2	28.4
14	620	1168	2116	2193	73.1	62.3	58.4	55.1	9.5	12.3	7.5	6.2	3.1	7.0	5.1	2.3	2.4	4.2	3.9	3.1	11.9	14.1	25.2	33.2
15	534	1630	2229	1660	70.4	55.7	54.0	50.9	12.4	15.4	9.6	6.0	5.1	7.7	5.2	2.8	3.6	5.8	4.2	2.4	8.6	15.5	26.9	38.0
16	3047	2249	2881	1826	72.2	63.1	53.0	50.9	15.4	13.2	11.1	6.6	4.4	6.4	5.7	2.7	2.3	2.9	2.7	1.6	5.8	14.4	27.6	38.2
17	853	1567	2286	1664	81.0	70.6	51.4	41.7	13.5	9.6	10.7	7.5	1.4	5.6	5.8	3.7	0.6	1.0	2.6	1.5	3.5	13.2	29.4	45.7
18	119	2133	1888	650	5.0	7.3	14.0	22.9	0.0	0.8	2.6	3.2	1.7	0.9	1.4	0.9	0.0	0.0	0.3	0.0	93.3	91.0	81.7	72.9
21	1266	875	1575	2392	74.7	74.4	70.4	65.0	11.6	11.9	6.5	4.3	3.9	4.2	3.1	1.7	8.2	5.3	4.3	3.1	1.6	4.2	15.7	26.0
22	621	655	1405	2216	76.3	67.8	60.7	60.0	11.4	11.6	8.5	5.4	3.7	5.5	5.7	2.4	5.0	6.1	4.3	3.1	3.5	9.0	20.8	29.1
23	127	390	1292	2765	78.7	71.0	59.7	58.1	8.7	7.9	10.0	6.0	2.4	5.9	5.2	3.4	3.9	3.8	4.0	4.1	6.3	11.3	21.1	28.4
24	543	1201	2107	1843	71.6	62.4	56.5	56.0	9.8	11.2	9.8	5.3	3.1	8.5	5.2	2.6	2.6	4.4	3.5	2.4	12.9	13.6	25.0	33.7
25	528	1567	2184	1564	67.2	56.4	52.8	54.5	13.4	15.3	11.5	5.1	5.7	7.1	4.8	2.6	4.2	6.8	4.6	2.6	9.5	14.4	26.3	35.1
26	2712	2263	2791	1706	72.3	63.3	53.2	47.0	16.1	12.8	12.3	6.7	3.5	7.2	5.9	3.0	2.0	3.4	2.8	1.6	6.1	13.4	25.8	41.6
27	884	1579	2272	1660	81.6	68.6	49.3	43.3	13.2	10.6	10.2	6.5	1.5	5.0	6.3	3.3	0.0	1.6	3.1	1.4	3.7	14.2	31.1	45.5
28	128	2226	1902	619	4.7	7.2	13.6	18.7	0.0	1.3	2.8	3.1	0.0	0.6	1.6	1.8	0.0	0.0	0.1	0.2	95.3	90.8	81.9	76.3
31	160	118	408	1592	75.6	63.6	57.4	58.2	6.3	12.7	5.4	2.0	3.8	8.5	2.2	1.9	6.3	9.3	4.4	1.5	8.1	5.9	30.6	36.3
32	82	89	344	1795	73.2	66.3	54.9	57.9	7.3	11.2	5.8	2.8	3.7	7.9	3.2	1.7	4.9	3.4	2.6	1.8	11.0	11.2	33.4	35.7
33	39	97	489	2443	87.2	80.4	68.9	63.5	7.7	9.3	5.1	4.4	0.0	3.1	2.2	2.9	0.0	1.0	2.2	3.1	5.1	6.2	21.5	26.2
34	157	338	1143	2654	78.3	71.0	70.8	63.9	5.1	10.1	4.9	3.9	1.3	5.3	3.3	2.4	1.9	1.2	1.6	2.3	13.4	12.4	19.4	27.5
35	306	898	1698	2420	76.5	64.3	64.2	62.4	5.9	13.7	6.5	4.9	4.6	6.6	4.0	2.5	2.9	3.2	2.8	2.1	10.1	12.2	22.5	28.0
36	3599	2813	3047	1405	69.7	57.3	49.6	49.2	16.1	13.8	12.8	8.2	4.3	7.8	6.1	4.3	1.7	4.1	3.1	2.1	8.2	17.0	28.4	36.2
37	1477	2172	2758	1793	77.0	64.8	52.3	46.2	15.2	11.6	10.8	7.5	2.3	6.0	6.9	4.1	0.7	1.2	2.4	1.3	4.8	16.4	27.6	40.9
38	355	2739	2519	1062	2.3	10.6	17.3	26.4	0.6	1.4	3.8	5.3	0.3	1.3	2.8	2.6	0.0	0.0	0.0	0.5	96.9	86.7	76.1	65.3
41	172	138	410	1552	75.6	67.4	59.0	57.1	7.0	12.3	5.1	2.3	2.9	9.4	3.7	1.4	6.4	7.2	4.1	1.7	8.1	3.6	28.0	37.5
42	96	110	336	1678	84.4	79.1	56.5	54.9	5.2	7.3	3.3	3.6	0.0	1.8	2.1	2.0	3.1	6.4	1.8	2.6	7.3	5.5	36.3	37.0
43	47	114	475	2224	80.9	85.1	62.1	62.5	10.6	4.4	5.9	4.0	0.0	0.9	2.7	2.3	0.0	4.4	3.2	2.6	8.5	5.3	26.1	28.6
44	159	352	1129	2565	76.7	75.0	68.0	64.0	3.8	6.0	5.4	4.1	0.6	5.7	4.0	2.3	0.6	1.4	2.0	1.9	18.2	11.9	20.5	27.7
45	368	929	1884	2327	72.8	64.6	63.1	61.2	8.7	11.1	6.7	4.3	4.9	6.1	5.2	2.7	3.8	3.4	3.5	2.0	9.8	14.7	21.5	30.0
46	3587	3003	3137	1551	69.6	55.4	49.0	49.5	16.9	15.1	12.2	8.6	3.8	8.7	6.8	3.8	2.1	4.2	3.1	2.0	7.6	16.7	29.0	36.2
47	1429	2132	2714	1796	76.3	66.5	51.3	46.3	15.9	10.8	11.1	7.1	2.7	5.8	6.7	3.6	1.3	2.2	2.4	1.9	3.8	14.8	28.5	41.0
48	379	2748	2540	1063	2.9	10.2	18.8	27.8	0.3	2.3	3.9	4.5	0.0	1.2	3.2	2.0	0.0	0.0	0.1	0.3	96.8	86.4	73.9	65.5
	26,210	40,350	56,002	60,092	70.9	50.3	50.4	55.0	13.4	9.7	8.4	5.1	3.4	5.3	4.8	2.6	2.6	2.8	2.8	2.4	9.7	31.9	33.6	34.9

The extent of restorations performed and the type of refoundation, depending on tooth number, are summarized in Table 4. Single- and two-surface restorations were the most frequently performed. In the majority of mandibular teeth, single-surface restorations predominated. In contrast, maxillary teeth, particularly anterior and premolars, showed a preference for two-surface restorations. Notably, commercial restorations were more frequently chosen for maxillary premolars with two-surface cavities. Multi-surface restorations were the least common overall, but within this group, more than one-third were commercial, especially in the maxillary anterior teeth.

Table 4. Percentage distribution of performed restorative procedures depending on the tooth number, the extent of the procedure, and the kind of refoundation.

oth	*n*	Single-Surface				Two-Surface				Multi-Surface			
		Commercial	Refunded	*p*-Value	Sum	Commercial	Refunded	*p*-Value	Sum	Commerc al	Refunded	*p*-Value	Sum
1	4311	5.3	28.0	<0.001 *	33.2	6.2	41.6	<0.001 *	47.9	5.2	13.7	<0.001 *	18.9
2	3094	5.1	35.4	<0.001 *	40.5	6.2	41.6	<0.001 *	47.8	4.5	7.2	<0.001 *	11.7
3	2754	6.0	41.1	<0.001 *	47.1	6.7	38.6	<0.001 *	45.4	3.1	4.4	0.014 *	7.5
4	3625	5.5	32.9	<0.001 *	38.3	13.0	37.1	<0.001 *	50.1	3.3	8.3	<0.001 *	11.6
5	3333	5.9	25.0	<0.001 *	30.9	14.4	41.9	<0.001 *	56.3	3.7	9.1	<0.001 *	12.8
6	6073	5.5	40.6	<0.001 *	46.1	6.5	34.6	<0.001 *	41.1	5.8	7.0	0.008 *	12.8
7	3668	6.8	38.3	<0.001 *	45.1	7.4	34.3	<0.001 *	41.6	6.2	7.1	0.134	13.3
8	575	8.5	33.0	<0.001 *	41.6	6.3	41.9	<0.001 *	48.2	3.5	6.8	0.016 *	10.3
1	4260	5.1	28.5	<0.001 *	33.6	6.1	41.1	<0.001 *	47.2	4.8	14.4	<0.001 *	19.2
2	3100	5.8	35.3	<0.001 *	41.1	6.6	40.9	<0.001 *	47.5	4.6	6.8	<0.001 *	11.4
3	2755	7.2	41.9	<0.001 *	49.1	6.1	37.1	<0.001 *	43.2	3.1	4.6	0.005 *	7.7
4	3361	6.0	30.9	<0.001 *	37.0	13.0	39.4	<0.001 *	52.3	2.6	8.1	<0.001 *	10.7
5	3245	5.4	24.6	<0.001 *	30.0	14.9	43.2	<0.001 *	58.2	3.5	8.3	<0.001 *	11.8
6	5681	4.9	39.0	<0.001 *	44.0	7.4	34.9	<0.001 *	42.3	6.7	7.0	0.551	13.7
7	3643	6.5	38.0	<0.001 *	44.4	7.9	33.8	<0.001 *	41.7	6.6	7.2	0.335	13.9
8	541	6.8	37.9	<0.001 *	44.7	8.5	35.1	<0.001 *	43.6	3.1	8.5	<0.001 *	11.6
1	1357	6.9	55.8	<0.001 *	62.7	2.1	27.6	<0.001 *	29.8	1.2	6.3	<0.001 *	7.5
2	1348	5.7	54.6	<0.001 *	60.3	3.2	31.8	<0.001 *	34.9	1.1	3.6	<0.001 *	4.7
3	2000	7.4	53.2	<0.001 *	60.6	3.6	30.9	<0.001 *	34.4	1.5	3.6	<0.001 *	5.1
4	2868	9.1	50.7	<0.001 *	59.8	6.6	27.1	<0.001 *	33.8	1.6	4.9	<0.001 *	6.5
5	3412	8.4	38.7	<0.001 *	47.1	11.0	33.1	<0.001 *	44.1	3.0	5.7	<0.001 *	8.7
6	6325	6.3	44.6	<0.001 *	50.9	6.6	30.2	<0.001 *	36.8	5.0	7.3	<0.001 *	12.3
7	4816	7.4	41.1	<0.001 *	48.5	8.9	30.9	<0.001 *	39.8	4.7	7.0	<0.001 *	11.7
8	1015	8.0	36.7	<0.001 *	44.7	11.4	32.8	<0.001 *	44.2	4.2	6.8	0.013 *	11.0
1	1351	6.4	56.6	<0.001 *	63.0	2.7	27.6	<0.001 *	30.3	1.0	5.8	<0.001 *	6.7
2	1279	5.9	51.1	<0.001 *	57.0	2.7	33.2	<0.001 *	35.9	1.3	5.8	<0.001 *	7.1
3	1821	7.2	51.8	<0.001 *	59.0	4.2	31.3	<0.001 *	35.5	1.5	4.0	<0.001 *	5.5
4	2796	9.1	50.2	<0.001 *	59.3	6.3	27.2	<0.001 *	33.5	2.0	5.2	<0.001 *	7.2
5	3479	8.5	36.9	<0.001 *	45.5	11.0	33.7	<0.001 *	44.7	3.0	6.9	<0.001 *	9.9
6	6463	5.9	44.9	<0.001 *	50.8	6.0	30.9	<0.001 *	36.9	5.0	7.3	<0.001 *	12.3
7	4730	6.9	38.7	<0.001 *	45.6	10.1	32.6	<0.001 *	42.7	5.3	6.4	0.025 *	11.8
8	1064	8.6	34.7	<0.001 *	43.3	10.8	33.6	<0.001 *	44.4	3.9	8.5	<0.001 *	12.3
	100,143	6.4	39.2	<0.001 *	45.7	8.0	34.9	<0.001 *	42.8	4.2	7.3	<0.001 *	11.5

Legend: *, significant differences in Z test for independent proportions.

Surgical extractions were the most frequently performed surgical procedures, as shown in Table 5. These primarily involved molar teeth, with mandibular wisdom teeth being the most commonly extracted.

Based on univariate logistic regression modeling, the odds ratios for surgical procedures compared to conservative procedures were assessed depending on personal factors (Table 6). Maxillary teeth were significantly less likely to be qualified for extractions. Molar teeth had the highest odds of extraction, in contrast to incisors, which had the lowest. Among demographic factors, females were 8.5% less likely to decide on tooth extractions compared to males. On the other hand, regarding age, teeth were most frequently extracted in patients over 51 years of age, with odds for extraction being 6% higher than in the 18–30 age group.

Table 5. Percentage distribution of performed surgical procedures depending on the tooth number and the extent of the procedure.

Tooth	n	Simple Extraction	Surgical Extraction	p-Value
11	953	37.0	63.0	<0.001 *
12	983	31.6	68.4	<0.001 *
13	1072	27.1	72.9	<0.001 *
14	1500	23.8	76.2	<0.001 *
15	1527	25.3	74.7	<0.001 *
16	1993	19.6	80.4	<0.001 *
17	1670	22.9	77.1	<0.001 *
18	4069	14.1	85.9	<0.001 *
21	928	36.4	63.6	<0.001 *
22	1017	34.2	65.8	<0.001 *
23	1109	30.0	70.0	<0.001 *
24	1380	23.5	76.5	<0.001 *
25	1399	25.5	74.5	<0.001 *
26	1901	18.3	81.7	<0.001 *
27	1720	21.1	78.9	<0.001 *
28	4174	12.7	87.3	<0.001 *
31	723	50.1	49.9	0.981
32	774	46.8	53.2	0.014 *
33	752	40.6	59.4	<0.001 *
34	1014	30.5	69.5	<0.001 *
35	1201	29.6	70.4	<0.001 *
36	2148	16.6	83.4	<0.001 *
37	1922	21.4	78.6	<0.001 *
38	5327	5.0	95.0	<0.001 *
41	716	52.9	47.1	0.032 *
42	756	44.8	55.2	<0.001 *
43	769	36.5	63.5	<0.001 *
44	1014	29.3	70.7	<0.001 *
45	1276	27.5	72.5	<0.001 *
46	2244	15.5	84.5	<0.001 *
47	1880	18.3	81.7	<0.001 *
48	5314	5.5	94.5	<0.001 *
	55,225	20.6	79.4	<0.001 *

Legend: *, significant differences in Z test for independent proportions.

Table 6. Odds ratios for surgical procedures vs. conservative procedures (restorative and endodontic procedures) depending on site, tooth type, gender, and age.

	Reference	Beta	SE	p-Value	OR	−95%CI	+95%CI
site: maxilla	mandible	−0.185	0.010	<0.001 *	0.831	0.814	0.848
tooth: incisor	molar	−0.796	0.015	<0.001 *	0.451	0.438	0.465
tooth: canine	molar	−0.648	0.020	<0.001 *	0.523	0.503	0.544
tooth: premolar	molar	−0.664	0.013	<0.001 *	0.515	0.501	0.528
gender: female	male	−0.088	0.010	<0.001 *	0.915	0.897	0.934
age: <18	18–30	−1.468	0.024	<0.001 *	0.230	0.220	0.241
age: 31–50	18–30	0.059	0.014	<0.001 *	1.061	1.032	1.091
age: >51	18–30	0.060	0.014	<0.001 *	1.062	1.034	1.092

* significant ratio for univariate logistic regression modeling.

Multidimensional correspondence analyses were conducted to graphically represent the relationship between individual factors and clinical decisions regarding the type of dental procedure. Based on scree plot evaluation, a two-dimensional analysis was selected for both demographic and personal oral factors (Figure 2).

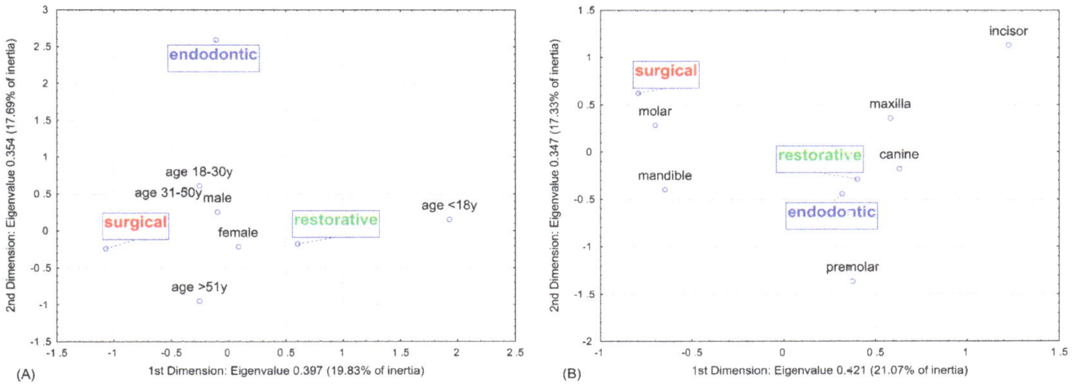

Figure 2. Multidimensional correspondence analysis for impact of (**A**) sociodemographic factors (i.e., age and gender) and (**B**) personal oral factors (i.e., tooth type and site) on the spectrum of dental procedures—2-dimensional plot.

The results revealed that males over 50 years of age were most likely to choose surgical procedures. In contrast, females—especially those under 18 years of age—more frequently opted for restorative procedures. Interestingly, males aged 18–30 years were the group most likely to undergo endodontic treatment.

In terms of tooth type and location, the analysis confirmed that mandibular molars were the most predisposed to extraction. Conversely, maxillary teeth—particularly canines and premolars—were more commonly selected for conservative procedures. Detailed parameters of the analysis are presented in Tables S1 and S2.

4. Discussion

A total of 182,654 medical records of patients treated at the University Center of Dentistry and Specialized Medicine in Poznan (Poland) between 2017 and 2023 were analyzed. During this period, two significant global events heavily influenced the number of dental services provided. The first quarter of 2020 saw the largest decline in dental services due to the rapidly spreading COVID-19 pandemic, which exposed the unpreparedness of healthcare systems worldwide. In response to the crisis, our center, following the recommendations of leading medical and dental societies, restricted its services to emergency care only during the early months of the pandemic [15–17]. This decision resulted in a drastic reduction in the number of patients admitted during this period [13,18–20]. In turn, on 24 February 2022, the war in Ukraine triggered a massive influx of refugees into neighboring Poland, driven by both the country's geographical proximity and cultural and linguistic similarities. In response, Polish authorities swiftly implemented mechanisms to assist those in need, including access to reimbursed medical services. This policy led to the largest recorded increase in dental services provided, as many refugees sought dental care at our center [21–23].

In addition to these global events, a long-term trend in Poland has also impacted the provision of dental services. Each year, an increasing number of dental practices previously offering treatments reimbursed by public funds have been closed or privatized. This shift is driven by factors such as the rising costs of maintaining dental clinics and acquiring materials, as well as the increasing expectations of patients, who demand higher-quality and more personalized services [24]. In this changing landscape, our center has emerged as the largest medical referral center providing specialist dental care reimbursed by the National Health Fund in central Poland. As a result, it has attracted a growing number of patients seeking free treatment, which is often no longer available in their local areas. Consequently, our center has experienced a steady upward trend in the number of procedures performed, reflecting its critical role in meeting the dental care needs of both Polish residents and refugees.

4.1. Sociodemographic Factors (i.e., Gender and Age)

Looking closely at the details of the procedures performed over these seven years, the clear dominance of females stands out across the entire study period and in every age group analyzed. The literature frequently highlights females' more frequent use of medical services, including dental care, which aligns with the study's findings [3–6,9]. This phenomenon reflects well-documented gender patterns. Furuta et al. suggest that oral health behaviors are influenced by various factors such as knowledge, attitude, lifestyle, stress, education level, and socioeconomic status, with the first three showing notable differences between genders [7]. Females tend to perceive a stronger connection between oral health and their quality of life, including mood, appearance, and overall well-being. This awareness translates into more frequent check-ups and adherence to recommended treatments, even when financial barriers are reported [3,5–7].

These conclusions are supported not only by survey data but also by the widely used DMF index, a key indicator of dental health in epidemiological studies. Among females, the F (filled) component is often dominant, indicating a higher likelihood of undergoing dental treatment for caries, while the M (missing) component is typically smaller, reflecting a lower tendency to remove teeth due to decay [1,4,25–27]. In this study's analysis, females were more likely to choose restorative dental treatments, particularly those under 18 years of age. This aligns with findings from the report "Monitoring the Oral Health Status of the Polish Population in 2016–2020". According to this report, the conservative treatment indicator—which reflects not only the availability and accessibility of preventive and therapeutic services but also patients' own concern for their oral health—was higher among females in both the 35–44 and 65–74 age groups [1].

The available literature clearly demonstrates that females tend to have greater knowledge, a more positive attitude, and a generally healthier lifestyle, which translates into better oral hygiene. This is evidenced by more frequent and thorough tooth brushing, interdental flossing, and less tobacco product use [3,5–7,28]. Consequently, females tend to have a healthier periodontium, yet paradoxically, they still experience higher rates of tooth decay [4,6,9,25–28]. Although some studies present a different perspective, they remain a clear minority [5]. Anthropologists attribute this paradox to three primary factors: earlier eruption of teeth in girls, leading to longer exposure to a cariogenic oral environment; easier access to food supplies and frequent snacking during food preparation; and the physiological and behavioral changes associated with pregnancy [9]. However, Lukacs et al. emphasized that anthropologists tend to focus on social issues while downplaying the less-documented impacts of hormonal factors [4].

Conversely, researchers like Ferraro and Vieira reported limited evidence supporting the idea that earlier tooth eruption significantly contributes to caries development [9]. Instead, growing attention has turned to the role of hormones, particularly estrogen, which fluctuates during puberty, menstruation, and pregnancy. These hormonal changes alter the biochemical composition of saliva, leading to a lower flow rate of both unstimulated whole saliva and stimulated parotid saliva in females. This reduction in saliva flow creates a more cariogenic oral environment due to diminished mechanical washing, buffering, and remineralization benefits provided by saliva [6,9,10,28]. Additionally, factors such as diseases, medical procedures, and medications (e.g., hormone replacement therapy and birth control pills) can further affect the composition and flow rate of saliva [10]. Pregnancy, in particular, has a profound impact on females' bodies and daily behaviors. It can lead to immune suppression, hormonal fluctuations, cravings, and salivary alterations, all of which contribute to a higher risk of caries [9,28,29]. Studies also indicate that males have higher concentrations of IgA immunoglobulin in their saliva, aiding in defense against cariogenic pathogens [30,31]. Moreover, females tend to have a deficient amelogenin gene and lower levels of amelogenin protein, which are critical for forming enamel matrix and may contribute to increased caries susceptibility [32,33].

Salivary composition, which is regulated by hormonal and biochemical factors, also differs between genders and may influence caries risk. Considering these biological differences, personalized treatment approaches could improve oral health outcomes. For a deeper exploration of gender as a biological variable in oral diseases, the recent review by Sangalli et al. provides valuable insights into these mechanisms [34].

There is also the other side of the coin. Males generally use healthcare services less often, including dental care, and when they do, it is typically for acute problems, such as dental pain, rather than for preventive care [5,6]. This pattern is also evident in this study's analysis. At our center, males were more likely to report with toothaches, often resulting in emergency procedures. Notably, the group of males aged 18–30 was found as the most likely to undergo interventional endodontic procedures. Males also more frequently opted for surgical procedures, which are often performed during pain visits. This tendency may stem from a lack of willingness to pursue conservative treatment or from the extent of tooth damage, where tooth extraction becomes the only viable option. Unfortunately, the study dataset lacks more detailed information on the underlying reasons for these choices.

The tendency to postpone treatment seems to be linked to "traditional masculine behavior", "masculinity beliefs", and the association of illness with a loss of masculinity. However, Galdas et al. suggested that occupational and socioeconomic status likely have a greater influence on these behaviors than gender alone, highlighting the need for further investigation [35,36]. Males are also characterized by less knowledge of proper oral hygiene practices. They tend to use harder toothbrushes, brush with excessive force, and are less likely to use recommended fluoride toothpaste or floss interdental spaces. These habits can lead to gingival damage and recession, contributing to the development of root caries [6,37]. This is supported by the observations of Su et al., who found that males are more prone to root caries, noncarious root lesions (such as erosions or abrasions), and root restorations [5].

Age appears to be another important factor influencing the choice of treatment method. As patients age, the percentage of teeth treated conservatively decreases (70.9% vs. 55%), while the number of teeth removed increases (9.7% vs. 34.9%), consistent with other reports [1,26,27,38]. With age, the percentage of third molars removed decreases, although it remains the highest among all tooth groups (65.3–76.3%). Endodontic procedures, however, were very rare across all age groups.

According to the report "Monitoring the Oral Health of the Polish Population in 2016–2020", the incidence of caries in children in Greater Poland rises from 21% in the group up to 3 years old to 89% by the age of 18. Treatment needs in this age group most often involve single- and two-surface fillings, while the demand for endodontic treatment and tooth extractions peaks at 9.2% in 10-year-olds. During the mixed dentition period, one in three children require tooth extraction. The report highlights the low conservative treatment rate for primary teeth (0.31 in 3- and 10-year-olds), indicating that treatment needs are insufficiently met. This rate increases 2.5 times for permanent teeth by the age of 18 (0.84) [1].

In Poland, among individuals aged 35–44, the prevalence of caries remains at an alarmingly high level of 98.7%. In Greater Poland, unfavorable changes in the conservative treatment index were observed, decreasing from 0.64 in 2010 to 0.56 in 2017. Among older adults aged 65–74, the percentage of edentulous individuals dropped to 18.8%, while the percentage of people with at least 20 preserved teeth increased from 8% to 27%. Despite these improvements, the DMFT index for seniors remains at a very high level of 24.9. However, the conservative treatment index rose to 0.67 nationally and 0.8 in the Greater Poland province [1].

Zilinskaite-Petrauskiene et al. described differences in factors influencing endodontic treatment between elderly and young patients. In older patients, a significantly higher proportion presented with necrotic pulp and required both endodontic and prosthetic treatment. With age, the difficulty of performing endodontic procedures increases due to challenges such as achieving proper access and locating root canal orifices. However, there were no significant differences between the two groups in terms of the number of treatment visits, the technical quality of root fillings, pain sensation, esthetic outcomes, or masticatory function [39].

The most common general reason for tooth extraction remains dental caries. Among younger patients, orthodontic indications are cited more frequently, whereas in older patients, periodontal disease becomes a more prevalent cause. This topic is explored in more detail later [38,40–44].

Socioeconomic factors significantly influence dental patients' decisions between conservative and surgical procedures. Individuals with higher income and education levels, as well as those residing in urban areas, often have better access to dental care and greater awareness of oral health, leading them to prefer conservative treatments. Conversely, those with lower socioeconomic status may face barriers such as cost and limited access, resulting in delayed care and a higher likelihood of requiring surgical interventions [45]. Occupational factors also play a role in treatment choices. For instance, individuals in demanding jobs or with irregular work schedules may opt for quicker solutions like extractions to minimize time away from work, whereas those in professions that prioritize esthetics may choose conservative procedures to maintain their appearance [46]. Future research should delve deeper into these socioeconomic and occupational influences to develop targeted strategies that improve access to and utilization of conservative dental care, particularly among vulnerable populations.

4.2. Personal Oral Factors (i.e., Tooth Group, Site, or Procedure Extent)

The vast majority of dental procedures performed across all dental groups at our center were dental restorations, with the notable exception of wisdom teeth, where extractions were the predominant treatment. In Poland, there has been a positive trend in recent years toward increasing the conservative treatment rate—defined as the ratio of teeth with properly made restorations to the total number of teeth filled and those requiring treatment [1]. This trend is somewhat encouraging, reflecting an improvement in access to and prioritization of restorative care. According to the medical records we analyzed, restorative treatment was most commonly performed on maxillary teeth, particularly on canines and premolars. In the mandible, single-surface restorations were more frequent, while in the maxilla, two-surface restorations were more common, especially in the anterior teeth and premolars.

There are reports indicating that permanent dental caries in children primarily affects molars, often appearing shortly after their eruption. For example, the first molar is affected in children as young as 5 years old, while the second molar tends to show caries in 12-year-olds [1]. Pizzo et al. reported that 44% of current active caries foci were found in the first molars of 6–7-year-olds based on the analysis of 742 subjects [47]. Similarly, Alves et al. found 17.2% of current active caries foci in second molars among 983 examined 12-year-olds [48].

The early onset of caries brings significant consequences in adulthood. Once a tooth is drilled, it often enters what is known as the "death spiral of restoration" or the "tooth cycle of death" [49]. This cycle involves repeated restorations, gradually leading to the loss of more tooth tissue until, eventually, endodontic–prosthetic treatment is required on the dental pillar, or in extreme cases, implant–prosthetic treatment after the tooth has been extracted. The sooner the "first drilling" occurs, the sooner the tooth may ultimately require removal. This process is associated with rising treatment costs. Unfortunately, under the National Health Fund in Poland, endodontic treatment is only covered for anterior teeth ("from canine to canine"), and fixed prosthetics are not reimbursed at all [50,51]. The long waiting times for refunded treatments, combined with the risk of pain or swelling from untreated teeth, add to the difficulty for patients [24]. Those with issues concerning posterior teeth, which often require more advanced or specialized care, are left dependent on commercial treatment if they wish to preserve their teeth. Additionally, the microscopic magnification of dental procedures, especially for molars with multiple roots (3–4) compared to the fewer roots (1–2) of front teeth, has been highlighted [52–55]. This approach not only increases treatment complexity but also raises the cost of the service. The subsequent need for the prosthetic reconstruction of crowns destroyed by caries adds to the financial burden. Many patients simply cannot afford these treatments [24].

On the other hand, tooth extractions are fully reimbursed, including the surgical removal of impacted teeth. Studies have shown that wealthier individuals tend to have higher treatment rates and higher F components in the DMF (decayed, missing, filled) caries index, while those with lower incomes are more likely to experience a higher M component, indicating a preference for extraction over attempts to preserve teeth. This disparity clearly suggests that many people with limited financial resources opt to extract teeth rather than invest in treatments to save them [1,25,27,56].

According to the study results, endodontic procedures, which are the last resort to preserve one's own teeth, were significantly less common compared to other dental services. These interventional procedures were most frequently performed in the 18–30-year age group. However, in the case of teeth with root canals that were ultimately filled, the percentage was notably small, with minimal differences across the age groups studied (2.6% vs. 2.6% vs. 2.8% vs. 2.8%). This procedure primarily involved the anterior and premolar teeth of the maxilla, with a slight gender difference (2.8% in males vs. 2.4% in females). The dominance of endodontic procedures in these two groups of teeth contrasts with the findings of other researchers, who typically report molars as the teeth most predisposed to root canal treatment, sometimes alongside premolars [57–60]. These studies also generally indicated a predominance of endodontic treatment in females [57,59]. Although these studies were conducted on relatively small research groups compared to this study's extensive database, it is believed that economic factors may have influenced the notably low percentage of endodontic procedures in this analysis. Unfortunately, due to the retrospective nature, the study lacks data on factors such as the economic status of patients, which could have further supported this hypothesis.

When surgical procedures are taken into account, the highest percentage of teeth removed in this study concerns molars, particularly lower molars in adults, which aligns with numerous other studies [25–27,40–42,61]. Surgical extractions were performed more frequently (79.4% vs. 20.6%) across all tooth groups, except lower teeth. This can be explained by the nature of our facility as a reference center, where more complex cases requiring specialized care are referred. In their reviews, Gotfredsen et al. and Elias et al. emphasize that the loss of anterior teeth has the greatest impact on esthetic and psychological issues, while the preservation of premolars tends to have a greater impact on patient satisfaction than the preservation of molars [62,63]. In contrast, the loss of posterior teeth does not appear to have significant subjective effects for patients. Older adults with shortened dental arches, meaning they have remaining anterior and premolar teeth, maintaining masticatory function, occlusal support, and dental arch stability [25].

In numerous studies, dental caries is identified as the primary cause of tooth extraction [40–44]. It is possible that the high percentage of molar extractions in adulthood is related to the early appearance of carious lesions shortly after the eruption of these teeth and the early onset of the so-called "death spiral" of tooth restoration. Multi-rooted teeth, such as molars, may seem more difficult to extract compared to single- or two-rooted teeth, so the specialized nature of our center may also be a contributing factor. McCaul et al. indicated molars as the most frequently extracted teeth in adults up to the age of 50. Before the age of 21, it was primarily premolars, especially the first upper premolars, and after the age of 50, more anterior than posterior teeth were extracted [41].

Dental caries was identified as the main cause of tooth extraction for nearly all tooth groups. The exceptions were the lower incisors, which were extracted for prosthetic reasons (other than caries or periodontitis), and premolars in people under 21, where the primary reason was orthodontic. Other researchers have also noted similar reasons for tooth extraction in various tooth groups [38,40,43]. The reason for the loss of front teeth at a later age has been explained by esthetic factors, easier access to conservative and endodontic treatments, and their greater resistance to caries, but less resistance to periodontal diseases, which tend to manifest later in life. This study dates back to 1999, and at that time, the authors observed a rise in interest in orthodontic treatments, leading to an increase in the number of premolar extractions compared to 1984 in younger people. There is currently an ongoing debate between the extraction vs. non-extraction of premolars in orthodontic treatments. At present, there is no conclusive evidence supporting the superiority of either method [64]. However, contemporary studies indicate a decreasing trend in the tendency to extract premolars before orthodontic treatment [65–67]. For example, Dardengo et al. analyzed this topic over a broad period from 1980 to 2011 and observed a reduction of about 20% in the frequency of cases requiring tooth extraction over the last 32 years [65]. Additionally, Fleming et al., based on surveys, noted a significant reduction—approximately 95%—in the tendency to prescribe orthodontic extractions over the past 5–10 years among British Orthodontic Society members [67]. In this study, the percentage of premolars removed was significantly lower in the <12, 18–30, and 31–50 age groups compared to the >51 group. This suggests a slight tendency to extract premolars for orthodontic reasons in the study population.

As previously mentioned, the largest percentage of services was tooth restorations, with the exception of wisdom teeth, which were most frequently removed (75.4–88.3%). These teeth were also the most commonly extracted across all age groups studied—removals outnumbered those of individual first molars by more than double. This result is not surprising. Dental caries is commonly cited as the primary cause for the extraction of these teeth [40,41,43,60]. Their position in the oral cavity is undoubtedly a contributing factor: located at the back of the dental arch, often tilted toward the cheek and frequently only partially erupted, they are difficult for patients to clean effectively. This makes them prone to the accumulation of food debris, which serves as a breeding ground for cariogenic bacteria. Conservative treatment is also challenging for dentists for similar reasons. Inadequate cleaning of these teeth promotes the stagnation of calculus, leading to periodontal disease, which is another common reason for their removal [68–71].

Furthermore, third molars often experience complete or partial impaction due to insufficient space in the dental arches. This can result in conditions such as pericoronitis, mandibular angle fractures, cysts, tumors, or damage to the adjacent molars, which may prompt clinicians to recommend prophylactic removal, even though there is currently no evidence to support the routine extraction of asymptomatic impacted teeth in adults. It is worth noting that impaction is seven times more common in the lower third molars. The tendency for impaction is attributed to the progressive agenesis of these teeth, due to their limited functionality in modern chewing physiology [68,70,71].

Adeyemo et al., based on an analysis of 1763 cases of third molar extractions, reported that caries was the primary cause for removal in 63.2%, recurrent pericoronitis in 26.3%, and periodontitis in 9.2%, with only 0.6% of extractions being prophylactic. The study emphasized that patients who had third molars removed due to caries were statistically younger than those who had them extracted due to periodontitis, but older than those with extractions due to pericoronitis [68]. Moreover, Ventä et al., based on an analysis of 6082 panoramic radiographs, identified third molars (both maxillary and mandibular) as the most commonly missing teeth up to the age of 80. They reported agenesis of all four wisdom teeth at a rate of just 3.4%, with at least one wisdom tooth missing in 22.6% of the cases [61]. Their findings were consistent with the results of a 1999 study, which examined a massive database of 100 million dental procedures among 7.5 million patients in the United States [72].

However, Baqain et al. indicated that upper wisdom teeth were extracted the least frequently [40]. It is important to note that this study was conducted at an oral surgery teaching clinic, where many extractions of third molars may have been excluded from the analysis due to the need for greater operator experience, which could have influenced the final outcome. When reviewing the literature, it is crucial to consider whether third molars were excluded from the analysis entirely.

4.3. Study Strengths, Limitations, and Future Directions

This study boasts several strengths, including the analysis of an extensive dataset comprising 182,654 medical records collected over a 7-year period (2017–2023). This timeframe covers critical global events, such as the COVID-19 pandemic and the outbreak of the Russia–Ukraine war, allowing for a comprehensive evaluation of long-term changes in dental healthcare.

However, the study also has its limitations. Key socioeconomic factors, such as patients' wealth, place of residence, and education level, were not available in the dataset, which restricted a more in-depth analysis of these important determinants. As the largest dental facility in central Poland, our center provides care to a diverse patient population, encompassing individuals from urban and rural areas as well as various socioeconomic backgrounds. However, this single-center setting may limit the generalizability of the study results. Additionally, the study did not include all clinics operating within the University Center of Dentistry and Specialized Medicine because several departments interrupted their services during the first wave of COVID-19.

Future research should aim to address these limitations by incorporating a more comprehensive dataset that includes socioeconomic factors such as income, education level, and place of residence. A multicenter approach involving other dental facilities across different regions would enhance the generalizability of the findings. Further studies should delve deeper into the socioeconomic, educational, and occupational influences to develop targeted strategies that improve access to and utilization of conservative dental care, particularly among vulnerable populations.

5. Conclusions

Consistent with the existing literature, this study's findings confirm that females and younger individuals are more likely to seek preventive and conservative services, while males are more likely to undergo interventional endodontic and surgical procedures. The frequency of surgical treatments increased with age, whereas conservative procedures declined. Restorative dentistry services were the most frequently performed procedures, particularly single- and two-surface restorations in maxillary teeth. Among surgical procedures, surgical extractions were more commonly performed than simple extractions, most frequently involving mandibular molars.

These results underscore the need for targeted interventions to improve oral health outcomes, particularly among males and older individuals, who are less likely to engage in preventive care. Strengthening efforts to promote conservative treatment and expanding access to guaranteed dental services are essential for reducing disparities and ensuring equitable oral healthcare for all socioeconomic groups.

Supplementary Materials: The following supporting information can be downloaded at https://www.mdpi.com/article/10.3390/jcm14051508/s1: Table S1: Detailed parameters of determined points in multidimensional correspondence analysis for the impact of sociodemographic factors (i.e., age and gender) on the spectrum of dental procedures; Table S2: Detailed parameters of determined points in multidimensional correspondence analysis for the impact of personal oral factors (i.e., tooth type and site) on the spectrum of dental procedures.

Author Contributions: Conceptualization, K.Ł. and K.N.; methodology, K.Ł. and K.N.; formal analysis, K.Ł. and K.N.; investigation, K.Ł., M.O., K.C., J.J. and K.N.; data curation, K.Ł. and K.N.; writing—original draft preparation, K.Ł. and M.O.; writing—review and editing, K.N.; visualization, K.N.; supervision, K.N. All authors have read and agreed to the published version of the manuscript.

Funding: This research received no external funding.

Institutional Review Board Statement: Ethical review and approval were waived for this study due to the retrospective character of performed analyses (The Bioethical Committee of the Poznan University of Medical Sciences, Decision no. KB-724/24, 29 October 2024).

Informed Consent Statement: Patient consent was waived due to the retrospective character of performed analyses (The Bioethical Committee of the Poznan University of Medical Sciences, Decision no. KB-724/24, 29 October 2024).

Data Availability Statement: The original contributions presented in the study are included in the article; further enquiries can be directed to the corresponding authors.

Conflicts of Interest: The authors declare no conflicts of interest.

References

1. Olczak-Kowalczyk, D.; Turska-Szybka, A.; Kaczmarek, U.; Mielczarek, A.; Adamczyk, K.; Rusyan, E. (Eds.) *Monitorowa Stanu Zdrowia Jamy Ustnej Populacji Polskiej w Latach 2016-2020: Choroba Próchnicowa i Stan Tkanek Przyzębia Populacji Polsk Podsumowanie Wyników Badań z Lat 2016–2019*; Sekcja Druków Warszawskiego Uniwersytetu Medycznego: Warszawa, Pola 2021; ISBN 978-83-7637-555-7.
2. Piotrowska, D.E.; Jankowska, D.; Huzarska, D.; Szpak, A.S.; Pędziński, B. Socioeconomic Inequalities in Use and Non-Use Dental Services in Poland. *Int. J. Public Health* **2020**, *65*, 637–647. [CrossRef] [PubMed]
3. Sfeatcu, R.; Balgiu, B.A.; Mihai, C.; Petre, A.; Pantea, M.; Tribus, L. Gender Differences in Oral Health: Self-Reported Attituc Values, Behaviours and Literacy among Romanian Adults. *J. Pers. Med.* **2022**, *12*, 1603. [CrossRef] [PubMed]
4. Lukacs, J.R. Sex Differences in Dental Caries Experience: Clinical Evidence, Complex Etiology. *Clin. Oral Investig.* **2011**, 649–656. [CrossRef] [PubMed]
5. Su, S.; Lipsky, M.S.; Licari, F.W.; Hung, M. Comparing Oral Health Behaviours of Men and Women in the United States. *J. De* **2022**, *122*, 104157. [CrossRef] [PubMed]
6. Lipsky, M.S.; Su, S.; Crespo, C.J.; Hung, M. Men and Oral Health: A Review of Sex and Gender Differences. *Am. J. Mens Hea* **2021**, *15*, 15579883211016361. [CrossRef]
7. Furuta, M.; Ekuni, D.; Irie, K.; Azuma, T.; Tomofuji, T.; Ogura, T.; Morita, M. Sex Differences in Gingivitis Relate to Interaction Oral Health Behaviors in Young People. *J. Periodontol.* **2011**, *82*, 558–565. [CrossRef]

Carrillo-Diaz, M.; Crego, A.; Romero-Maroto, M. The Influence of Gender on the Relationship between Dental Anxiety and Oral Health-Related Emotional Well-Being. *Int. J. Paediatr. Dent.* **2013**, *23*, 180–187. [CrossRef] [PubMed]
Ferraro, M.; Vieira, A.R. Explaining Gender Differences in Caries: A Multifactorial Approach to a Multifactorial Disease. *Int. J. Dent.* **2010**, *2010*, 649643. [CrossRef] [PubMed]
Lukacs, J.R.; Largaespada, L.L. Explaining Sex Differences in Dental Caries Prevalence: Saliva, Hormones, and "Life-history" Etiologies. *Am. J. Hum. Biol.* **2006**, *18*, 540–555. [CrossRef] [PubMed]
Nydell Helkimo, A.; Rolander, B.; Koch, G. Dental Fear in School Children and Young Adults Attending Public Dental Health Care: Prevalence and Relationship to Gender, Oral Disease and Dental Treatment; Trends over 40 Years. *BMC Oral Health* **2022**, *22*, 146. [CrossRef] [PubMed]
Piuvezam, G.; de Lima, K.C. Self-Perceived Oral Health Status in Institutionalized Elderly in Brazil. *Arch. Gerontol. Geriatr.* **2012**, *55*, 5–11. [CrossRef] [PubMed]
Nijakowski, K.; Cieślik, K.; Łaganowski, K.; Gruszczyński, D.; Surdacka, A. The Impact of the COVID-19 Pandemic on the Spectrum of Performed Dental Procedures. *Int. J. Environ. Res. Public Health* **2021**, *18*, 3421. [CrossRef]
Łaganowski, K.; Ortarzewska, M.; Czajka-Jakubowska, A.; Surdacka, A.; Nijakowski, K. Long-Term Impact of the COVID-19 Pandemic on Dental Care Delivery in Poland: A Single-Center Retrospective Analysis. *Int. Dent. J.* 2025, *accepted*.
World Health Organization. *COVID-19: Operational Guidance for Maintaining Essential Health Services During an Outbreak: Interim Guidance, 25 March 2020*; World Health Organization: Geneva, Switzerland, 2020.
Polskie Towarzystwo Stomatologiczne. *COVID-19 a Praca Lekarza Dentysty: Wytyczne PTS Uaktualnione*; Polskie Towarzystwo Stomatologiczne: Wrocław, Poland, 2020.
American Dental Association. *What Constitutes a Dental Emergency?*; American Dental Association: Chicago, IL, USA, 2020.
Kranz, A.M.; Chen, A.; Gahlon, G.; Stein, B.D. 2020 Trends in Dental Office Visits during the COVID-19 Pandemic. *J. Am. Dent. Assoc.* **2021**, *152*, 535–541.e1. [CrossRef] [PubMed]
Takeda, A.; Tomio, J.; Fukuda, H.; Ando, Y.; Yokoyama, T. Trends in Dental Visits during the State of Emergency for COVID-19 in Japan: A Retrospective Observational Study. *BMJ Open* **2022**, *12*, e064666. [CrossRef] [PubMed]
Walter, E.; von Bronk, L.; Hickel, R.; Huth, K.C. Impact of COVID-19 on Dental Care during a National Lockdown: A Retrospective Observational Study. *Int. J. Environ. Res. Public Health* **2021**, *18*, 7963. [CrossRef] [PubMed]
Prusaczyk, A.; Bogdan, M.; Vinker, S.; Gujski, M.; Żuk, P.; Kowalska-Bobko, I.; Karczmarz, S.; Oberska, J.; Lewtak, K. Health Care Organization in Poland in Light of the Refugee Crisis Related to the Military Conflict in Ukraine. *Int. J. Environ. Res. Public Health* **2023**, *20*, 3831. [CrossRef] [PubMed]
Ociepa-Kicińska, E.; Gorzałczyńska-Koczkodaj, M. Forms of Aid Provided to Refugees of the 2022 Russia-Ukraine War: The Case of Poland. *Int. J. Environ. Res. Public Health* **2022**, *19*, 7085. [CrossRef] [PubMed]
Jankowski, M.; Lazarus, J.V.; Kuchyn, I.; Zemskov, S.; Gałązkowski, R.; Gujski, M. One Year On: Poland's Public Health Initiatives and National Response to Millions of Refugees from Ukraine. *Med. Sci. Monit. Int. Med. J. Exp. Clin. Res.* **2023**, *29*, e940223. [CrossRef]
Tomaszewski, M.; Matthews-Brzozowska, T. Dental Services Market in Poland and Its Impact on the Health Decisions of Patients and Doctors. *Eur. J. Paediatr. Dent.* **2022**, *23*, 225–229. [CrossRef]
Nguyen, T.C.; Witter, D.J.; Bronkhorst, E.M.; Truong, N.B.; Creugers, N.H. Oral Health Status of Adults in Southern Vietnam—A Cross-Sectional Epidemiological Study. *BMC Oral Health* **2010**, *10*, 2. [CrossRef] [PubMed]
Zhang, Q.; Witter, D.J.; Bronkhorst, E.M.; Creugers, N.H. Dental and Prosthodontic Status of an over 40 Year-Old Population in Shandong Province, China. *BMC Public Health* **2011**, *11*, 420. [CrossRef] [PubMed]
Damyanov, N.D.; Witter, D.J.; Bronkhorst, E.M.; Creugers, N.H.J. Dental Status and Associated Factors in a Dentate Adult Population in Bulgaria: A Cross-Sectional Survey. *Int. J. Dent.* **2012**, *2012*, 578401. [CrossRef] [PubMed]
Russell, S.L.; Gordon, S.; Lukacs, J.R.; Kaste, L.M. Sex/Gender Differences in Tooth Loss and Edentulism. *Dent. Clin. N. Am.* **2013**, *57*, 317–337. [CrossRef] [PubMed]
Steinberg, B.J.; Hilton, I.V.; Iida, H.; Samelson, R. Oral Health and Dental Care During Pregnancy. *Dent. Clin. N. Am.* **2013**, *57*, 195–210. [CrossRef] [PubMed]
Eliasson, L.; Birkhed, D.; Osterberg, T.; Carlén, A. Minor Salivary Gland Secretion Rates and Immunoglobulin A in Adults and the Elderly. *Eur. J. Oral Sci.* **2006**, *114*, 494–499. [CrossRef]
Jankowski, J.; Nijakowski, K. Salivary Immunoglobulin a Alterations in Health and Disease: A Bibliometric Analysis of Diagnostic Trends from 2009 to 2024. *Antibodies* **2024**, *13*, 98. [CrossRef]
Patir, A.; Seymen, F.; Yildirim, M.; Deeley, K.; Cooper, M.E.; Marazita, M.L.; Vieira, A.R. Enamel Formation Genes Are Associated with High Caries Experience in Turkish Children. *Caries Res.* **2008**, *42*, 394–400. [CrossRef] [PubMed]
Deeley, K.; Letra, A.; Rose, E.K.; Brandon, C.A.; Resick, J.M.; Marazita, M.L.; Vieira, A.R. Possible Association of Amelogenin to High Caries Experience in a Guatemalan-Mayan Population. *Caries Res.* **2008**, *42*, 8–13. [CrossRef] [PubMed]

34. Sangalli, L.; Souza, L.C.; Letra, A.; Shaddox, L.; Ioannidou, E. Sex as a Biological Variable in Oral Diseases: Evidence and Fut Prospects. *J. Dent. Res.* **2023**, *102*, 1395–1416. [CrossRef] [PubMed]
35. Galdas, P.M.; Cheater, F.; Marshall, P. Men and Health Help-seeking Behaviour: Literature Review. *J. Adv. Nurs.* **2005**, *49*, 616– [CrossRef] [PubMed]
36. Westbrook, M.T.; Mitchell, R.A. Changes in Sex-Role Stereotypes from Health to Illness. *Soc. Sci. Med.* **1979**, *13*, 297–302.
37. Ioannidou, E. The Sex and Gender Intersection in Chronic Periodontitis. *Front. Public Health* **2017**, *5*, 189. [CrossRef] [PubMe
38. Panasiuk, L.; Kosiniak-Kamysz, W.; Horoch, A.; Paprzycki, P.; Karwat, D. Tooth Loss among Adult Rural and Urban Inhabita of the Lublin Region. *Ann. Agric. Environ. Med.* **2013**, *20*, 637–641. [PubMed]
39. Zilinskaite-Petrauskiene, I.; Haug, S.R. A Comparison of Endodontic Treatment Factors, Operator Difficulties, and Perceived O Health–Related Quality of Life between Elderly and Young Patients. *J. Endod.* **2021**, *47*, 1844–1853. [CrossRef]
40. Baqain, Z.H.; Khraisat, A.; Sawair, F.; Ghanam, S.; Shaini, F.J.; Rajab, L.D. Dental Extraction for Patients Presenting at Oral Surg Student Clinic. *Compend. Contin. Educ. Dent.* **2007**, *28*, 146–150. [PubMed]
41. McCaul, L.K.; Jenkins, W.M.M.; Kay, E.J. The Reasons for the Extraction of Various Tooth Types in Scotland: A 15-Year Follow *J. Dent.* **2001**, *29*, 401–407. [CrossRef]
42. Aljafar, A.; Alibrahim, H.; Alahmed, A.; AbuAli, A.; Nazir, M.; Alakel, A.; Almas, K. Reasons for Permanent Teeth Extractic and Related Factors among Adult Patients in the Eastern Province of Saudi Arabia. *Sci. World J.* **2021**, *2021*, 5534455. [CrossR [PubMed]
43. Broers, D.L.M.; Dubois, L.; De Lange, J.; Su, N.; De Jongh, A. Reasons for Tooth Removal in Adults: A Systematic Review. *Dent. J.* **2022**, *72*, 52–57. [CrossRef] [PubMed]
44. Lindahl, O.; Ventä, I. Level of Difficulty of Tooth Extractions among Roughly 100,000 Procedures in Primary Care. *Clin. C Investig.* **2023**, *27*, 4513–4520. [CrossRef] [PubMed]
45. Nurminen, M.; Blomgren, J.; Mikkola, H. Socioeconomic Differences in Utilization of Public and Private Dental Care in Finla Register-Based Evidence on a Population Aged 25 and Over. *PLoS ONE* **2021**, *16*, e0255126. [CrossRef]
46. Bertoldi, C.; Lalla, M.; Pradelli, J.M.; Cortellini, P.; Lucchi, A.; Zaffe, D. Risk Factors and Socioeconomic Condition Effects Periodontal and Dental Health: A Pilot Study among Adults over Fifty Years of Age. *Eur. J. Dent.* **2013**, *7*, 336–346. [CrossRe
47. Pizzo, G.; Matranga, D.; Maniscalco, L.; Buttacavoli, F.; Campus, G.; Giuliana, G. Caries Severity, Decayed First Permanent Mol and Associated Factors in 6-7 Years Old Schoolchildren Living in Palermo (Southern Italy). *J. Clin. Med.* **2023**, *12*, 4343. [CrossR [PubMed]
48. Alves, L.S.; Zenkner, J.E.A.; Wagner, M.B.; Damé-Teixeira, N.; Susin, C.; Maltz, M. Eruption Stage of Permanent Molars a Occlusal Caries Activity/Arrest. *J. Dent. Res.* **2014**, *93*, 114S–119S. [CrossRef]
49. Desai, H.; Stewart, C.A.; Finer, Y. Minimally Invasive Therapies for the Management of Dental Caries—A Literature Revi *Dent. J.* **2021**, *9*, 147. [CrossRef] [PubMed]
50. Obwieszczenie Ministra Zdrowia z Dnia 12 Października 2021 r. w Sprawie Ogłoszenia Jednolitego Tekstu Rozporządze Ministra Zdrowia w Sprawie Świadczeń Gwarantowanych z Zakresu Leczenia Stomatologicznego. Available online: htt //isap.sejm.gov.pl/isap.nsf/DocDetails.xsp?id=WDU20210002148 (accessed on 6 January 2025).
51. Malkiewicz, K.; Malkiewicz, E.; Eaton, K.A.; Widström, E. The Healthcare System and the Provision of Oral Healthcare European Union Member States. Part 6: Poland. *Br. Dent. J.* **2016**, *221*, 501–507. [CrossRef] [PubMed]
52. Bud, M.G.; Pop, O.D.; Cîmpean, S. Benefits of Using Magnification in Dental Specialties—A Narrative Review. *Med. Pharm. R* **2023**, *96*, 254–257. [CrossRef]
53. Bahcall, J.K. Visualization in Endodontics. *Eur. J. Gen. Dent.* **2013**, *2*, 96–101. [CrossRef]
54. Ganesan, S.; Basheer, S.N.; Kumar, O.N.; Chohan, H.; Murugesan, S.; Subramani, S.K. Enhancing Precision in Endodon Procedures: An In Vitro Investigation of Magnification and Enhanced Visualization. *J. Pharm. Bioallied Sci.* **2024**, *16*, S2697–S26 [CrossRef]
55. Das, P. Dental Operating Microscope in Endodontics—A Review. *IOSR J. Dent. Med. Sci.* **2013**, *5*, 1–8. [CrossRef]
56. Krustrup, U.; Petersen, P.E. Dental Caries Prevalence among Adults in Denmark—The Impact of Socio-Demographic Factors a Use of Oral Health Services. *Community Dent. Health* **2007**, *24*, 225–232.
57. Hollanda, A.C.B.; Alencar, A.H.G.D.; Estrela, C.R.D.A.; Bueno, M.R.; Estrela, C. Prevalence of Endodontically Treated Teeth i Brazilian Adult Population. *Braz. Dent. J.* **2008**, *19*, 313–317. [CrossRef]
58. Khan, S.; Khabeer, A.; Al Harbi, F.; Arrejaie, A.; Moheet, I.; Farooqi, F.; Majeed, A. Frequency of Root Canal Treatment amo Patients Attending a Teaching Dental Hospital in Dammam, Saudi Arabia. *Saudi J. Med. Med. Sci.* **2017**, *5*, 145. [CrossR [PubMed]
59. Scavo, R.; Martinez Lalis, R.; Zmener, O.; DiPietro, S.; Grana, D.; Pameijer, C.H. Frequency and Distribution of Teeth Requir Endodontic Therapy in an Argentine Population Attending a Specialty Clinic in Endodontics. *Int. Dent. J.* **2011**, *61*, 257–2 [CrossRef] [PubMed]

Wigsten, E.; Jonasson, P.; EndoReCo; Kvist, T. Indications for Root Canal Treatment in a Swedish County Dental Service: Patient- and Tooth-specific Characteristics. *Int. Endod. J.* **2019**, *52*, 158–168. [CrossRef] [PubMed]
Ventä, I.; Snäll, J.; Rice, D.P.; Suominen, A.L. Is the Third Molar the Most Frequently Extracted Tooth? A Population-Based Study Utilizing Dental Panoramic Radiographs in Adults. *Clin. Oral Investig.* **2024**, *28*, 443. [CrossRef]
Gotfredsen, K.; Walls, A.W.G. What Dentition Assures Oral Function? *Clin. Oral Implant. Res.* **2007**, *18*, 34–45. [CrossRef] [PubMed]
Elias, A.C.; Sheiham, A. The Relationship between Satisfaction with Mouth and Number and Position of Teeth. *J. Oral Rehabil.* **1998**, *25*, 649–661. [CrossRef]
Benson, P.E.; Alshawy, E.; Fenton, G.D.; Frawley, T.; Misra, S.; Ng, T.; O'Malley, P.; Smith, G. Extraction vs. Nonextraction of Premolars for Orthodontic Treatment: A Scoping Review Examining the Extent, Range, and Characteristics of the Literature. *Am. J. Orthod. Dentofacial Orthop.* **2023**, *164*, 368–376. [CrossRef] [PubMed]
Dardengo, C.D.S.; Fernandes, L.Q.P.; Capelli Júnior, J. Frequency of Orthodontic Extraction. *Dent. Press J. Orthod.* **2016**, *21*, 54–59. [CrossRef] [PubMed]
Jackson, T.H.; Guez, C.; Lin, F.-C.; Proffit, W.R.; Ko, C.-C. Extraction Frequencies at a University Orthodontic Clinic in the 21st Century: Demographic and Diagnostic Factors Affecting the Likelihood of Extraction. *Am. J. Orthod. Dentofac. Orthop.* **2017**, *151*, 456–462. [CrossRef] [PubMed]
Fleming, P.S.; Cunningham, S.J.; Benson, P.E.; Jauhar, P.; Millett, D. Extraction of Premolars for Orthodontic Reasons on the Decline? A Cross-Sectional Survey of BOS Members. *J. Orthod.* **2018**, *45*, 283–288. [CrossRef]
Adeyemo, W.; James, O.; Ogunlewe, M.; Ladeinde, A.; Taiwo, O.; Olojede, A. Indications for Extraction of Third Molars: A Review of 1763 Cases. *Niger. Postgrad. Med. J.* **2008**, *15*, 42. [CrossRef] [PubMed]
Santos, K.K.; Lages, F.S.; Maciel, C.A.B.; Glória, J.C.R.; Douglas-de-Oliveira, D.W. Prevalence of Mandibular Third Molars According to the Pell & Gregory and Winter Classifications. *J. Maxillofac. Oral Surg.* **2022**, *21*, 627–633. [CrossRef] [PubMed]
Themkumkwun, S.; Sawatdeenarunat, S.; Manosuthi, P. Surgical Removal of Third Molars in a Young Adult: Review of Indications and Surgical Techniques. *J. Korean Assoc. Oral Maxillofac. Surg.* **2023**, *49*, 184–191. [CrossRef] [PubMed]
Ghaeminia, H.; Nienhuijs, M.E.; Toedtling, V.; Perry, J.; Tummers, M.; Hoppenreijs, T.J.; Van Der Sanden, W.J.; Mettes, T.G. Surgical Removal versus Retention for the Management of Asymptomatic Disease-Free Impacted Wisdom Teeth. *Cochrane Database Syst. Rev.* **2020**, *5*, CD003879. [CrossRef] [PubMed]
Eklund, S.A.; Pittman, J.L. Third-Molar Removal Patterns in an Insured Population. *J. Am. Dent. Assoc.* **2001**, *132*, 469–475. [CrossRef] [PubMed]

MDPI AG
Grosspeteranlage 5
4052 Basel
Switzerland
Tel.: +41 61 683 77 34

Journal of Clinical Medicine Editorial Office
E-mail: jcm@mdpi.com
www.mdpi.com/journal/jcm

www.ingramcontent.com/pod-product-compliance
Lightning Source LLC
Chambersburg PA
CBHW041949260926
51850CB00019B/2231
9783725865826